T0260199

Leeuwenhoek's Legatees and Beijerinck's Beneficiaries

Leeuwenhoek's Legatees and Beijerinck's Beneficiaries

A History of Medical Virology in the Netherlands

Gerard van Doornum
Ton van Helvoort
Neeraja Sankaran

Amsterdam University Press

The publication of this book has been made possible by financial contributions from:
- Beijerinck Virology Fund of the KNAW
- Stichting Historia Medicinae
- Stichting Pathologie, Onderzoek en Ontwikkeling

The funds bear no responsibility for the content.

Cover illustration: Edvard Munch, *Self-Portrait with the Spanish Flu*, 1919
It is a sick and enfeebled artist who meets our gaze in *Self-Portrait with the Spanish Flu*.
Edvard Munch became ill at the turn of the year 1918-1919, having apparently contracted the
Spanish flu, which became a serious worldwide epidemic, taking the lives of many millions
of people in the years from 1917 to 1920. In a series of studies, sketches and paintings, Munch
followed the various stages of the illness, illustrating how close death came to life.
The painting was donated to the National Gallery by Charlotte and Christian Mustad in 1937.
Source: Nasjonalmuseet, Oslo, http://samling.nasjonalmuseet.no/en/object/NG.M.01867,
latest access August 2019

Cover design: Coördesign, Leiden
Typesetting: Crius Group, Hulshout

ISBN   978 94 6372 011 3
e-ISBN   978 90 4854 406 6 (pdf)
DOI   10.5117/9789463720113
NUR   685

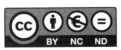

To the memory of Jan van der Noordaa
A true legatee and beneficiary of Leeuwenhoek and Beijerinck
Nestor of Dutch medical virology

Jan van der Noordaa (1934-2015)

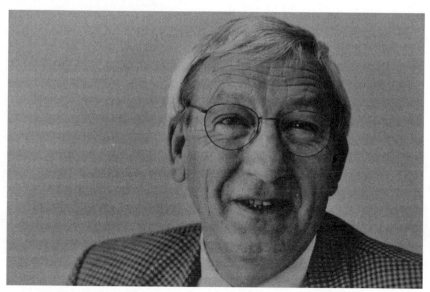

By courtesy of E. van der Noordaa

Table of Contents

List of illustrations

Acknowledgements

The authors would like to express their sincere thanks to the foundations M.W. Beijerinck Virology Fund of the Royal Netherlands Academy of Arts and Sciences and the Foundation Historia Medicinae, respectively, which made it possible to publish the book.

Additional funding was received for copy-editing and proofreading from the Foundation Pathology Research and Education SPOO that is related to the DDL.

The British historian M. Worboys worked on the field of the history of tropical medicine and acknowledged that he was drawing almost entirely on the work of other historians. Likewise, in the event of scarcity of original sources we had to do the same. Of course, we apologize for any misinterpretations of the work of our forebears.

During the long period it has taken to research and write this book we approached a great number of persons for information or comment. Perhaps their help is already forgotten by now, but we hasten to acknowledge our debt to their information, comments or feedback. With their help many amendments were made to original versions of the book. Their support was very valuable in helping us sort out the forest from the trees.

As it is impossible to specify everyone's contributions, we limit ourselves to thanking the people below for their help:

C. Aitken, H.G.A.M. van der Avoort, W. Beekhuizen, E.P. Beem, P.A.J. Bentvelzen, K. van Berkel, H. Bijlmer, D. M. Birkenhäger-Frenkel, H.P.J. Bloemers, R.J.F. Burgmeijer, R.A. Coutinho, G. Dekker, A.M. Dingemans-Dumas, A.J. van der Eb, B.E. Fabius-Vleghert, T. Ferwerda, P.K. Flu, R.A.M. Fouchier, J. Galama, J. Goudsmit, P.D. Griffiths, C. Haarnack, B. Hofman, E. Houwaart, J. Huisman († 2016), J.C. de Jong († 2017), M. de Jonge, P. Kager, J.C. Kapsenberg, A.E. Kersten, A.C. Koppen-Murk, A.C.M. Kroes, J. Leeuwenburg, M. van Lieburg, L. van Lieshout, A.M van Loon, P.J. van der Maas, C.R. Madeley, A.E. Marble, C. van Maris, W. Maruanaya, J. Meijer, R. Meloen, P. P. Mortimer, R.P. Mouton, E. van der Noordaa, J. van der Noordaa († 2015), R. Nusse, E. Ombre, A.D.M.E. Osterhaus, M.F. Peeters († 2011), R. Plasterk, A.M. Polderman, J.D. Querido, W.G.V. Quint, J. Rahamat-Langendoen, W. Rakhorst, M. van Ranst, P.J.M. Rottier, E.J. Ruitenberg, H.C. Rümke, J. ter Schegget, J. Schirm, P. Schröder, A.H.W.M. Schuurs, K.W. Slaterus († 2014), G.L. Smith, S.K. Somerwil-Ayrton, P.C. van der Vliet, H.J.C. de Vries, D. van Waarde, C. Walboomers-van Rijn, E.D. Waleson-Mollinger († 2016), B. van Weemen, K. Weijer, H.T. Weiland, G.J.S. Wilde († 2019), R. Woudenberg, B.A.M. van der Zeist.

Nevertheless, a special thanks to the reviewers who have commented on the manuscript on behalf of the M.W. Beijerinck Virology Foundation of the KNAW, and to those who have commented on versions of chapters (in whole or in part) of the book at the request of the authors: H.G.A.M. van der Avoort, E.P. Beem, H.P.J. Bloemers, R.J.F. Burgmeijer, A.M. Dingemans-Dumas, R.A.M. Fouchier, J. Huisman, P. Kager, J.C. Kapsenberg, A.C.M. Kroes, J. Leeuwenburg, A.M. van Loon, J. van der Noordaa, A.D.M.E. Osterhaus, J. ter Schegget, J. Schirm, D. van Waarde, and B.A.M. van der Zeist. Of course, the authors of the book remain responsible for any ambiguities or inaccuracies that remain. We apologize for any errors or omissions and if contacted, the authors will be pleased to rectify them at the earliest opportunity.

Our main sources of information have been articles of scientists who published in the past on their work. We are grateful to the Erasmus MC Medical Library and the Central Medical Library of the University Medical Centre Groningen for the numerous deliveries of articles we have asked for.

We would also like to thank Inge van der Bijl and Julie Benschop-Plokker, our editors at the Amsterdam University Press, for their help, and Leslie Reperant of Pikado for correcting our usage of the English language in Chapters 4, 7, 8, 9 and 10 of the manuscript.

A final acknowledgment is to the Van der Noordaa family with regard of our dedication of the book to the memory of Jan van der Noordaa, the pater familias of Dutch medical virologists through the last quarter of the twentieth century.

Gerard van Doornum
Ton van Helvoort
Neeraja Sankaran

Abbreviations

AAI	Accelerating Access Initiative
ACS	Amsterdam Cohort Studies on HIV infection and AIDS
AFP	Acute flaccid paralysis
AIDS	Acquired immunodeficiency syndrome
AMC	Amsterdam Medical Center (Academisch Medisch Centrum), since 2018 location AMC of Amsterdam UMC
Amsterdam UMC	Amsterdam University Medical Center, locations AMC and VUmc
ASM	American Society for Microbiology
AvL	Antoni van Leeuwenhoek Hospital (Antoni van Leeuwenhoek Ziekenhuis)
AZL	Academisch Ziekenhuis Leiden
AZR	Academisch Ziekenhuis Rotterdam
AZU	Academisch Ziekenhuis Utrecht
CLB/Sanquin	Central Laboratory of the Blood Transfusion Service of the Netherlands Red Cross, since 1998 Sanquin (Centraal Laboratorium van de Bloedtransfusiedienst van het Nederlandse Rode Kruis)
CMV	Cytomegalovirus
COTG	Central Organ Tariffs Healthcare (Centraal Orgaan Tarieven Gezondheidszorg)
CPE	Cytopathic effect
CVI Lelystad	Central Veterinary Institute, Lelystad
DAVS	Dutch Annual Virology Symposium
DDL	Delft Diagnostic Laboratories, moved to Rijswijk in 2003
DTA	Direction of Technical Assistance of the Ministry of Foreign Affairs
DTaP/IPV	Diphtheria, tetanus, acellular pertussis, inactivated poliovirus
DTaP/IPV/Hib	Diphtheria, tetanus, acellular pertussis, inactivated poliovirus, *Haemophilus influenzae* type B
DTP	Diphtheria, tetanus, pertussis
EAVRI	East African Virus Research Institute
EBV	Epstein-Barr virus
EGRVD	European Group for Rapid Viral Diagnosis
EIA	Enzyme immunoassays
ELISA	Enzyme-linked immunosorbent assay
EMBO	European Molecular Biology Organization
ERL	Epidemiological Research Laboratory, London
EHNRI	Ethiopian Health and Nutrition Research Institute
ENARP	Ethiopian-Netherlands HIV/AIDS Research Project

Erasmus MC	Erasmus Medical Center, Rotterdam
ESAVD	European Association against Virus Diseases
ESCMID	European Society of Clinical Microbiology and Infectious Diseases
ESCV	European Society for Clinical Virology
ESV	European Society for Virology
FUNGO	Fundamental Medical Research
GG&GD Amsterdam	Municipal Health Service, Amsterdam
GGD Amsterdam	Municipal Health Service Amsterdam, since 2005
GHI	Health Inspectorate, until 1995
GNGH	Society for the Advancement of Science, Medicine and Surgery (Genootschap ter bevordering van Natuur- Genees- en Heelkunde)
GPLN	Global Polio Laboratory Network
GR	Health Council of the Netherlands (Gezondheidsraad Nederland)
HAV	Hepatitis A virus
HBV	Hepatitis B virus
HCV	Hepatitis C virus
HIV	Human immunodeficiency virus
HMPV	Human metapneumovirus
HPV	Human papillomavirus
IGZ	Health Inspectorate, since 1995 (Inspectie voor de Gezondheidszorg)
IPV	Inactivated polio virus vaccine (Salk)
KEMRI/KMRI	Kenyan Medical Research Institute
KIT	Royal Tropical Institute (Koninklijk Instituut voor de Tropen)
KNAW	Royal Netherlands Academy of Arts and Sciences
KNMG	Royal Netherlands Medical Association (Koninklijke Nederlandsche Maatschappij tot Bevordering der Geneeskunst)
KNMP	Royal Dutch Pharmacists Association (Koninklijke Nederlandse Maatschappij ter bevordering der Pharmacie)
KNVM	Royal Netherlands Society for Microbiology (Koninklijke Nederlandse Vereniging voor Microbiologie)
KWF	Queen Wilhelmina Fund (Netherlands Cancer Society)
LCI	National Coordination Structure for Infectious Diseases (Landelijke Coördinatiestructuur Infectieziekten)
LHV	National Association of General Practitioners (Landelijke Huisartsen Vereniging)
LUMC	Leiden University Medical Centre
Maastricht UMC	Maastricht University Medical Center
MTI	Mammary tumour inciter
MMTV	Mouse mammary tumour virus

MRC	Medical Research Council, London
MSM	Men having sex with men
NASBA	Nucleic acid sequence-based amplification
NATEC	National Antiviral Therapy Evaluation Centre, at AMC
NHI	Netherlands Institute of General Practitioners (Nederlands Huisartsen Instituut)
NIH	National Institutes of Health, USA
NIPG	Netherlands Institute for Preventive Medicine, Leiden
NKI-AVL	Netherlands Cancer Institute-Antoni van Leeuwenhoek Hospital (Nederlands Kanker Instituut-Antoni van Leeuwenhoek Ziekenhuis)
NMG	Nederlandse Maatschappij tot Bevordering der Geneeskunst
NTvG	Netherlands Journal of Medicine (Nederlands Tijdschrift voor Geneeskunde)
NVTG	Netherlands Society for Tropical Medicine (Nederlandse Vereniging voor Tropische Geneeskunde)
NWO	Dutch Research Council (Nederlandse Organisatie voor Wetenschappelijk Onderzoek)
NVI	Netherlands Vaccine Institute, RIVM, Bilthoven
NVLA	Netherlands Society of Laboratory Medical Doctors (Vereniging van Laboratorium Artsen)
NVMM	Netherlands Society for Medical Microbiology
NVvB	Netherlands Society for Biochemistry
NVvM	Netherlands Society for Microbiology, since 2011 designation Royal
NWKV	Dutch Working Group for Clinical Virology (Nederlandse Werkgroep Klinische Virologie)
OPV	Oral poliovaccine (Sabin)
PAGRVD	Pan American Group for Rapid Viral Diagnosis
PCR	Polymerase chain reaction
PHLS	Public Health Laboratory Service, UK
QCMD	Quality Control for Molecular Diagnostics
Radboudumc	Radboud University Medical Centre
R.I.T.	Recherche et Industrie Therapeutique, Rixensart, Belgium
RIV	National Institute of Public Health (Rijks Instituut voor de Volksgezondheid), relocated from Utrecht through 1953-1965 to Bilthoven
RIVM	National Institute for Public Health and the Environment (Rijksinstituut voor Volksgezondheid en Milieu), since 1984
RVP	National immunization programme (Rijksvaccinatieprogramma)
RSV	Respiratory syncytial virus
SARS	Severe acute respiratory syndrome

SAZU	Stads- en Academisch Ziekenhuis Utrecht, since 1971 AZU, and since 1999 UMC Utrecht
SGM	Society for General Microbiology
SIIL	Serum Institute of India Ltd
SIV	Simian immunodeficiency virus
SKML	Foundation for the Quality Control of Medical Laboratory Diagnostics (Stichting Kwaliteitsbewaking Medische Laboratoriumdiagnostiek)
SKMM	Foundation for the Quality Control of Medical Microbiology (Stichting Kwaliteit Medische Microbiologie)
SSDZ	Foundation of Collaborating Delft Hospitals (Stichting Samenwerkende Delftse Ziekenhuizen)
SVM	Foundation for the Advancement of Public Health and the Environment (Stichting tot Bevordering van de Volksgezondheid en Milieuhygiëne)
SVOI	State Veterinary Research Institute (Staatsveterinair Onderzoekingsinstituut)
TMD	Tobacco mosaic disease
TMV	Tobacco mosaic virus
TNO	Netherlands Organisation for Applied Scientific Research (Nederlandse Organisatie voor Toegepast-Natuurwetenschappelijk Onderzoek)
TNO-NGO	Netherlands Organisation for Applied Scientific Research: Health Organisation, or Dutch Health Organisation
TNO-RVO	Netherlands Organisation for Applied Scientific Research: Defence, Safety and Security
UICC	Union Internationale contre le Cancer
UMC	University Medical Centre
UMCG	University Medical Center Groningen
UMC Utrecht	University Medical Centre of the University of Utrecht
UVRI	Uganda Virus Research Institute
VOC	Dutch East India Company (Vereenigde Oostindische Compagnie)
VRL	Virus Reference Laboratory, PHLS, London
VUmc	VU University Medical Center, Amsterdam
WHO	World Health Organization
WIC	Dutch West India Company (West-Indische Compagnie)
WMDI	Working Group for Molecular Diagnosis of Infectious Diseases (Werkgroep Moleculaire Diagnostiek van Infectieziekten)
ZWO	Netherlands Organisation for Pure Scientific Research (Nederlandse Organisatie voor Zuiver-Wetenschappelijk Onderzoek)

Preface

> To me it seems most desirable that the collaborative character of these
> investigations should be understood, not solely for personal reasons but because
> much of all modern medical research is conducted in this way.
>
> – *John F. Enders (1961)*

The title of the book pays tribute to two Dutch scientists without whom virology would arguably not exist today, at least not in its present guise. The first is Antony van Leeuwenhoek, whose reports of microscopic discoveries in the early eighteenth century aroused interest in the world of invisible creatures. His findings laid the basis for a theory of a particulate cause of infectious diseases, but, as George Rosen wrote, without any tangible results in support of the theory (1993/1958, pp. 84-85). Some 250 years later Martinus Willem Beijerinck launched the discipline of virology with his idea that tobacco mosaic disease (TMD) was caused by a living contagious fluid or filterable living pathogen.

When asked why he wanted to climb Mount Everest, George Mallory famously replied, "Because it's there" (New York Times. 1923. Climbing Mount Everest is work for supermen. New York Times, 18 March). Our answer to the question of why we decided to write a book about the history of medical virology in the Netherlands is : Because there isn't one. Although there are a fair number of books about the history of medical, experimental, animal, or plant virology in the Western world more generally (Booss and August, 2013; Calisher and Horzinek, 1999; Chastel, 1992; Grafe, 1991; Waterson and Wilkinson, 1978), only a few talk about virology in the Netherlands. A lacuna surely, considering that it was the birthplace for the discipline; the place where Beijerinck first characterized the principle '*contagium vivum fluidum*'. Even with the publication of Bos's and Thung's histories of plant virology in the Netherlands (Bos, 2000; Thung, 1957) and Offringa's history of the veterinary faculty of the University of Utrecht (1971, 1981), a history of Dutch medical virology is still lacking. This is why we decided to make it our focus in this book.

Travelling through Dutch virology we compared the developments in the Netherlands with other Western countries; this voyage may also give insight in the connections and communication between scientists in former days. Travelling companions were medical doctors, self-taught

Figure 2   Antoni van Leeuwenhoek (1632-1723)

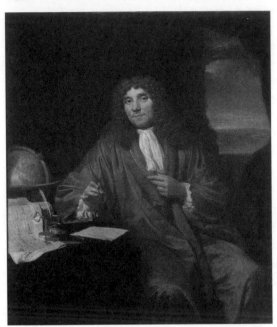

Portrait by Jan Verkolje, c. 1680-1686
Reproduction by courtesy of Rijks Museum, Amsterdam

scientists, biologists, graduate engineers, veterinarians, biochemists, physicists, epidemiologists, and molecular biologists. As the Nobel Prize winner John F. Enders (1961) wrote in a commentary on a for him very laudatory editorial about his accomplishment in developing a vaccine against measles: 'To us it seems most desirable that the collaborative character of these investigations should be understood, not solely for personal reasons but because much of all modern medical research is conducted in this way.'

The work of Dutch researchers during the last decades of the twentieth century, such as that of R.A. (Roel) Coutinho, J. (Jaap) Goudsmit, F. (Frank) Miedema, S.A. (Sven) Danner, and J.M.A. (Joep) Lange in the Amsterdam Cohort Studies on HIV infection and AIDS, was made possible by building on the tradition of J.J. van Loghem and A. Charlotte Ruys from the first half of the century. R. (Roel) Nusse, a biologist at the NKI, could use the laboratory mice which were introduced in the Netherlands by R. Korteweg in 1931. Nusse continued his career in the USA, when he joined the laboratory of Harold Varmus at the University of California. A.D.M.E (Albert) Osterhaus could proceed in Rotterdam on the influenza track beaten earlier by J. Mulder in

Groningen, who moved to Leiden in 1946, and by N. Masurel from the late 1950s in Leiden and since 1967 in Rotterdam.

Of course, we are aware that connections between the various fields of virology, which persist to this day, mean that we will often have to cross the borders between them. For instance, Martinus W. Beijerinck, the father of the virus concept, made his seminal discoveries through his experiments on tobacco plants and not on any human disease. About a hundred years later, vectors that were developed towards the end of the twentieth century for delivering genes to mammalian cells were derived from the work of among others investigators at the Wageningen University, such as R.W. Goldbach, J.M. Vlak and A. van Kammen on recombinant baculoviruses from invertebrate hosts during the last decades of the twentieth century. In the 1930s the veterinarian H.M. Frenkel worked together with medical doctor H.W. Julius to improve the continuous flow cell culture instrument of J. de Haan; later, after 1945 Frenkel initiated among others the medical doctors J. Huisman and J.G. (Cootje) Kapsenberg into the secrets of virology. The veterinarian J.D. Verlinde was head of the Department for Medical Microbiology of the Netherlands Institute for Preventive Medicine and professor at the Medical Faculty in Leiden, and likewise his student H.A.E. van Tongeren who was also a veterinarian became professor at the Free University in Amsterdam. Several of the scientific students or co-workers of the veterinarian M. Horzinek were appointed at medical faculties in the Netherlands: A.D.M.E. Osterhaus, W.J.M. Spaan, H.G.M. Niesters, B.A.M. van der Zeijst, M.P.G. Koopmans. Not only do virologists cross borders, but as we know, viral pathogens in humans can be transmitted by animals without causing disease in the intermediary reservoirs or vice versa. The interspecies transmission plays an important role in emerging viral diseases.

According to the medical historian Michael Worboys, the case for a Bacteriological Revolution in late-nineteenth-century medicine in Britain remains unproven (Worboys, 2000, 2007). Although Worboys restricted his argument to Britain on the grounds that the rate and extent of change might have been different in other countries, we believe that similar forces were operative for development of virology as scientific discipline and medical specialism in the Netherlands as well. When was the start of medical virology? Was it a revolution or an evolution? Which people were involved in medical virology?

We should note that although the terms 'human', 'medical' or 'clinical virology' are often used interchangeably in the wider medical literature, in this book we have used the term 'clinical virology' more specifically to represent that part of virology directly involved in patient care, namely the fields of diagnostic and therapeutic virology. Medical virology encompasses the study of human virus infections in a much broader sense and includes basic research, vaccine technology, tumour virology, research on antiviral drugs, and epidemiology, in addition to clinical virology.

The objective of this book is to give a chronicle of medical virology in the Netherlands in a wider, international context. We approached the project with the idea that most chapters would give factual, chronological accounts of the environment in which medical virology developed – i.e. the main institutions and laboratories in the Netherlands – combined with short biographical notes on leading figures. Unfortunately, we came across the fact that primary sources are very scant. Luckily, that problem could be overcome by information in medical journals, obituaries, reports of conferences or meetings of learned societies, commemorative books, historical records, and annual scientific reports of the Netherlands Cancer Institute-Antoni van Leeuwenhoek Hospital (NKI-AVL).[1] In addition, different editions of textbooks published from the late 1930s to the late 1950s provided information on the international position of Dutch virology in the first half of the twentieth century. The following textbooks were used for insight in the international developments: Van Rooyen and Rhodes, *Virus diseases of man* (1948, rev. ed.); Doerr and Hallauer, *Handbuch der Virusforschung* (1938-1950); Gildemeister, Haagen and Waldmann, *Handbuch der Viruskrankheiten* (1939); Rivers and Horsfall, *Viral and rickettsial infections of man* (1959). The *Reflections on a life in medicine and science* of Tom Rivers and prepared by Samuel Benison were also very useful. An update for the period until 1980 was provided by Frank Fenner and Adrian Gibbs who published *Portraits of viruses: A history of virology* in 1988. The author of the first mentioned textbook, Clennel Evelyn van Rooyen, is a descendent of a Dutch ancestor, who travelled in the service of the Dutch East India Company (VOC) to Ceylon (Halifax Chronicle Herald, 1989).

Some chapters are built around specific themes, such as the reception and redefinition of virus concept in Dutch medical circles, the Dutch Working Group for Clinical Virology, Dutch virology in the tropics, tumour virology, contributions from the Netherlands to technical innovations, and immunizations.

As we were interested in the circumstances under which virology in the Netherlands began, we have explored nineteenth-century notions about five infectious diseases which came later to be recognized as viral diseases: smallpox, measles, rabies, poliomyelitis, and influenza. Therefore, the first

---

1   Netherlands Cancer Institute-Antoni van Leeuwenhoek Hospital (NKI-AVL).

chapter begins in the nineteenth century – even the eighteenth century in the case of smallpox – and describes the understanding of and measures against these diseases. The pathway from the first insights into the nature of viruses at the end of the nineteenth century to medical virology was a long and protracted one. It is not surprising that the relatively recent science of virology has been considered as part of modern medicine built on foundations established in the nineteenth century. The origins of virology are various, and the discipline stems more from botany and veterinary medicine than from human medicine.

The second chapter deals with the concept of virus as put forward by M.W. Beijerinck in 1898, the reception of this concept among medical circles in the Netherlands, and also with redefinition of concepts of virus or bacteriophages by other Dutch researchers later in the twentieth century. Were they but spectators while the action took place in Germany, France, United Kingdom, or the United States?

In the third chapter we have attempted to describe the developments in the first half of the twentieth century – of institutes, research and diagnostic facilities in the laboratories – interspersed with short biographical details of the leading figures. Scientific research in the Netherlands was conducted almost exclusively in three venues: university laboratories, the laboratory of the NKI, and the institutes for tropical hygiene which were connected with the universities in Amsterdam and Leiden, respectively.

Chapter four is concerned with the general developments in virology and the organization of virologists over the latter half of the twentieth century. In common with developments in other countries, medical virology in the Netherlands really began to take off sometime in the middle of the twentieth century, with the practice of diagnostic virology gradually taking hold in general hospitals after the 1970s. There is consensus that the advance of virology in the 1950s can be ascribed to the application of the monolayer cell culture as first described by Enders, Weller and Robbins in their pivotal paper of 1949 (Enders et al., 1949; Mortimer, 2009; Booss and August, 2013). This development in cell culture technique was readily introduced into the Netherlands in the 1950s and contributed strongly to the commencement of clinical virology in the Netherlands. However, diagnostic virology remained from 1950 until 1970 of limited practical use for the patient. This chapter then pursues the development of clinical virology in the 1960s and 1970s when diagnosing virus infections started to be executed in a timely manner to benefit the management of the treatment of patients. Before the application of cell culture techniques, use of animals and tissues for virus identification was very cumbersome and in practical terms the results were often too late to help the patient. The development of immunofluorescence techniques in the 1960s and enzyme-linked immunosorbent assay (ELISA) techniques and further fruits of immunology (such as the monoclonal antibodies) were introduced in the 1970s. This caused a rapid and decisive step forwards in the 1970s. During the 1980s and, in particular, during the 1990s the spectacular advances in molecular biology together with the rise of information technology facilitated the expansion of diagnostic virology in the last decades of the twentieth century. This growth encompassed epidemiology, diagnosis and treatment, and viro-immunology research of new emerging virus infections. With the epidemic of human immunodeficiency virus infections, the application of antiviral therapy proceeded with rapid strides from the 1980s after a hesitant start.

The chapter continues with the way in which virologists organized themselves. The Virology section within the Royal Netherlands Society for Microbiology[2] deals with the activities of the different branches of virology: fundamental research, medical virology, plant virology, and veterinary virology. The Section organizes the successful "Dutch Annual Virology Symposium". The Dutch Working Group for Clinical Virology of which the epidemiologist M.F. Polak of the National Institute of Public Health[3] was the initiator, is part of the Netherlands Society for Medical Microbiology. This working group played an important role in the 'devolution' of virus diagnostic work from some specialized virology, public health laboratories to general hospital microbiological laboratories. The position of medical virology within the national as well international virology and microbiology community is ascertained on the basis of the history of the Dutch Working Group for Clinical Virology, the DAVS, and the annual General Spring Meeting of both Societies.

Chapter 5 pays attention to the institutes where medical virology was practised in the second half of the twentieth century. Over the first decades of this period the leading laboratories were in Amsterdam, Leiden and Utrecht. The authors also focus on the Amsterdam Cohort Studies in the discussion on the institutes in Amsterdam. The Laboratory of Virology of the Central Public Health Laboratory of RIV in Utrecht and since 1958 in Bilthoven, the Department of Bacteriology and Experimental Pathology of the Netherlands Institute for Preventive Medicine in Leiden, and the Laboratory for Hygiene in Amsterdam played important roles in the 1950s and 1960s. This picture changed with the establishment of four new medical faculties:

2   Nederlandse Vereniging voor Microbiologie (NVVM).
3   Rijksinstituut voor de Volksgezondheid (RIV).

the new medical faculties at the existing Free University in Amsterdam and Radboud University in Nijmegen in the 1950s, and thereafter the medical faculties at the new universities in Rotterdam and Maastricht, in 1964 and 1974, respectively. In addition to the university laboratories, some municipal public health laboratories and, later, the larger general hospitals offered diagnostic virological services. At the end of the chapter attention is paid to a number of commercial companies that produce vaccines or diagnostic kits or offer other services related to medical virology.

The core theme in Chapter 6 is the Dutch contributions in a variety of technical developments. It covers the phase-contrast microscope, the electron microscope, enzyme-linked immunosorbent assays, agar gel electrophoresis, the introduction of DNA in mammalian cells, the various methods using synthetic peptides (Pepscan), and nucleic acid purification.

Chapter 7 traces the Dutch contribution to medical virology in the tropics. This chapter does not provide a comprehensive picture of medical virology in the tropics, but is rather confined to a short overview of control and public health measures as well as the laboratory facilities for diagnostics of virus infections in the former Dutch colonies. The chapter also covers Dutch activities in the field of virology in Africa from the 1960s onwards.

Chapter 8 is again thematic and deals with tumour virology and persistent virus infections. This chapter encompasses the environment of the NKI and the academic centres which played a substantial role in tumour virology throughout the twentieth century. The rise and fading of the Working Group on Persistent Virus Infections and Oncogenesis is also described. Concurrent with the vanishing of this working group was the rise of molecular biology and cell biology.

Chapter 9 explores the organization of national immunization programmes with regard to viral infections polio, rubella, measles, mumps, hepatitis B, influenza, and human papilloma virus. The role of the Central Laboratory of the National Institute of Public Health in the production of vaccines will get attention, of course.

The book ends with conclusions and short summaries. Each written history has an end, and we decided to limit ours to the close of the twentieth century. Nevertheless, as movements and developments do not always occur in synchronicity, sometimes we had to cross over into the twenty-first century. We hope that others will do further research on the revolution that is still unfolding, thanks to such developments in next-generation sequencing, immunology, vaccines, epidemiology and antiviral drugs.

1 Origins in the dark

Virus diseases in the Netherlands before the discovery of viruses

The golden age [of microbiology] was thus characterized by advances not only in laboratory techniques and demonstration of specific microbial causes of infections but also in the means to prevent those infections. [...] Notably absent from the list were advances about the scourges that we now know as viral diseases.
– *Booss and August (2013, p. 8)*

However violent your attacks, sir, they will remain without success. Confidently await the results that virus attenuation holds in reserve to help mankind in its struggle against the onslaught of disease.
– *Louis Pasteur (letter to Robert Koch, 1882, in Girard, 1988, quoted in Porter, 1973)*

The history of medical virology is inextricably bound up with laboratories. Indeed, as medical historians Andrew Cunningham and Perry Williams claim, the transition to laboratory medicine that took place in nineteenth century was a revolution at least as great as the transition to hospital medicine that preceded it (Cunningham and Williams, 1992, p. 3). What the famed Claude Bernard proclaimed for medicine in general is especially relevant to virology, a sub-discipline whose very existence originated with laboratory discoveries:

Medicine does not end in hospitals, as is often believed, but merely begins there. In leaving the hospital, a physician, jealous of the title in its scientific sense, must go into his laboratory; and there, by experiments on animals, he will seek to account for what he has observed in his patients, whether about the action of drugs or about the origin of morbid lesions in organs or tissues. There, in a word, he will achieve true medical science. (Claude Bernard, 1865, quoted in Cunningham and Williams, 1992, p. 3)

The laboratory revolution in most of Western Europe occurred in two waves. The first wave occurred between the 1820s and 1840s and was characterized by the rise of physiology, theories and methods of which were linked to chemistry, physics and anatomical pathology (Lenoir, 1992). The microscope appeared to be a helpful instrument to differentiate between normal and

pathological tissues and cells. A second wave of laboratory medicine occurred between the 1860s and the 1880s when laboratories for anatomy,
pathology and physiology were institutionalized within medical faculties.
The laboratory thus became the dominant space in which modern medicine
was conducted and the first steps were taken towards the direction of the
great institutes of Louis Pasteur and Robert Koch, where the propositions of
the germ theory of diseases would be demonstrated (Cunningham and Williams, 1992, p. 3). One of the first clear statements of the idea of a *contagium
vivum or contagium animatum* – i.e. a 'living' or animated contagium – as
the origin of infectious diseases came from Koch's teacher Jacob Henle in
1840; although his concept too, was based on thoughts and observations of
predecessors and contemporaries (Winkelstein, 1995; Ackerknecht, 2009, p. 7;
Gradmann, 2014). Henle summarized the characteristics of the *contagium
animatum* responsible for the occurrence and transmission of epidemic
and endemic diseases as follows:

> The contagious agent is a substance which in the course of a disease
> is excreted by the sick organism, and which communicated to healthy
> individuals produces the same disease in them. [...] It is easy to prove
> that contagions [...] actually multiply within the diseased organisms.
> An atom of pox poison can produce a rash over the entire body. [...] The
> symptoms of the disease do not appear directly after the entry of the
> contagious agent but rather after a certain period, which varies in the
> different contagions. (Henle, 1840, quoted in Winkelstein, 1995)

The public health specialist and historian of social medicine George Rosen
(1910-1977) translated the ideas formulated in the first chapter of Henle's
book *Pathologische Untersuchungen* (1840), entitled 'Concerning miasmata
and contagion'. According to Rosen the theory that infectious diseases were
caused by the growth of germs in the body was still new and therefore unac-
ceptable to many capable physicians and others in the scientific world during
the mid-nineteenth century. The English surgeon Joseph Lister combined
his ideas on the problem of wound infection with the findings of Pasteur,
who had shown the ubiquity of bacteria in the air and that putrefaction was
due to contamination with such organisms (Rosen, 1993/1958). As Rosen put
it aptly, the antiseptic principle, first applied by Lister on 12 August 1865,
had a chequered career; acceptance of the antiseptic techniques and the
underlying principle was neither rapid nor widespread in the 1850s and
1860s. Lister's predecessors in solving the mystery of wound infection were
Ignaz Semmelweis and Oliver Wendell Holmes, who independently showed

the cause of puerperal fever. Both came up a wall of resistance; Holmes resorted to literature, and Semmelweis was driven mad and died ironically enough of a septic wound of the finger several days after admission into an asylum. Luckily, Lister persevered in spite of being widely criticized; he was amply honoured later in life. As a consequence, the means for controlling infectious diseases in the nineteenth century were limited, with empirical experience and epidemiology making up the cornerstones of the measures taken (Rosen, 1993/1958, p. 293).

The development of this second wave in the Netherlands specifically has been covered by H. Beukers in his study on the laboratories of physiology, histology and chemistry at the Dutch universities during the nineteenth century (Beukers, 1986). The University of Groningen was the first to appoint I. van Deen as professor of physiology in 1852, followed by universities in Amsterdam and Utrecht where A. Heinsius, a physiologist trained by F.C. Donders, and the same Donders, a physiologist and also ophthalmologist, were appointed in 1858 and 1862, respectively. Leiden was last in 1866, when Heinsius moved there from Amsterdam. Although the first appointment, Van Deen did not open a laboratory in Groningen for fourteen years, while Donders had to wait four years until he could use his. In comparison, laboratories of newer disciplines, such as bacteriology, serology and parasitology, were established within laboratories for tropical hygiene only after the 1880s. Pursuant to the Higher Education Act of 1876, each university was mandated to appoint a professor holding the chair of medical police and hygiene. But the first appointments were a surgeon (J.E. van Iterson) in Leiden; a military doctor and hygienist (G. van Overbeek de Meijer) in Utrecht, a general practitioner (A.P. Fokker) in Groningen, and a hygienist (J. Förster) in Amsterdam (De Knecht-van Eekelen, 1991).

Evident in this second phase of laboratory medicine is a split in beliefs about disease causation and transmission between two sides that we may designate as contagionists and epidemiologists. Diseases such as smallpox or measles were considered to be contagious as they were transmitted from person to person, whereas others (such as cholera and yellow fever) were considered to be epidemic – used in the Hippocratic sense of a disease influenced by air, season, water, soil or sanitation as well as by mode of life – or miasmatic, i.e. caused by the state of the atmosphere or by poor sanitary conditions (Joly, 1964a, pp. 75-87; Joly, 1964b, pp. 71-74; Müri, 1986; Houwaart, 1991, p. 55; Thomassen à Thuessink, 1822). Interestingly, control measures based on contagionist principles resulted in practices such as isolation and quarantine instead of sanitary improvement, whereas the sanitary measures adopted as a result of the miasmatic principle – a questionable

Figure 3   Louis Pasteur (1822-1895)

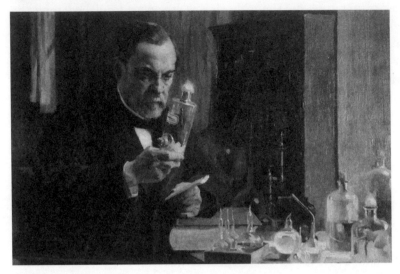

Detail of Albert Edelfelt's 1886 painting showing Louis Pasteur (1822-1895) in his laboratory at
the École normale supérieure in 1885, holding a bottle containing the spinal cord of a rabbit
inoculated with the rabies virus.
Reproduction by courtesy of © Institut Pasteur/Musée Pasteur
Photo: François Gardy

assumption that was never shown to be true – did in fact, help in controlling
large epidemics, such as cholera and malaria. Both diseases were prevalent
in the Netherlands, but the association between foul drinking water and
cholera was only admitted – reluctantly at that – towards the end of the
nineteenth century (Verdoorn, 1981/1965, p. 46). Thanks, however, to the
construction of waterworks in Amsterdam in 1854 for unrelated reasons,
the capital was less stricken by the cholera epidemic that ravaged the rest
of the country in 1866.

From the late 1850s on the investigations of Pasteur, and later of Koch and
others provided a stronger rationale for the connection between microbes
and infectious diseases. Microbiology – consisting mainly of bacteriology
and parasitology – emerged as one of the new medical disciplines over the
1880s and 1890s, and this laboratory-based germ theory established the basis
for epidemiology as a discipline and for various public health measures. By
the mid-1890s the Pasteur Institute in Paris and Robert Koch's Institute for
Infectious Diseases in Berlin had become the most prestigious microbiological
research laboratories in Western Europe (Weindling, 1992, pp. 170-188). We
will not detail the controversy between Pasteur's 'microbiology' school and
Koch's 'bacteriology' school, already masterfully outlined by others (Mollaret,

1983; Brock, 1988; Geison, 1995). But we will highlight one pertinent aspect of the controversy: that of the difference between the styles of approach of the two schools. As Thomas D. Brock observed, Pasteur 'was a champion of immunization methods, whereas Koch favoured public health measures for the control of disease' (1988, p. 177). Koch's Berlin school reacted negatively to Pasteur's rabies vaccine, which had been developed in 1885 without isolating the causative agent, and so the Germans had to oppose its use. As saliently noted by H.A. Lechevalier and M. Solotorovsky (1974, p. 280), in their authoritative *Three centuries of microbiology*, Pasteur's method must have smelled, at first, of charlatanism to the dogmatic Koch. But in the face of its success, he too adopted Pasteur's techniques within a few years in order to organize an anti-rabies vaccination service (Brock, 1988, p. 177). When in 1890, Koch in his turn announced the discovery of tuberculin – to which he ascribed not only diagnostic, but also therapeutic properties – Pasteur and the heads of the departments of the Pasteur Institute sent to Koch 'all their best congratulations for his great discovery' (Brock, 1988, p. 205). That the first trials using tuberculin did not reveal it to be the much anticipated curative agent after all, was an unfortunate sequel to this early episode in the history of microbiology, but not germane here as tuberculosis is not a viral disease.

Events unfolded somewhat differently in places other than France and Germany. In late Victorian era Britain, for example, changes in disease theories and medical practices associated with germs and bacteriology, although equally profound, were evolutionary rather than revolutionary (Worboys, 2007). It is the latter pattern that the Netherlands appears to have paralleled as well in the development of germ theory and its incorporation into public health measures.

The Dutch medical historians E.S. Houwaart and J.A. Verdoorn addressed the ways how in the Netherlands medical doctors as well as national and municipal authorities handled general problems of containing contagious diseases for which the causes were imperfectly understood in the nineteenth century (Houwaart, 1991; Verdoorn, 1981/1965). Houwaart gives an overview of the hygienic movement and the influence of the 'hygienists' on public health in the Netherlands during the period from 1840 to 1890. Verdoorn wrote an authoritative book on public health in Amsterdam during the nineteenth century. The discoveries of Pasteur, Koch and others were not applied to the protection measures of community health by the medical doctors of the Health Inspectorate until 1890. In an address at the 1881 meeting of the Netherlands Society of Medicine,[4] for instance, C.H. Kuhn,

4   Nederlandse Maatschappij voor Geneeskunst (NMG), since 1949 KNMG.

professor in pathological anatomy, expressed his doubts about whether infectious diseases were caused by bacteria (Houwaart, 1991, pp. 159, 157). Germ theories were absorbed slowly by Dutch doctors, who for a long time held a wait-and-see attitude. Facilities of medical microbiology research in the Netherlands were only established, and hesitantly at that, in the last decades of the nineteenth century (Van Lieburg, 1986). Of course, this development paralleled the protracted process of the acceptance of the germ theory in medicine in the Netherlands (Houwaart, 1991, p. 159; Verdoorn, 1981/1965).

In this chapter we probe in greater detail, the ideas and practices used in the nineteenth century by the medical profession in the Netherlands in response to such highly contagious diseases – now all known to be caused by viruses – as smallpox, measles, rabies, poliomyelitis and influenza. Recognized by their clinical symptoms, these diseases cover the spectrum from the highly contagious and symptomatic, e.g. smallpox, to contagious and highly asymptomatic, e.g. poliomyelitis. The latter disease is undoubtedly contagious, but only 0.1 to 1 per cent of the infected persons would develop paralytic disease, whereas 90 to 95 per cent would remain asymptomatic (Kapsenberg, 1988b, p. 693). Clearly, of the latter, only the symptomatic cases of influenza or poliomyelitis could be diagnosed without any definite knowledge about microbial causes. Nevertheless, epidemiological data on communicable diseases are relatively reliable as mandatory notification for cholera, typhoid, measles, scarlet fever, diphtheria, and pertussis was introduced in the Netherlands in 1865, and definitions of notifiable diseases must be interpreted in the light of the understanding in that period (Verdoorn, 1981/1965, p. 44). We have restricted ourselves to five diseases – smallpox, measles, rabies, poliomyelitis and influenza – and explored the development of ideas about them in an era before it was known that they were caused by viruses, or indeed, what viruses even were. In each case we have also looked at public health interventions taken at the time as well as then current 'ordinary' treatments for individual patients. Were these diseases already recognized by medical doctors; what was known of their epidemiology? It is our hope that by the book's end readers will have a better awareness about such issues.

Definition of virus

Infectious units (obligate intracellular parasites) consisting of either RNA or DNA enclosed in a protective coat. Viruses contain no functional ribosomes [for protein synthesis] or other cellular organelles and no energy-producing enzyme systems, although many viruses contain enzymes involved in nucleic

acid transcription. They cannot grow in size but their nucleic acid contains the necessary information for their replication in a susceptible host cell. This cell may provide some of the enzymes necessary for viral replication but its main function is to provide the energy-producing systems. The host cell may or may not be destroyed in the process of viral replication and release.
– *Brian W.J. Mahy (1997)*

Smallpox, public health measures and immunization

We start with smallpox, characterized by Willibrord Rutten in his social and demographic history of this disease in the Netherlands as that 'most horrible of all harpies' (1997). It is generally accepted that smallpox was very destructive all across Western Europe, the Netherlands inclusive, during the eighteenth century, with the last severe outbreak occurring in Europe and the Netherlands in 1870-1871 during the Franco-Prussian War (Fenner et al., 1988, p. 231; Rutten, 1997). Although outbreaks of smallpox in children occurred frequently during this period and the death rates among children in Amsterdam and Rotterdam were quite high, there was a remarkable reduction in child mortality after 1810, presumably due to the containment of smallpox. For instance, in 1780 child mortality (aged 0-9 years) in Amsterdam was about 480 per 1,000 live births of which smallpox accounted for approximately 20 per cent; the share of smallpox decreased to 1-2 per cent between 1810 and 1820 and since then the infant mortality rate remained between 350-400 per 1,000 live births (Rutten, 1997, p. 372). As smallpox is a 'crowding disease', it is spread over the countryside depended on the rate of vaccination – already a known practice by this time – and population density. Other factors contributing to the provincial level of smallpox mortality included the distance from the focus of infection – usually a larger urban centre – and health condition of sub-population in the affected area. Rutten has calculated that vaccination rate and population density explained up to 42 per cent and 52 per cent, respectively, of the variation in the smallpox mortality per province.

Although not common knowledge in eighteenth-century Europe, the prevention of smallpox by the administration of pustular fluid of patients via a scratch on the skin of healthy persons was a centuries-old practice in other parts of the world. It was first reported independently in China and India not before the fourth century AD and seventh century AD, respectively, and in the tenth century AD in south-western Asia, and then introduced in Egypt and other parts of North Africa. This method of inoculation of material of smallpox pustules, known as variolation, caused a less severe disease than did natural airborne infection, and upon recovery the person was immune to further infection. But variolation also had a major disadvantage that was already known then because the viruses used in this method were not attenuated and could therefore still cause severe disease and had a death toll of 1 in 48 to 60 cases. But this figure was much lower than the death toll of 20-30 per cent of naturally acquired smallpox (Fenner et al., 1988, pp. 246 and 255). The English Lady Mary Wortley Montagu promoted the introduction of variolation to Western Europe after she encountered the method in 1717 in Turkey, and decided to apply it to her children. Her desire to do so was likely the result of her own experience – her elegant appearance forever marred by pockmarks from having herself suffered from smallpox in England in 1715 at the age of 26 years. Whereas variolation became an accepted method in the English countryside, medical, ethical and religious objections hampered the adoption of this practice in the rest of Europe for some decades to come (Rutten, 1997, p. 25; Eriksen, 2013). It gradually gained acceptance, beginning, likely for economic reasons, in the higher circles of society, where the expensive regimens to prepare children for inoculation were affordable. The famous Herman Boerhaave, also known as the 'Dutch Hippocrates', never recommended inoculation to prevent smallpox, although he devoted a positive aphorism about this subject in 1728 (Hillen, 2017). In his 'Aphorismen' Boerhaave wrote in 1728: 'Prophylaxis insitiva videtur satis certa, tutaque.'[5] Boerhaave's student, the Swiss-born Amsterdam-based physician T. Tronchin, was the first person to introduce inoculation in the Netherlands, when he administered it to his son in 1748 (Endtz, 1986). Thomas Schwencke, professor of anatomy and surgery at the Hague Medical School, performed the first inoculation there in 1754 (Hillen, 2017).

The fate of the recipients of variolation was inconsistent and unpredictable. A particularly famous case is that of the family of the highborn Isabella Agneta Elisabeth van Tuyll van Serooskerken, who became later famous under the pen name Belle van Zuylen (Endtz, 1986; Wolff, 1986). Following the example of Tronchin's son, first in 1754 two of her brothers and then in 1755 Isabella herself, were inoculated successfully against smallpox without complications. Unfortunately, their mother would not fare so well. More than a decade later, probably driven by the serious smallpox epidemic in Europe in 1768, she was inoculated by the English inoculator J.S. Williams

5   In Dutch, translated by Love: inenting komt mij zeker en heilzaam genoeg ter voorbehoeding tegen pokken voor (Prophylaxis by scarification appears to me salutary and safe enough).

Figure 4   Jan Ingen Housz (1730-1799)

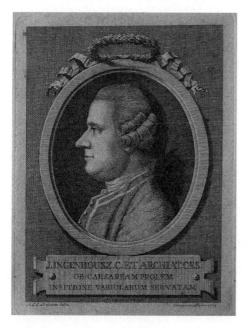

Portrait by Jan Verkolje, c. 1680-1686
Reproduction by courtesy of Rijks Museum, Amsterdam

in Utrecht. Her daughter Isabelle wrote a letter on 28 October 1768 to her friend Constant d'Hermenches: 'Ma mère se prepare pour l'inoculation.'[6] On November 15, she wrote again to report that after the treatment her mother had the smallpox without being seriously ill and that they were confident of a rapid convalescence. Seventeen days after the inoculation the vesicles were dried in. Unfortunately, however, the patient suffered from respiratory symptoms with fever and died on 4 December 1768. The professors of the Medical Faculty in Utrecht reprimanded Williams, who defended himself by publishing the course of the illness with interpretation of the symptoms and the therapeutic considerations wherein he concluded that the patient died of a then prevailing serious cold. Whatever the truth of the matter, it is no surprise that this fatal accident did not prove beneficial for the success of an inoculation campaign against smallpox in the Netherlands.

Meanwhile, the ever-capricious outcomes of the inoculations decided the fates of physicians and patients in other parts of Europe as well. In 1768, for instance, Jan Ingen Housz, a Dutch medical doctor and scientist who

6   My mother is being prepared for the inoculation.

lived in London, went to Vienna. In response to a plea from Empress Maria Theresa to King George III, Ingen Housz was recommended by the royal physician Sir John Pringle (Ingen Housz et al., 2005; Jenkins, 1999; Walvoort, 2006). He arrived in May and after the successful inoculation of the royal children in September was rewarded by the Empress with an appointment as court physician and councillor, together with a life-long annual pension of 5,000 florins. He was then requested to travel to Florence to inoculate the Emperor Joseph's brother, Leopold, Grand Duke of Tuscany, and his family, and to teach the art of inoculation in the Habsburg dominions. A biography of this remarkable medical doctor was recently published by a descendant of one of his brothers (Ingen Housz et al., 2005). Ingen Housz started his career as a general practitioner in Breda in the south of the Netherlands, where he had been born in 1730. After a decade he moved in 1767 to England to learn smallpox inoculation, which in time, led to his adventures and accolades as described above. After serving the royal family for several years in Vienna, he dedicated his later life to scientific experimentation, notably revealing the fundamentals of photosynthesis and the motion of particles in a medium, which was published 43 years before Robert Brown described this phenomenon that got his name to honour him (Ingen Housz et al., 2005; Van der Pas, 1971). In 1789 Ingen Housz left Vienna and continued his scientific experiments in England.

In a report on his journey to Holland in 1768, Denis Diderot, the famous Encyclopaedist, noted that whereas variolation was introduced in some Dutch cities as method of controlling the disease, it was forbidden in other places where it was considered to be prejudicial (Benot, 2013). Diderot's main source for this information was in all likelihood the Dutch physician and scientist Petrus Camper, whom he had met in The Hague (Benot, 2013, p. 41). Camper was an influential figure who had been professor of medicine first in Amsterdam, then Franeker and eventually in Groningen (Van Berkel and Ramakers, 2015, pp. 9-16). In 1774 Camper demonstrated his knowledge and experience as an inoculator in his answer in a competition of the Académie Royale des Sciences, Inscriptions & Belles Lettres de Toulouse (Camper, 1774). He also executed studies on inoculation to combat rinderpest (cattle plague), which had been sweeping across Dutch livestock since 1740 (Huygelen, 1997). Camper and his colleague Van Doeveren were asked by the municipality of Groningen to study the inoculation in cattle using nasal mucus of sick animals as infective material. The experiments were performed in cooperation their colleague Munniks and with Geert Reinders, a clever farmer who later received prizes from two learned societies, the Amsterdam Society for the Advancement of Agriculture[7] and the Holland Society of Sciences[8] in Haarlem (Bruins, 1951; Tersteeg, 1998). Although the results were rather meagre, Reinders persevered and inoculation of calves instead of yearlings or heifers was more successful.

Also, in 1776, the learned Batavian Society of Empirical Philosophy[9] in Rotterdam held a competition on strategies for spreading the word about variolation among the general public both in cities and the countryside (Van Lieburg, 1985, pp. 52 and 115). Unfortunately, the lack of further documented information about this event prevents us from discussing the effects of the competition meaningfully, but it shows that variolation was perceived as much less dangerous as smallpox and those efforts were made to make it more acceptable to society.

Meanwhile among English farmers in the eighteenth century, the insusceptibility of milkmaids to variolation gave rise to a 'vague opinion' about the protective value of cowpox (Fenner et al., 1988). This opinion was famously put to the test when the country doctor Edward Jenner demonstrated that the inoculation of humans with material from eruptions upon teats of cows protected humans against smallpox as well. Jenner arrived at the idea of using the fluid of cowpox vesicles as inoculum based on the following observations:

> Among those whom in the country I was frequently called upon to inoculate, many resisted every effort to give them the Small Pox. These patients I found had undergone a disease they called the Cow Pox, contracted by milking cows affected with a peculiar eruption on their teats. (Jenner, 1801, quoted in Bazin, 1999, p. 180)

The fluid that Jenner used was called vaccine or vaccinia after the Latin word *vacca* for cow and inoculation using vaccinia acquired the label 'vaccination' by which we know it today. He conducted his first successful experiments demonstrating protection against smallpox by inoculating a lad named James Phipps with cowpox material on 14 May 1796.

Soon after the 1798 publication of Jenner's *Inquiry into the causes and effects of variolae vacciniae*, the aforementioned Ingen Housz wrote the first of a series of letters informing Jenner about a farmer who caught

7   Amsterdamsche Maatschappij ter bevordering van den Landbouw.
8   Hollandsche Maatschappij der Wetenschappen (today: Koninklijke Hollandsche Maatschappij der Wetenschappen).
9   Het Bataafsch Genootschap der Proefondervindelijke Wijsbegeerte.

cowpox by milking an infected cow (Beale and Beale, 2005). When the farmer was later inoculated with smallpox, serious symptoms developed; as Ingen Housz described, 'a great many Small pox came out, and he communicated the infection to his father, who died of it.' In the exchange of letters that followed, Ingen Housz and Jenner argued over whether infection with cowpox conferred protection against smallpox. Then on Thursday 19 September 1799, the front page of the *Bath Chronicle* carried an advertisement for 'improved inoculation' in which Mr Henry Jenner, Surgeon, of Berkeley in Gloucestershire, announced that he would be attending the White Lion Inn, weekly 'for the purpose of inoculating [...] in the milder way [...] those who wish to escape the Small-Pox'. Henry Jenner was Edward Jenner's nephew, assistant, and erstwhile apprentice. Here then, was Jenner's success in action. But on an inside page of the very same newspaper was a brief and more poignant notice: 'Saturday, died at Bowood-park, Dr Ingenhousz, physician to his Imperial Majesty, and member of several learned societies.' Thus, as Beale and Beale (2005) concluded wryly, 'the Ingen Housz-Jenner correspondence was most certainly at an end'.

In 1799 Levie Salomon Davids, a physician in Rotterdam, received from John Walker, an English physician who sojourned in Leiden, some vaccine material which had been dried onto cotton threads. When Davids administered the vaccine to a two-year-old boy on 17 October 1799, he became the first person to attempt vaccination in the Netherlands (Rutten, 2010; Veldhuyzen, 1957). Previously, he had tried using some vaccine dried on glass slides which he received from Paris, but this material had proven ineffective. It seems quite probable that the effective vaccination material provided by Walker had come from William Woodville, director of the London Small-Pox and Inoculation Hospital, and possibly contained a mixture of cowpox and smallpox virus (Fenner et al., 1988; Rutten, 1997, pp. 214-216). Evidently, despite the French Revolution and the constitution of the Batavian Republic in 1795, there was still some freedom of movement between England and the continent. Anyway, it was not until five months after the preparation of the thread in England before Davids vaccinated the two-year-old boy. Thus, it might be possible that the vaccine was expired and had lost activity, and then vaccination should be expected to be ineffective. After an incision was made by a barber-surgeon Davids put the cotton thread with vaccine in the wound. When the boy got fever at the seventh day, the thread was removed and a lesion was present. A second lesion developed and both lesions healed after fourteen days. To prove later the success of the operation, Davids administered again a dose of natural smallpox agent to the boy, who appeared immune – resistant – because he neither fell ill nor developed any lesions (Rutten, 1997, p. 211).

In 1801 the Executive Committee of the Batavian Republic decreed smallpox as Public Enemy Number One. Even so, authorities were hesitant at first about using vaccination and adhered to the variolation using material from smallpox lesions to appease fears of transmission of cowpox back to cattle. But after 1806, vaccinations using cowpox fluid were widely adopted in all the urban centres of the Netherlands. The acceptance of vaccinations in the rural areas took a little more time. When in 1806, the Batavian Republic was changed into the Kingdom of Holland by Napoleon Bonaparte, his brother Louis Napoleon became King of Holland. In 1808 Louis Napoleon promulgated a decree which laid the foundation for the vaccination campaigns for decades to come. Now, inoculation using cowpox was advocated, and the older method of variolation only allowed after specific permission of the municipal authorities. After the fall of Napoleon Bonaparte and the return of William Frederik, Prince of Orange-Nassau, the Kingdom of the Netherlands, was proclaimed in 1813. Nevertheless, the 1808 smallpox immunization policy of Louis Napoleon was continued under the reign of King William I and his successors until 1872, when the Law on Provisions against contagious diseases,[10] also known as Law on Epidemics, was introduced.

The aim of the Law on Provisions was to vaccinate all infants on a voluntary basis. The subjects were preferably healthy children between the age of one to two years and parents were obliged to come back with the child on the third, eighth and eleventh days after the first vaccination for revision of the results of the inoculation before a certificate was issued. The lymph from the lesions of these children was collected during their later visits and used for vaccination of other subjects. From the early 1820s onward, children missing a vaccination certificate were supposed to be excluded from primary school. But these regulations proved easy enough to evade, for example, vaccination was obligatory only for children of the poor. When an original vaccination certificate needed for admittance to school was missing, authenticated copies were easily provided by municipal authorities because they knew that there were serious lacunae in the records (Rutten, 1997, pp. 419-420). The vaccinations were executed mainly by medical doctors who were organized in societies for the advancement of cowpox inoculation with the purpose of maintaining a chain of cowpox virus in humans. The number of doctors reporting figures on numbers of vaccinations performed per

10 Wet tot voorzieningen tegen besmettelijke ziekten.

quarter to municipal or provincial authorities varied, and fell, for example, to 70 per cent or lower in Amsterdam in the latter half of the 1840s (Rutten, 1997, p. 298). Penalties for non-compliance established by the minister had to be withdrawn on sentence pronounced by a judge.

The history of the control and prevention of smallpox in the nineteenth century can also be found in the works of the above-mentioned societies that were founded soon after the introduction of inoculation with cowpox in the Netherlands, e.g. the Society for the Advancement of Cowpox Inoculation under the device 'Ne pestis intret vigila' (Be watchful that the pestilence does not come in)[11] in Rotterdam in 1799 or the Amsterdam Society for the Advancement of Cowpox Inoculation for Those of Limited Means[12] in 1803. As cowpox was a sporadic disease, there was a shortage of cowpox material derived from cattle, but the arm-to-arm vaccination in humans was practised to overcome shortages and an effective vaccine could thus be produced for decades after hundreds of passages of cowpox.

Alongside compulsory vaccinations movements from 1820 onward, opposition to vaccination was growing and led by young intellectuals of the so-called Réveil movement, a religious circle founded by the poet and savant Willem Bilderdijk, who had fought against ideas of the Enlightenment and the French Revolution (Rutten, 1997, pp. 284-288). Leading figures in the opposition to vaccinations included the poet Isaac da Costa, medical doctor Abraham Capadose, and Willem and Dirk van Hogendorp, sons of the influential politician Gijsbert Karel van Hogendorp. As a young doctor Capadose had performed vaccinations in Amsterdam when he worked with his uncle, Dr I. Capadose, who as court physician of King Louis Bonaparte devoted himself to encourage vaccination. Both Capadose and Da Costa were descendants of prominent Portuguese Jewish families, but both converted later to Dutch Reformed religion. The brothers Van Hogendorp were vaccinated in their childhood, as their father was an advocate of cowpox inoculation. The attitude towards vaccinations of both brothers at adult age was in sharp contrast not only to the view of their father but also to the standpoint of their grandfather Willem van Hogendorp who was the author of a book published in 1779 and titled *Sophronisba: of, de gelukkige moeder door de inëntinge van haare dochters* (Sophronisba; or, The happy mother who had her daughters inoculated) in which he recommended variolation.

About half a century after the introduction of vaccination using cowpox, the learned Society for the Advancement of Science, Medicine and Surgery

---

11   Genootschap tot Bevordering der Koepokinenting, onder de zinspreuk *Ne pestis intret vigila.*
12   Het Amsterdamsch Genootschap ter Bevordering der Koepokinenting voor Minvermogenden.

paid attention to the problem of smallpox and the prevention by vaccination. An obvious explanation as to why it did not act earlier is that the society started in 1795 only for chirurgeons – barber-surgeons – who were not involved in the vaccination practice, and only in 1845 medical doctors too were included in the membership. At that time a committee was appointed to study several aspects of variola, cowpox and the immunization by means of a standard form that could be used by the members to gather information on clinical aspects of smallpox, duration of protection by cowpox inoculation, the appropriate age to administer the (re)vaccination, and contraindications of vaccination (GNGH, 1845).

The human arm-to-arm method for the production of the infectious material for vaccinia inoculations was beset with problems. For one there was the risk of transmitting symptomatic bacterial infections while transmission by blood of syphilis or hepatitis B was unknown in those days. In addition, the method proved inadequate when the human arm-to-arm chain was broken for some reason and new, fresh material from infected cows was not available to rejuvenate the cycle of production. To address such problems of shortage, Gennaro Galbiati and Michele Troja, two physicians in Naples, developed a method of continuous production of cowpox in calves (Buonaguro et al., 2015). As early as 1803 they were able to prove that cowpox could be transferred from cowpox-vaccinated people to calves and that the lymphatic material recovered from these calves had not lost their effectiveness in preventing smallpox. The production of the so-called animal lymph in Naples was taken up and continued by physicians/researchers Ferdinando Palasciano and Giuseppe Negri in 1844. In 1861, Negri successfully took on the task of producing the vaccine at his own expense and established manufacturing facilities in Paris and Lyon, too.

As with the vaccination, the idea of using calf – that is to say animal – lymph to inject into humans was slower to gain acceptance in the Netherlands than in Italy and France. Animal-derived vaccines were first introduced in quick succession in Rotterdam and Amsterdam in 1868 and 1869 with the foundation of the Parcs Vaccinogènes, associated with one of the vaccination clinics at these cities (Veldhuyzen, 1957, p. 42). In fact, cowsheds for some calves were built against the building of the clinic. Over the course of the next decade from 1871 to 1883, such vaccination clinics with adjoining Parc Vaccinogène for the large-scale vaccine production were established in The Hague, Utrecht, Dordrecht, Haarlem, 's-Hertogenbosch, Groningen, Arnhem, Leeuwarden, Middelburg, Maastricht, and the last in Nijmegen in 1889. Eventually there were a total of thirteen vaccination government-recognized clinics nationwide. The Parcs Vaccinogènes accommodated a waiting room, consultation room, administrative office, and separate cowsheds for some calves. The calves were used as a source of vaccination material; the fluid from the pocks on the fifth day after inoculation was expressed and suspended in the preservative glycerol, which was considered to be a convenient bactericidal solvent that also prevented ice-formation. There was, however, one drawback to this method for at temperatures above 0°C glycerol could inactivate vaccinia virus rather rapidly.

Despite the large-scale vaccinations against smallpox since the beginning of the nineteenth century, a big epidemic of smallpox occurred in Amsterdam in 1871. Verdoorn has attributed this outbreak to the laxity of the medical doctors and the indolence of the inhabitants with regard to vaccination (Verdoorn, 1981/1965, pp. 182-185). But as mentioned above, there was an additional factor that might have played a role in the epidemic: Since the beginning of the nineteenth century certain Calvinist groups strongly opposed vaccinations on religious grounds, and it is possible that their opinions carried more weight among the potential recipients. Thus, there would have been a significant disparity between the availability of the vaccine versus the number of people who actually received them. Adriaan M. Ballot, a medical doctor in Rotterdam who published on sanitary problems, compared the death rates attributable to smallpox in the Netherlands during the great 1870-1871 epidemic against figures from London, where vaccination was compulsory. He was a general practitioner in Rotterdam, and he was a protagonist for the public health interests of his fellow citizens (Thomas and Ballot, 1918). According to his calculations, had London relied on the type of voluntary vaccination applied in the Netherlands, the number of deaths there during the months of the epidemic should have been increased to 3,000 per week rather than the actually observed number of 286. Based on these figures he pleaded for a compulsory vaccination of all children in the Netherlands (Ballot, 1871). In 1872, following Ballot's report, Dutch officials passed a law that obliged all children and teachers to be vaccinated before they entered school. Since school attendance was mandatory, such an indirect measure might have been the best approach to achieve their ends without inciting resistance.

In summary then, the immunization programmes and preventive measures to control epidemics of smallpox in the nineteenth century were based on practical insights and empirical observations gained from experiments with fluid scraped from the lesions that appeared after inoculation. Fundamental knowledge about the nature of the agents that caused either smallpox (variola) or cowpox was still lacking, but at a practical level, not essential for successful prevention or containment of the disease. Nevertheless, speculative ideas about the nature of the mysterious agents existed widely.

According to W.F. Veldhuyzen, Europeans in the eighteenth century still adhered to the view of smallpox causation first suggested by the Arab physician Rhazes in the tenth century AD (Veldhuyzen, 1957, p. 43). Comparing the bodily process to that of the fermentation of wine, Rhazes explanation for the cause of smallpox was that:

> Small-Pox arises when the blood putrefies and ferments, so that the superfluous vapours are thrown out of it, and it is changed from the blood of infants, which is like must, into the blood of young men, which is like wine perfectly ripened: and the Small-Pox itself may be compared to the fermentation and hissing noise which take place in the must at that time. (Rhazes, 1848, p. 29)

It is evident from the 1776 doctoral thesis *De variolis* (On variola) of an Anglo-American student Eduardus Gautt, who defended his thesis at Leiden University, that he still held on to a version of this conception. But although he accepted the premise that smallpox poison (virus) 'works in the human body as ferment', he was unsure as to the nature of the fermentation. He wrote: 'I cannot determine which type of fermentation it concerns: as in wine, or vinegar, or septic, or is it fermentation in itself?' In the original Latin this read as: 'Agit hoc virus in corpus humanum ad instar fermenti. Sed quae species fermentationis hic contingat, utrum vinosa? An acetosa an septica? An potius sit fermentatio sui generis? Ego quidem mihi determinandum non sumo' (Veldhuyzen, 1957, p. 43).

Fermentation – both practically and theoretically – would in fact prove fundamental to the emergence of the entire discipline of microbiology. The general knowledge about the actual process would be broadened by the studies in the nineteenth century by Antoine Lavoisier, Joseph Louis Gay-Lussac, and Louis Jacques Thenard. But it was left to Louis Pasteur, who began his studies of fermentation in 1854, to bring together the practical knowledge of the problem of fermentation together with its significance as a metaphor in explanations of disease causation. In his opinion, ferment – or the active principle of fermentation – was a living entity. Convinced that putrefaction was a kind of fermentation due to microbial activity, in 1863 he informed Napoleon III that his ambition was to arrive at the knowledge of the cause of putrid and contagious diseases (Dubos, 1986/1950; Rosen, 1993/1958).

The implications of Pasteur's ideas and findings on fermentation for understanding the cause of diseases such as smallpox would not be realized for some decades to come. It is clear in hindsight that such a realization required knowledge of the fundamental differences between agents such as bacteria and viruses, a difference whose significance is sometimes overlooked even today. Thus, despite the knowledge that living bacteria caused infections, a disease such as smallpox was not attributed to such living causes. This gap in understanding is evident from talks at the 1881 meeting of the Amsterdam Society for the Advancement of Cowpox Inoculation for Those of Limited Means, where the treatment of human lymph with antiseptics to prevent contamination was a prominent topic of discussion. In a session on vaccination, the lecturers reported results of a study showing that the addition of a 3 per cent solution of carbolic acid to the human cowpox lymph did not disturb the action of the vaccine, but killed living organisms or bacteria (Veldhuyzen, 1957, p. 43). The explanation, offered by the chairman of the meeting and president of the society, J. van Geuns, was that being a chemical ferment, the vector of the vaccine agent was left intact, while living organisms were killed by the carbolic acid. Based on such events Veldhuyzen is probably justified in his conclusion that almost a century after Jenner the concept of virus was still in its infancy. Indeed, such a state of affairs persisted well into the 1930s. In his lecture 'Life's fringes', the famous microbiologist A.J. Kluyver observed, even at that late date, that 'many investigators were inclined to regard viruses – and this applies to the bacteriophages as well – as something produced by the infected cell which has been designated variously as an enzyme, a metabolic disturber, a lethal factor, hereditary factor or simply gene' (Kluyver, 1937).

Measles, lack of prevention?

Measles is a common, highly contagious disease of childhood, which like smallpox has likely existed in humans since antiquity. It shares many similar features with smallpox and indeed for centuries appears to have been regarded as an alternative, somewhat milder, form of the same disease. The first documented recognition that these two diseases were different appears in the tenth-century treatise by Rhazes on smallpox and measles, a book that was reprinted about forty times in Europe between 1498 and 1866. A larger part of the book is devoted to smallpox, but Rhazes pointed out various differences in the seasonality, type of patients most prone to the disease, actual symptoms and prognoses of the two diseases (Kaadan, 2000). Despite this knowledge, well into the nineteenth century, measles had to be differentiated from other diseases with rash characterized as so-called maculopapular eruptions: not only smallpox but also scarlet fever, and rubella. For much of the period under consideration here, measles was considered as a mild disease although the frequency of serious complications is much higher than we would expect today in times of vaccines. Nowadays, the rate of serious complications due to measles in unvaccinated children is about 10 per cent in the developed world, and between 10-20 per cent in developing countries, depending on the age of the child and the specific country (Anderson and May, 1992). Prevention and containment were often difficult for as we now know, measles exanthema typically appears only about fourteen days after exposure to the virus, whereas patients are already highly infectious from the eighth day after infection during the so-called prodromal phase.

The old and respected *Netherlands Journal of Medicine*[13] contains some interesting reports on the changing epidemiologic pattern of measles in the late eighteenth and nineteenth century. In 1871, the Rotterdam physician Ballot, who had presented data on smallpox, also compared the death rates attributed to smallpox, scarlet fever and measles over three consecutive 30-year periods in his city: from 1778-1807, 1808-1840 and 1841-1870. Whereas smallpox showed a steep decline in incidence from 333 cases per 100,000 inhabitants in the first period to 80 and to 44 over the latter two, figures were much smaller and less variable for scarlet fever: 66, 55 and 6.5 deaths per 100,000 people. In contrast the figures for measles appeared to increase rather than decrease, albeit by small numbers – 32, 74, and 81 deaths per 100,000 people, respectively – in the same three periods (Ballot, 1871). Based on this data he attributed the sharp decrease in the death toll of smallpox to vaccinations. As the numbers indicate, scarlet fever had ceased to be an epidemic by the third period. The almost tripling of deaths attributed to measles meant that towards the middle of the nineteenth century measles became a more important cause of death in Rotterdam than either smallpox or scarlet fever. More recently, Verdoorn who analysed the death rates attributed to measles in Amsterdam over the latter half of the nineteenth century found that after an initial dip from 260 to 120 between 1855 and 1880, there was an increase to 210 in 1890 and a sharp increase the following year to 278 total deaths. He seems to attribute the higher figures for Amsterdam to the bad housing conditions and overcrowding (Verdoorn, 1981/1965, p. 53).

Since the 1860s, members of the hygiene movement had held high positions at the provincial health inspectorates or health councils, and made efforts to regulate the municipal and provincial sanitary regulations by

13   Nederlands Tijdschrift voor Geneeskunde (NTvG).

national law (Houwaart, 1991, p. 266). Although government and parliament could agree with these proposals, both institutions were hesitant to restrict municipal autonomy. In this regard it is of importance that over the period 1866 to 1872 there were epidemics of cholera, typhoid fever, and, most relevant here, smallpox epidemics. With the passage of the 1872 the Law on Provisions against contagious diseases mentioned earlier, measles was included in the list of notifiable diseases besides cholera, typhoid fever, smallpox, scarlet fever, diphtheria and whooping cough. By this law, all children with measles and anyone in contact with them had to be excluded from school. The introduction of this law encountered much resistance from the medical doctors who were afraid of intrusions into the doctor-patient relationship. Furthermore, such measures were seen as impractical and even unnecessary because of the relatively mild symptoms of the disease and the absence of preventive measures, such as inoculation. The argument that measles posed no serious threat may seem remarkable today, but in 1861 a report on the complication of pneumonia after measles was published in the NTvG (Drielsma, 1861; Catrin, 1891 and 1897). High mortality rates depending on the epidemic, age, and social class were also reported (Haakma Tresling, 1872, 1893; Hanlo 1880).

Measles was removed from the notification list in 1900. The arguments that convinced members of the House of Representatives were the overall lack of hygienic measures and indications that exclusion from school was not effective anyway (Netherlands Staten-Generaal, 1889). The discussion on whether to institute measures and what they needed to be for the prevention of measles had its share of both proponents and opponents, sometimes embodied in the same person. In a publication in the NTvG, the medical doctor A.O.H. Tellegen, for example, favoured the inclusion of measles in the notification law, but at the same time also proposed other measures for its prevention. Remarkably, he pointed out that since measles was already very infectious in the prodromal stage, its exclusion from schools would not be particularly effective as it would have already spread. Also he argued that contracting measles at an earlier age would protect children against new infections later. At the same time, he pleaded for keeping children between six months to three years of age from attending their nursery schools during epidemics, in the absence of other measures, because the mortality due to the disease was highest in that age group (Tellegen, 1879). It would be a long time before anti-measles immunization could be employed. The first measles vaccines only became available in the 1960s; general vaccination against measles was included in the national Dutch immunization programme in 1976.

Rabies, treatment and public health measures

Rabies is a horrifying disease that is transmitted to humans through the bite of an animal harbouring the infectious virus. This disease was recognized in ancient times (Baumann, 1924). Of the disease itself the famous first-century physician and medical writer Celsus wrote in *De medicina*, 'The Greeks call it hydrophobia, a most wretched disease, in which the sick person is tormented at the same time with thirst and the fear of water, and in which there is but little hope' (Mutinelli et al., 2004). After an incubation period from less than 30 days to sometimes more than one year, the early, general symptoms reported were fever, malaise, nausea and vomiting, and in case the wound is still present, paraesthesia, or pain at the wound. The most common clinical picture was furious rabies with hydrophobia – beginning with difficulty in swallowing liquids and increasing to spasms in the pharynx that spread to the respiratory muscles; the other was a paralytic disease without hydrophobia (Bleck and Rupprecht, 2005). In any case, once established, the disease was (and is) invariably fatal.

Compared to the outbreaks of plague and smallpox sweeping Europe, however, rabies never claimed large numbers of victims, even in epidemic situations (Wilkinson, 1977). Knowing what we now do about the virus and disease, we think that one reason for this pattern could be that the disease is rarely transmitted from human to human. The virus is harboured in the salivary glands of the animal and humans are typically infected when bitten by an infected animal. The most common important animal reservoirs include the domestic dog, the wolf, fox and, in some regions, several species of bats. Symptoms of the fatal disease develop over an extended period, varying from days, weeks or even months. The disease is ultimately fatal and, to this day, there is no cure against the disease save vaccination.

At the end of the eighteenth century public health measures against rabies were directed towards efforts at controlling – i.e. capturing and isolating – the rabid animal. The reporting of animals known to have bitten a person or showing suspicious signs to the local authorities was compulsory. If clearly rabid, the dogs had to be placed in custody for observation or killed, and the body disposed of safely to prevent contamination due to the spread to other animals (Ali Cohen, 1864a and 1864b). Then, a municipal ordinance had to be promulgated and dogs had to be tethered at home and at the yard; of course, dogs were not allowed to roam the public streets. Furthermore, stray dogs had to be dealt with by police and even civilians, who were allowed kill stray dogs or bring them to the police (Baron, 2006).

Twenty-seven such ordinances were issued in the city of Groningen, with peaks in 1806, 1814-1815 and 1838-1840.

Initiatives to institute provincial measures against rabies – as reported by the hygienist L. Ali Cohen, health inspector of the provinces of Groningen and Friesland, for example – were not successful. In the 1850s and 1860s Cohen and other Dutch public health workers published reports on governmental measures against rabies in France and Germany in the NTvG. The measures taken against the rabid animal in France and Germany were similar to those in the Netherlands. Meanwhile, treatment measures of the wounded persons were drastic. For instance, the rapid burning – cauterization – of the wound using a red-hot iron within one hour of being bitten appeared to offer the best chances to survive. Over a period of ten years (1852-1862) there were 195 deaths due to rabies of which 111 did not receive this treatment, 45 were treated too late and 39 treated insufficiently. Thirty-five of the 63 people who remained free of disease had been treated within one hour of being bitten. It is no small wonder that Ali Cohen was discouraged enough to comment on a French report that there was no treatment available for this horrible disease (1864b). He sighed: 'With regard to her nature, to the causes of her spontaneous appearance, to her treatment, to all these points, we did not make nowadays absolutely any progress since the beginning.'[14]

In 1867 an international congress of veterinarians was organized in Vienna, where among the many issues discussed was the question of the most effective measures that could be taken by the governments to prevent or at least to minimize the detrimental effects of rabies (Hekmeijer, 1867). Of the 170 participants at congress, 54 were official representatives of their government. But although the Dutch government was not represented for reasons unknown to Hekmeijer, a leading veterinarian who attended the congress, there seems to have been some transmission of information because legislative action based on recommendations of the congress was carried out in the Netherlands. In 1875, for example, the House of Representatives passed an act on provisions against rabies. Consequently, national measures, rather than local or municipal ordinances, were instituted, including measures to muzzle dogs, report rabid animals to the local authorities, and destroy rabid dogs and cats (Polak, 1964). One measure of how seriously the people took this disease is the establishment, even in advance of this law, of a

14   Met betrekking tot haren aard, tot de oorzaken van haar spontaan tevoorschijn komen, tot hare behandeling, op al deze punten zijn wij thans volstrekt niet verder gevorderd, dan men is geweest in aanvang der tijden.

stable for mad dogs (*dolle-honden stal*) built at the State Veterinary School (Rijks-Veeartsenij School) in Utrecht (Offringa, 1971, p. 133).

As for treatment, various makeshift home remedies were used to treat human patients for centuries. One measure apparently advocated in the province of Gelderland during the eighteenth century was the dosing of the patient with an herbal infusion containing a mixture of supposed medicinal herbs: *imperatori, artemisia, betonica, abrotanum, ruta, salvia, semper vivum majus, carduus felonum*, and *levisticum* (De Feyfer, 1928). It was also recommended that the same potion be used to wash the wound, which had to remain open by washing and scratching for as long as possible. Another preferable and, hopefully, more common treatment was the immediate cauterization of the bite wound with a red-hot iron, *ferrum candens* (Van Beverwijck, 1670, quoted in De Feyfer, 1928). In fact, cauterization had already been advised by Celsus in the first century AD, and would continue to be recommended by physicians well into the nineteenth century. Therapies against rabies attempted in the Netherlands by the nineteenth century did not differ significantly from those that were recommended in England as presented by K. Codell Carter (Braat, 1937; Codell Carter, 1982). On the other hand, there was a great diversity in the prophylactic and therapeutic measures that followed after the nineteenth century. As one physician observed: 'Every remedy which the terrors of the disease or the ingenuity of the physician could suggest has been tried.' (Codell Carter, 1982).

Scientifically, it is evident from articles that were published in the NTvG in the 1880s that the Dutch were not only aware of Pasteur's work, but also, that with the exception of some resistance in certain medical circles, regarded it very favourably. The year 1885 marked a complete change for the treatment of rabies, after Pasteur and his colleagues Émile Roux and Charles-Edouard Chamberland decided to treat Joseph Meister – a young man bitten by a rabid dog but still asymptomatic. The medical doctors E.F.A. Vulpian, member of the French rabies commission, and J. Grancher, clinical professor of children's diseases at the Parish Faculté de Médecine, examined the boy and concluded that he almost surely faced death from rabies (Geison, 1995). As Pasteur was not a medical doctor, Grancher administered the actual injections to Meister. Although this episode had a happy outcome, the historian Geison has charged that the scientists acted in a highly unethical manner, as they conducted an experimental trial of a live rabies vaccine on a human subject (Geison, 1995). True, the patient had an indeterminable chance of surviving without it, but compounded as it is with murkiness over issues of informed consent, such an experiment would certainly not meet with approval with any ethics review board anywhere in the world today. But at the time, Fortune smiled on both Pasteur and Meister. The new method – consisting of a series of thirteen injections containing increasing concentrations of the vaccine material – appeared successful, as the young Meister never developed the symptoms that typically followed when bitten by a presumably rabid dog. Despite their possibly premature decision to treat young Meister then, Pasteur and his colleagues became a famous and enduring medical legend!

Of course, Pasteur and Roux were hardly the only, or even the first researchers to study rabies. Other researchers in laboratories across Europe were also working, attempting to identify the cause. As early as 1804, for example, George Gottfried Zinke from Jena, Germany, proved that rabies was an infectious disease, by successfully transmitting it from a rabid to a healthy dog using saliva to inoculate the latter (Grafe, 1991; Johnson, 1959; Wilkinson, 1977). Much later, in 1879, Pierre Victor Galtier (1846-1908), professor at the Veterinary School of Lyon, experimenting on domesticated rabbits, reported that rabies could be transmitted from dogs to rabbits with a marked reduction of the incubation time of the disease. He also claimed that sheep could be rendered immune to rabies by intravenous injection of saliva from rabid dogs (Geison, 1995; Théodoridès, 1986, 1989). In 1896 Galtier published a book on the subject: *La rage envisagée chez les animaux et chez l'homme au point de vue de ses caractères et de sa prophylaxie* (Considerations on rabies in animals and humans from the viewpoint of symptoms and prophylaxis). Thereafter, however, he added nothing new to the development of a rabies vaccine, and hence disappears from history. Nevertheless, according to the medical historian Théodoridès, the work of Pasteur and his collaborators would not have been realized without Galtier's earlier fundamental work. While he relied heavily on Galtier's preliminaries, Pasteur referred only once in his copious publications on rabies to the latter's claim about experimental immunity. Mitigating this snub somewhat, his successor, Roux, in contrast, frequently mentioned the work of Galtier in his 1883 thesis *Des nouvelles acquisitions sur la rage* (Geison, 1995, p. 184; Théodoridès, 1986).

Based on previous work on chicken cholera and anthrax, in the early 1880s Pasteur and Roux tried to alter the virulence of rabies virus by sequential passages through living organisms that were susceptible to rabies infections. Galtier had already demonstrated that the rabbit was a suitable experimental model for rabies but later experimenters made an interesting discovery; they found that whereas serial passage through rabbits increased its virulence to both dogs and humans, the serial passage through monkeys had the opposite effect (Geison, 1995). They also found that the incubation period of the infective agent of rabies in *rabbits* could be reduced to about one week by prolonged serial passages. This stable or 'fixed' rabies virus (*virus fixe*) was still highly virulent. In 1884 they reported that the virus could be attenuated – i.e. altered for decreased virulence – for dogs by serial passages through monkeys. When the attenuated virus was injected dogs it never resulted in rabies. Sometimes, it did not even produce any effects when inoculated by the otherwise infallible intracranial route. Although secretive at first, Pasteur eventually revealed the crucial features of the method for attenuating the virulence of the *virus fixe*. Strips of infected rabbit spinal cords were desiccated by extracting moisture from filtered air by caustic potash. The dried cord turned out to be non-infectious but remained effective as a vaccine – i.e. in inducing immunity against the disease. In 1885 this substance was used for immunization of humans who were bitten by a rabid dog.

The success of the rabies vaccine offered to Pasteur the opportunity to organize a subscription; the donations together with subsidy of the state were sufficient to establish in 1888 an Institut Pasteur encompassing laboratories and a Service de Rage for treatment of rabies patients. Formally inaugurated in 1888, the service soon began to grow in reputation all over Europe, as people from a variety of places and countries who had been bitten by rabid dogs or wolves could be referred there for treatment.

In 1885, the daily paper *Het Nieuws van den Dag*[15] pursued a surprising action. The young R.H. Saltet, who would become in 1896 successor of Förster, the first professor of hygiene in Amsterdam, was sent to Paris to examine the fantastic discovery of Pasteur; his conclusion was that Pasteur's method ought to be made available to Dutch patients (Van Riemsdijk, 1928). Thereafter the Minister of the Interior, Theodoor Heemskerk, took the decision that Dutch citizens could be treated in Paris at the expense of the Dutch state, when deemed necessary by a district veterinarian in consultation with the district medical doctor of the inspectorate. The first person to have been granted permission to go to Paris for treatment was a man named L. Jooren, but records indicate that he changed his mind and preferred to go to a priest who treated him with incantations, prayers and exhortations to perform good works (Polak, 1964; Scheltema Beduin, 1886, p. 438). History does not record the result of this treatment, but meanwhile, J. Attema Czn, a student at the Veterinary School in Utrecht, whose finger had been bitten during his examination of a dog that might have been rabid, became the first Dutch patient to be treated in Paris in 1886 (Polak, 1964).

15   *Daily News.*

With the establishment by the Belgian microbiologist and immunologist Bordet of the Institut Antirabique in Brussels in 1907, Dutch exposed
individuals no longer had to travel to Paris for anti-rabies treatment. Bordet's
institute continued to offer the Dutch anti-rabies treatments closer to home
until World War I, when reaching Brussels from the Netherlands became
a problem. Immediately thereafter patients were sent to the Institut für
Infektionskrankheiten in Berlin for treatment, but after November 1914
Dutch patients could go to the Bacterio-Therapeutisch Instituut of Spronck
at the Pasteurstraat in Utrecht. The Dutch were not yet caught up in vaccine
preparation technology, however, because the vaccine that was used at the
Pasteurstraat in Utrecht was ironically obtained from Berlin.

In 1889 the NTvG published a series of 'Letters from Paris' written by M.
Straub, a physician (appointed later in 1895 as professor of ophthalmology
in Amsterdam) who was deeply interested in bacteriology. At government's
request Straub had studied the activities of the Service de Rage. In his letters
from Paris he described his three months stay in Paris and his work at the
Institute (Straub, 1889). His report contains descriptions of the lay-out of the
building and his daily routine in the institute, where he met figures, such
as Émile Roux, Charles Chamberland, and Elie Metchnikoff. Because he
was obliged to report on the rabies vaccine to the government, he was not
allowed to publish his conclusions on the vaccine in the NTvG. That same
year L. Ali Cohen, who had been inspector of the Health Inspectorate in the
northern provinces of the Netherlands, published the results of his analysis
of 'inoculation antirabique' of Pasteur in the NTvG. His conclusions were
that, although the theoretical basis was not fully understood, the efficacy of
the vaccine of Pasteur against rabies could not be denied (Ali Cohen, 1889).

In 1900, fifteen years after the treatment of young Joseph Meister, and
five years after the death of Pasteur, Christiaan Eykman, then professor of
hygiene in Utrecht, was invited by the editors of the NTvG to review the
new treatment for rabies. Eykman, who in 1929 would go on to receive a
Nobel Prize in Physiology and medicine for his work on the cause of beriberi,
visited the Institute Pasteur where Roux, the third director of the institute
after Pasteur's death in 1895, extended a warm welcome to him and also
offered him opportunity to study the medical records of patients who were
treated with the vaccine. In his review Eykman discussed the experimental
basis, the practice, and the statistical results of the method (Eykman, 1900).
He began the review with a reminder that although Pasteur had come up
for considerable criticism from many quarters, his method was ultimately
successful. Among opponents in France were the physician Professor Michel
Peter, who was in fact Pasteur's cousin by marriage, and the veterinarian

Professor Gabriel Colin. The most vociferous detractor was Dr Auguste Luteaud, editor of the *Journal de Médecine de Paris*, who accused Pasteur of giving his patient rabies rather than curing it ('M. Pasteur ne guérit pas la rage, il la donne'). In England the critics were mostly anti-vivisectionists and anti-vaccionists. But, although Eykman did not mention the fact in his report, no less a personage than T.H. Huxley had sallied forth against these opponents (Geison, 1995, pp. 218-220). In Germany and Austria, too, the medical world – in particular the influential surgeons Anton von Frisch and Theodor Billroth from Vienna and Robert Koch in Berlin – had at first stood aloof from Pasteur's method. But as Eykman pointed out, by 1898 clinics for vaccination according to Pasteur's method were opened in the Rudolf Hospital in Vienna and at the Institute for Infectious Diseases in Berlin; the very sites from where their extensive critiques had emerged just a few years earlier.

Reading the reports today, it seems remarkable that Eykman paid as much attention as he did to the crusade of anti-vivisectionist in the Netherlands against the Pasteur's rabies vaccine. But it must be noted that at the time it had been the activities of the Netherlands Association against Vivisection[16] that had led the editors of the NTvG to request him to write the review. The association had recently published a brochure entitled *De Genezing van hondsdolheid. Pasteur of Buisson?*[17] The introduction was written by the physician Dr G. Luchtmans, who recommended Buisson's hydrotherapy consisting of application of vapour bathes to prevent and cure hydrophobia. Eykman confined his attention to the debate in that brochure by referring to an 1888 book by J.R. Suzor on Pasteur's method which contained critiques and rebuttals in equal measure.

Meanwhile Eykman discussed the issue of the timing of Pasteur's administration of the vaccine with Roux, inquiring as to whether the decision to administer it to Meister had been taken before or after he had decisive experimental results with regard to the safety of the vaccine. Roux, who had executed the experiments together with Pasteur, assured Eykman that he himself had obtained promising results in unpublished experiments, in which he had administered the rabies vaccine to dogs that had been bitten. Roux's claims ran contrary to the results of Von Frisch, who had found that administration of the rabies vaccine after subdural administration of the rabies virus into the dog yielded negative results (Geison, 1995, p. 223). However, this last claim did not have much impact as in real life humans

16 Nederlandsche Bond tot Bestrijding der vivisectie.
17 *Therapy of rabies: Pasteur or Buisson?*

acquired rabies through a bitten arm or leg and not through the subdural route, after which the incubation time is too short to achieve immunity.

Eykman discussed also his doubts about the state of the virus in the vaccine – i.e. whether it was 'mutated' and hence less virulent, or merely diminished in quantity. He asked Roux about the methods for quantifying vaccine doses and, dissatisfied with the answers, proposed reassessing the doses using a more accurate dilution method developed by the Hungarian Enver Högyes. Roux was not in a position to comment on the objections, because he did not have the liberty to change the Pasteur-approved methods. Finally, after studying the medical records on the use of the vaccine, Eykman discussed the safety of the vaccine. Although critical of the statistics, his conclusion after he had reviewed the figures was that the treatment of humans with the rabies vaccine was effective enough in most cases. Although he acknowledged the drawback posed by the fact that the vaccine could occasionally cause rabies, he concluded that the frequency was too low to put forward as grounds for prohibiting the use of the vaccine. In other words, the advantages outweighed the disadvantages.

Poliomyelitis, the summer disease

Although there are indications that poliomyelitis (polio) has existed since ancient times – e.g. the findings of mummies dating to the early thirteenth century BC with signs of polio-like deformities of the leg – there are no definitive descriptions of the disease in any medical writings from antiquity (Galassi et al., 2017; Paul, 1971). Indeed, there is little verifiable documenta-tion on polio until the modern era. The first cases of infantile paralysis in Europe were described in 1734 by the physician Johannes Gothofredus Salzmann, defending his thesis in Strassbourg, and in 1789 by Michael Underwood, a London paediatrician. More widespread outbreaks were not reported until the nineteenth century (Rida, 1964; Paul, 1971; Melnick, 1988; Chastel, 1992). Even with these publications, information was scarce and, according to the famous polio virologist and historian John R. Paul, it is a 1840 monograph *Beobachtungen über Lähmungzustände der unteren Extremitäten und deren Behandlung* (Observations on paralytic conditions of the lower extremities and their treatment) by the German orthopaedic surgeon Jacob von Heine that stands out as a historical landmark in the history of polio (Paul, 1971). Heine described the paralytic conditions of the lower limbs and the therapeutic possibilities. He listed all the clinical features of infantile paralysis and concluded that the symptoms pointed to an affection of the central nervous system, and especially of the spinal cord (Heine, 1840 and 1860; Paul, 1971).

Despite Heine's substantial contributions to the clinical recognition of poliomyelitis, however, further knowledge proceeded slowly. Documentation on disease outbreaks and mortality rates in the Netherlands remained sparse before the twentieth century. For instance, even the application of a wide variety of search terms yielded only about seven publications possibly related to poliomyelitis in the NTvG through the entire nineteenth century (Van Doornum, not published). According to Paul (1971), the disease occurred mainly sporadically and even during epidemics was thought not to be contagious. Considered at first to be primarily a disease of infants and young children, polio was, however, also noticed to occur more frequently in older age groups by the end of the nineteenth century. One possible explanation for the shift in demographics might be that poliovirus became established and survived for centuries in an endemic manner. Epidemiologists have suggested that poliovirus infections changed in character and began to cause periodic epidemics due to the introduction of modern sanitation (Anderson and May, 1992, p. 99). Ironically, a higher standard of hygiene seemed to render a greater proportion of the juvenile and adult population more susceptible to the infection, and furthermore cause more serious complications, such as paralysis in these populations. There is, however, one communication from 1859 which reveals that physicians were aware that infantile paralysis in very young children was not as uncommon as previously believed (Van Campen, 1859). This communication referred to a single German publication by someone named Irtl on cases of infantile paralysis presented to the clinic (ambulatorium) of Prof. Schuh in Germany. The little patients were mostly under the two years of age and generally presented with paralysis of the lower limbs. In many instances, it would appear, the condition was overlooked by the parents until the age that children should have normally begun to walk. We assume that a similar pattern of incidence and detection of poliomyelitis must have also occurred in the Netherlands.

In the Dutch medical literature two reports were published by a general practitioner B.H. Stephan, who later became the medical director of a hospital, describing a cluster of four cases of infantile paralysis that occurred in Zaandijk in August 1869 (Stephan, 1885, 1895). This cluster of cases, which presented with cerebral symptoms after a period of fever, was actually observed by a local general practitioner, Mulder, who communicated this information to Stephan. Mulder suspected a contagious cause of the illness, because of the initial fever, the specific prodromal complaints and the cyclic pattern of the disease. He suggested also that the infecting agent might be located in the gastrointestinal tract, although he admitted that the infectious character of acute poliomyelitis was not generally recognized. In the latter of the two publications (1895) Stephan concluded that there was more evidence that acute poliomyelitis was an infectious disease. The occurrence of this cluster in August is consistent with later observations of the typical seasonal pattern of polio in temperate zones, where most viruses are isolated during summer and early autumn (Kapsenberg, 1988b, p. 717).

It is the Stockholm paediatrician Oskar Medin who deserves the credit for providing a definitive description of clinical features of poliomyelitis in the nineteenth century. In 1890 at the Tenth International Medical Congress in Berlin, Medin presented his clinical observations on an 1887 epidemic of infantile paralysis in Sweden (Axelsson, 2009). It was, incidentally, the same congress where Koch presented his premature speech on the use of tuberculin as a remedy against tuberculosis. Medin was the teacher of Ivar Wickman, who later described a second Scandinavian epidemic in 1905, and proposed the name Heine-Medin disease. The first communication in the NTvG referring to the Heine-Medin disease appeared in 1910, in which C.H. Hermanides described a 1906 outbreak among eight children in Noordwijk and pointed out that the disease was not harmless (Herderschêe, 1910; Hermanides, 1911). In 1906 the name 'poliomyelitis anterior acuta' was used for small epidemics during the summer in the region Achterhoek of the province Gelderland (Muntendam, 1909).

In conclusion, such outbreaks of poliomyelitis the Netherlands in the nineteenth century were small and infrequent, possibly due to herd immunity. Consequently, the clinical entity poliomyelitis did not attract much attention within medical circles in the Netherlands during that period.

Influenza, not just a common cold

A highly infective virus disease of the respiratory tract, influenza, nowadays more commonly known as the flu, is believed to be an ancient disease that might have spread to humans in prehistoric times, coinciding with the first settlements in farming or urban communities (Dobson, 2015; Dobson and Carper, 1996; Potter, 1998, p. 4). The earliest reports of a possible outbreak in 412 BC were recorded by both Hippocrates and Livius, but the first convincing description of an influenza epidemic goes back to 1173-1174 (Hippocrates, 1923; Nicholson et al., 1998). The disease has gone by many names in its long history, with the specific label of influenza derived from

Italian – *una influenza* – which translates as 'an influence' because the mysterious visitation of respiratory symptoms was thought to be the result some celestial influences. The term appears to have been imported into English sometime in the mid-eighteenth century and eventually became the label for the disease the world over. Another common historical name was *grippe* or *grip* – from the French verb *gripper* (to grab) – which was often used at the same time as influenza itself. Reports in the NTvG show that whereas the term 'influenza' was used more frequently in the Netherlands during the epidemic in 1889-1890, the term *griep* (*grippe*) was used more frequently in communications on the 1918 epidemic (G. van Doornum, personal communication, 2016). Physicians in the seventeenth and eighteenth and even early nineteenth centuries considered influenza to be 'a mysterious but not very dangerous disease', outbreaks of which affected the weak and the aged most of all (Dobson, 2015). Even though it could kill, it was not seen to be as dangerous or frightening as other epidemics – poxes (smallpox or syphilis) and plagues – of the past. This attitude would change the world over in the late nineteenth and early twentieth centuries.

The first appearance of influenza in the Dutch language appears to have been a description of a 1782 outbreak entitled 'Comment on the epidemic catarrh, which occurred mainly in the month June of the year 1782 in Amsterdam'[18] by a physician, Dr Jan Petersen Michell (Quanjer, 1921: 5). Then in 1800 a naval physician named Pieter van Woensel published *The lamplighter, being a complete treatise on influenza, i.e. public common cold.*[19] Van Woensel, who sojourned as a medical doctor in St Petersburg at the court of Catherine the Great from 1771 to 1778, was also a satirist. Using the pen name Amurath-Effendi Hekim-Bachi, he published an almanac-like series of satires under the title *De lantaarn* (The lantern) over the period from 1792 to 1801 (Nieuwenhuis, 2014). *The lamplighter* was actually a front for revealing himself as the anonymous author of an earlier (1800) edition of *De lantaarn*, which had been forbidden by the authorities of the Batavian Republic. Van Woensel used the term 'influenza' metaphorically as the prevalent 'epidemic' of patriotism caused by the British belligerency. On one hand, this publication might be interpreted to mean that influenza was considered as a possible threat in the life of individuals and the society at the beginning of the nineteenth century. On the other hand, as mentioned

18   Aanmerking over de zinking-koorts, welke voornamelijk in de maand Juni des jaar 1782, te Amsterdam geheerscht heeft. See also: Geist-Hofman et al., 1972.
19   De bijlichter, zijnde een uitgewerkte verhandeling over de influenza, dat is: publieke verkoudheid.

above, until 1889 influenza was generally not considered a threatening disease. As influenza notification to the authorities was not obligatory in the Netherlands, only sporadic reports of outbreaks are available to us today, e.g. reports of epidemics, in 1847/1848 in Friesland and Nijmegen and in 1855 in Haarlem (De Jong, 2010; Van Schevichaven, n.d.; Waardenburg, 1858).

The first influenza epidemic in the Netherlands to be described thoroughly was an outbreak that started in Russia in October 1889, spread over Europe and then to North America, took rather more than two months to reach the Cape, three months to reach South America, four months to reach India, five months to reach New Zealand and Australia, and eventually went as far as Iceland, Mauritius and some remote places in Africa and Asia (Parsons, 1891a and 1891b). It spread along the railway routes from Siberia into Western Europe; the speed of diffusion along the route was no faster than the speed of trains (Le Goff et al., 2009; Le Goff, 2011; Nolen, 1889; Rahamat-Langendoen, 2008). The initiative to gather factual information about the epidemic in the Netherlands was launched following similar initiatives in France, Belgium, England, Germany and Austria (Wertheim Salomonson and De Rooy, 1893). In March 1890 after the end of the outbreak, two hygienists – W.P. Ruysch, advisor at the Ministry of Health, and R.H. Saltet of the Health Inspectorate but acting in a personal capacity – decided to form a committee to describe the epidemiology and experiences of the epidemic. In close consultation with the Netherlands Society for the Advancement of Medicine Ruysch and Saltet designed a questionnaire which was distributed among all 562 members of the society in the Netherlands. It included sixteen questions on vital statistics, epidemiology, symptomology and treatment; the last question concerned the opinion on the mode of transmission of influenza. There was a delay in the handling of the data, but thanks to the appointment of C. de Rooy and J.K.A. Wertheim Salomonson to the committee as rapporteurs, a report was eventually published in 1893.

As per the report, the influenza epidemic had started in the Netherlands in October 1889 with sporadic cases, reached its acme in January 1890, and ended in February 1890 in the main cities in the west of Holland, and a month later in the countryside. Due to the design of the questionnaire – which contained open questions – results were not quite reliable. Nevertheless, morbidity was estimated to be 37.5 per cent of the population. The medical practitioners observed 4,282 deaths due to influenza being 2.7 per cent of the influenza patients who consulted their doctor. The estimated mortality of the population directly attributed to influenza was 1 per thousand. This figure was in accordance with the official death rate. The mortality rates of January 1890 for the age groups 20-40 years and 65-79 years increased by

67 and 202 per cent, respectively, compared to those from a year ago. The excess mortality – namely the risk of death posed by a particular disease as opposed to general mortality rates which take into account all possible causes of death – indirectly attributable to influenza in the Netherlands was about 9.7 per 10,000 inhabitants per annum. In the more densely populated city of Amsterdam the excess mortality was even 19.15 per 10,000 inhabitants per annum.

Remarkably, only 292 of the 562 medical doctors surveyed assumed that influenza was communicable via person-to-person transmission; 26 filled in miasmatic-contagious, 40 entered only miasmatic; four doctors thought that the infection was acquired in a way similar to malaria. Two hundred of the 562 (36 per cent) indicated that influenza was not contagious. Only one respondent mentioned the presence of bacteria upon microscopic examination of sputum smears. Almost prophetically, the authors stated that the agent had to be a virus that was transmitted by air or from person to person: in the medical terminology of the times therefore, influenza was a 'miasmatic-contagious' disease. A short comment on the Dutch report appeared in the *British Medical Journal* in 1894 in which the clinical symptoms classified under three distinct forms were mentioned (British Medical Journal, 1894). In a discussion on the possible cause of the cardiac complications and diabetes the words virus and toxic agent were used interchangeably.

By the time of the epidemic, the hitherto ignored influenza moved to centre stage in the Netherlands, even featuring in a dispute between a minister and a member of parliament in the Dutch House of Representatives in 1899. T. Heemskerk, the Minister of the Interior at the time, jeered in a diatribe at the theology faculties at the state universities, where modern (rather than classical) theology was dominant. Only recently converted from being an adherent of modern theology into a devotee of pietism, Heemskerk declared that he felt seasick and nauseous having to listen to the gospel preached by a modernist; he could not suppress a feeling of nausea. A member of parliament, F. Lieftinck, reproached the minister for orating against the dissenting modernists although he had used himself the same type of arguments just a few years earlier, saying: 'that attitude makes me feel indisposed, not seasick, but I am afraid of the approaching influenza, because I'm starting to sneeze' (F. Lieftinck, quoted in Bornebroek, 2006).[20]

---

20 Wanneer iemand hier zo extripode staat te oreeren over andersdenkenden als de heer Heemskerk, die betrekkelijk weinig jaren geleden zulke stellingen verdedigde', sprak Lieftinck, 'dan maakt mij dit ook onwel, niet zeeziek, maar dan word ik bang voor de naderende griep, omdat ik begin te niezen.

In 1892, Adrien Proust, professor of hygiene at the medical faculty of Paris, delivered an elaborate paper to the Académie de Médecine. Proust had chaired a committee that provided the French government with an extensive report on the 1889-1890 influenza epidemic (Proust, 1892). In fact, the report was based on a questionnaire distributed by the Secretary of the Interior, but only upon Proust's demands for one. In his paper he distinguished three clinical forms of influenza: i) a nervous influenza with intense cephalalgia, pain in the eye orbits, joints and muscles; ii) a pulmonary form; and iii) a gastric form. It is interesting to compare the morbidity and mortality figures shown in the Dutch and the French report. In the Netherlands at least 37.5 per cent of the population was affected and the official, direct mortality rate was about one per 1,000 inhabitants per annum. The French, who extrapolated the figures found for the army to the total population, estimated that about 50 per cent of the population acquired influenza. In the 40 most densely populated cities in France the mortality indirectly attributable to influenza was 18.1 per 10,000 inhabitants. As the mortality in the smaller cities and the rural areas was much lower, the total excess mortality in France was estimated to be 12.3 per 10,000 inhabitants per annum (Proust, 1892, p. 556). Remarkably, only 292 of the 539 (52 per cent) medical doctors in the Dutch report assumed that influenza was a communicable disease by person-to-person transmission. In contrast, the French report treated the issue of influenza as communicable and transmissible from human to human, as a given. The rapid spread was explained by the short incubation period of 48 hours or less.

It is also illuminating to compare the 1893 Dutch report to an 1891 report on English epidemics of 1889-1890 and 1891, and their distribution in England and Wales, by H. Franklin Parsons, vice-president of the Public Medicine section of the British Medical Association. Similar to the situatcion in the Netherlands, notification of influenza was not obligatory in England. Furthermore, with the exception of London, influenza was not included in the list of the causes of death recorded by the registrar-general (Parsons, 1891a and 1891b). An estimated 25 per cent of the persons employed in large offices in London and around one in eight of those employed out of doors were attacked by influenza in 1890. The mortality in London ascribed directly to influenza was 146 per million inhabitants or 1.46 per 10,000 inhabitants per annum. During the four-week period ending on 25 January 1890, which may be taken as the period over which the epidemic of that year lasted, the deaths registered in London from all causes taken together were 2,258 above the average of the corresponding weeks during the previous ten years. This excess was equal to a rate of 6,638 per million (66.38 per 10,000 inhabitants) per annum (Parsons, 1891a and b). Parsons pointed out that different parts of the country had suffered in different proportions so that an estimate based on London experience would probably give an exaggerated idea of the extent of the epidemic in the country at large. For example, the mortality directly attributed to influenza in Ireland was small, but the death/rate from all causes rose from 16.5 per 10,000 inhabitants per annum in the last quarter of 1889 to 245 in the first quarter of 1890; the latter being the highest death rate recorded since the establishment of registration (Parsons, 1891b, p. 13). The author noted that this high excess mortality regarded the class of the population requiring poor law medical relief. The mortality figures for the troops quartered in the three military districts in Ireland were much lower (Parsons, 1891b, p. 156).

The next great influenza epidemic – or one should say pandemic, given the global scale or the outbreak – would be the so-called Spanish influenza of 1918, which wreaked great havoc in populations the world over. The cause of the disease has remained unknown throughout the 1920s; initially after the Spanish influenza pandemic there was a belief that the rapid spread of the epidemic was caused by a virus and complications were due to secondary bacterial infections e.g. the species that had been isolated by a German bacteriologist Richard Pfeiffer, from the noses of flu-infected patients (1892a and 1892b). Tyrrell described nicely how three strands of of research in the USA and the United Kingdom came together in 1933 (Tyrrell, 1998, pp. 21-23). It wasn't until the 1930s that an American medical researcher named Richard Shope, working on an influenza-like disease of swine, definitely showed that a bacteria free filtrate produced a mild illness in swine and addition of the bacterium *Haemophilus influenzae suis* caused the full blown disease rather than bacterium was the cause of the primary infection (Shope, 1931a and 1931b). The other strands were the experiments carried out in England at institutes encouraged and funded by the Medical Research Council that had a policy to encourage research on viruses.

Human and animal medicine in the nineteenth century

The subject of the work of veterinarians relative to doctors' work is treated here because of the involvement of the medical profession in the epizootics as the cattle plague (rinderpest). Before about 1800 veterinary medicine was considered to be interwoven with human medicine. Only over the nineteenth century veterinary medicine became from an unreformed profession a separate and independent profession.

Of the diseases discussed in this chapter, rabies is a zoonotic or animal-borne disease which indicates the significance of the relationships between human and animal infections. Furthermore, as seen in the case of smallpox, the knowledge of such relationships has proved extremely useful for developing vaccines and treatments against the disease. We therefore turn next to a brief discussion of the ways in which between Dutch medicine and public health on the one hand and veterinary medicine on the other related to one another before the twentieth century.

The recognition of links between human and animal disease is evident from the fact that in the eighteenth century such leading physicians as Petrus Camper had declared in no uncertain terms that he considered the care for livestock to be the duty of medical doctors: 'It is the duty of medical practitioners to take care not only of the health of people, but also of their possessions, i.e. their cattle'[21] (Offringa, 1971, p. 16). Medical doctors were repeatedly appealed to for advice on how to prevent cattle plague or rinderpest, e.g. in 1744 by the state of South Holland on the medical faculty in Leiden, and in 1745 by the municipality of Utrecht on the medical faculty there (Offringa, 1971, pp. 15-16). During a later epizootic in 1768, the municipality of Groningen approached Camper and W. van Doeveren and requested them to study the disease and offer proposal for prevention and treatment of the disease (Offringa, 1971, p. 17; Tersteeg, 1998; Van Berkel, 2015, p. 83). According to Offringa this period can be seen as the first step of 'the long emancipatory way' of the profession as veterinarian. First, veterinary medicine was raised as *ars veterinaria* to the level of the *ars medicinae*. Animal medicine, however, remained the competence of medical science, which resulted in separation between theory and practice. Whereas medical scientists gathered information on the theoretical aspects of veterinary science, a diverse assortment of people, including farriers, flayers or skinners, cow leeches, knowledgeable farmers and 'veterinary quacks' and, after the 1820 founding of the veterinary school, its matriculates had hand-on practical experience working with infected animals. Then, it took some decades until by the second half of the eighteenth century when science and practice were united in the hands of the veterinaries. Eventually, in 1925 the Veterinary School became the Veterinary Faculty of the University of Utrecht.

The demand for a school dedicated to the veterinary sciences in the Netherlands had been recognized by Society for the Advancement of Agriculture in the late eighteenth century. Subjects such as liver rot in sheep and splenic

21   het is de plicht van de geneesheren niet alleen om over de gezondheid van den mensch te waken, maar ook over hun bezittingen, te weten het vee.

fever in cattle, both of which led to severe economic losses, received ample attention in the published lectures. In 1796, the society held a competition for viable ideas for a veterinary school (Offringa, 1971, p. 17). Jan Arnold Bennet, a medical doctor and later a professor of rural economy in Leiden, won the award in 1799. Although the society only published his submission in their proceedings in 1820, Bennet's ideas appear to have influenced in preparation to the establishment of a Dutch Veterinary School, which was inaugurated in Utrecht in 1821. This event signified a factual recognition of veterinary medicine, but unfortunately, this separation meant that the veterinary schools were slower than medical establishments to adopt the scientific approach to solving medical problems (Offringa, 1971, p. 87). Just how far apart the human and veterinary medicine had drifted is evident in an 1847 issue of the journal *Het Repertorium*, in which the editors declared that announcements about veterinary medicine should be published in the journal because human and veterinary medicine were reciprocal. The statement, however, was not repeated when a decade later this journal was merged with others to form the *Netherlands Journal of Medicine*. Meanwhile, the gradual shift in responsibilities of animal care from the medical to veterinary professionals is exemplified in an 1892 decree by the Dutch government that the Parcs Vaccinogènes for the production of cowpox vaccine contract a veterinary surgeon for the supervision of the care of the calves (Offringa, 1971, p. 87). Whether or not social position and incomes influenced the relationship between medical doctors and veterinary practitioners is open to question. For a more detailed discussion, we refer interested readers to Offringa's *Van Gildestein naar Uithof: 150 jaar diergeneeskundig onderwijs in Utrecht*, vols I and II, in which the emancipation of the veterinary profession is an important theme (Offringa, 1971, p. 345).

Progress from confluence: The meeting of public health and laboratory science

Although humans had successfully curbed some viral diseases even *before* the nature of viruses as the causal agents of infectious disease was in any way understood (Lechevalier and Solotorovsky, 1974), there can be no doubt that, as the historian William F. Bynum wrote, 'science was one of the important influences in shaping the structure of medicine in the nineteenth century'. To be sure, the impact of modern science in earlier eras covered in this book was more striking on the doctors' ability to diagnose and prevent infectious diseases, rather than on their therapeutic achievements (Bynum, 1994, p.

xii). But even the earlier public health measures were based on scientific principles – via such disciplines as medical geography, historical pathology and statistics. Although hygienists closely followed the developments in microbiology, statistics remained their preferred method for interpreting empirical data (Houwaart, 1991, p. 161). Germ theory and bacteriology could only be used to guide and legitimate preventive measures towards the end of the nineteenth century. With the exception of smallpox and rabies (after 1886) preventive measures against viral infection remained based on clinical and epidemiologic observations. It was only in the twentieth century after viruses were recognized as a class of pathogens distinct from bacteria and other microbes, and techniques were made available for properly isolate, identify and cultivate them, that there was any progress in developing effective therapies. Indeed, one might argue that even today, viral infections remain among the most notoriously difficult diseases to treat, and that the old adage 'prevention is better than cure' holds as true as it ever did in most of their cases. Nevertheless, in the chapters that follow we trace the history of various scientific developments and consider the impact of different theoretical and practical scientific advances – within the Netherlands especially, but also in other parts of the world – on the unfolding of Dutch medical virology.

2 Redefining viruses

The development and reception of the virus concept in the
Netherlands

> The [tobacco mosaic] infection is not caused by microbes,
> but by a contagium vivum fluidum.
> – *Martinus Beijerinck (1898)*

> Viruses are viruses.
> – *André Lwoff (1957)*

In the previous chapter we considered the history of viral disease in the
Netherlands in an era *before* anyone knew what a virus really was. Such
an approach naturally begs the question as to when such a thing became
known, but the answer is not straightforward at all. Much has been written
on this subject, and for full expositions, we refer readers to the classic works
of Sally Smith Hughes (1977) and A.P. Waterson and Lise Wilkinson (1978).
In this chapter we offer but a brief tour, highlighting those aspects of the
discovery and understanding of viruses that are most relevant to the history
of understanding viral disease in the Netherlands.

The word *virus* has been in use for a very long time, long before anything
was known about the existence of any sort of ultramicroscopic or even
microscopic, agent of infectious disease was discovered. It appears to have
been imported into the English language from Latin as a word for 'poison'
or 'venom' or noxious substance, sometime in the fifteenth or sixteenth
centuries (Waterson and Wilkinson, 1978, p. 3). Perhaps the best-known
reference is Edward Jenner's famous exposition on the prevention of smallpox
in 1798. The term 'virus' appears multiple times in this treatise, variously
representing the 'morbid matter' of the disease – i.e., the material from
the pustules of the pox – or the causative disease agent itself. After the
advent of the germ theory in the nineteenth century the word was used
rather non-specifically to denote agents of infectious disease. This idea is
implicit, for example, in Louis Pasteur's 1890 declaration: 'En résumé, tout
virus est un microbe.' This statement, which translates as 'In summary,
every virus is a microbe,' conveys his opinion that all infectious agents were
microscopic living entities. Since that time the term 'virus' has undergone
multiple 'variances' in meaning until various aspects were consolidated

Figure 5   M.W. Beijerinck (1859-1931)

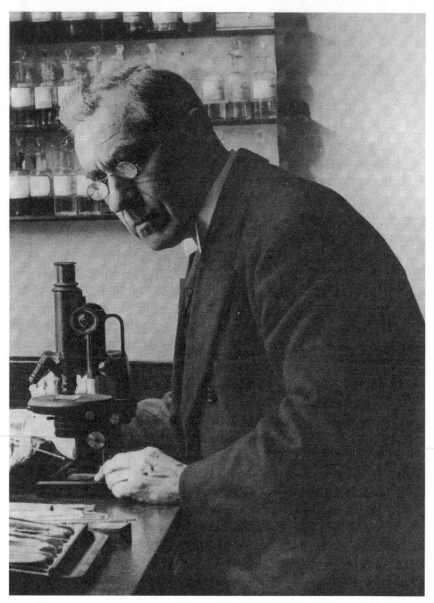

M.W. Beijerinck (1859-1931) shortly before his retirement from the chair in Delft, at the age of 70
Photo reproduced from G. van Iterson, L.E. den Dooren de Jong, A.J. Kluyver (eds), *Verzamelde
Geschriften van M.W. Beijerinck*, Zesde Deel, 1940

by the French microbiologist André Lwoff to denote an entity that was
an Aristotelian natural kind in its own right: an obligate parasite of living

host cells composed of a core of a single species of nucleic acid encased in a proteinaceous coat (Lwoff, 1957; Lwoff and Tournier, 1966; Löwy, 1990, p. 88; Van Helvoort and Sankaran, 2019).

The discovery of a remarkable anomaly

The Netherlands can justly claim a place of pride in the foundational chapter of the history of virology – not just medical virology but the discipline in its entirety – because the first person who suggested that viruses were different from other disease agents was Dutch. In 1886, German agricultural scientist Adolf Mayer, director of the Agricultural Experimental Station in Wageningen, the Netherlands, described a new 'mosaic' disease of tobacco plants (TMD), which he was investigating upon the request of Dutch farmers affected by losses due to this disease. Although he was unable to find the causative agent, he believed it to be an infectious disease of bacterial cause (Mayer, 1942/1886). A few years later a Russian graduate student studying the same disease reported that it appeared to be caused by an invisible and filterable entity, but like Mayer, was unable to isolate a causative bacterial agent (Ivanowski, 1942/1892).[22] Then in 1898, the Dutch microbiologist, Martinus Willem Beijerinck, Mayer's former colleague, by then in Delft, proposed an entirely new type of causative agent for the disease. He first presented his experiments and ideas in 1898 to the Koninklijke Nederlandse Akademie van Wetenschappen (the Royal Netherlands Academy of Sciences) – an enlarged[23] version of this lecture was published in German the following year – where he announced: 'We were dealing here with a disease which was caused by a *contagium* which was not a *contagium fixum* in the usual sense of the words' (Beijerinck, 1961/1899, p. 154). Instead, he described the tobacco mosaic agent as a *contagium vivum fluidum*, a Latin phrase conveying the meaning of a living and fluid infectious agent.

Beijerinck's phrase was something of a contradiction in terms. At the time, the conception of life entailed that any being deemed living – *vivum* – had

22   This researcher's name has been variously translated into English by different authors in different ways, e.g., Ivanovski, Ivanovsky, Ivanowski, and Iwanowsky. For the sake of convenience and consistency, the version used in the text here is Ivanowski, which was the spelling used in the *Phytopathological Classics* translation by J. Johnson, 1942. Direct quotes and titles of papers bearing his name, however, use the spelling used by the author of the publication quoted.
23   The English translation of the proceedings published by the KNAW was a verbal translation of the Dutch text. In contrast, the German version contained a translation of an enlarged text that was used by J. Johnson for the translation published in *Phytopathological Classics* 7 (1942).

to be organized, which meant it was corpuscular or particulate (*fixum*) and therefore certainly not fluid! Although the translation for the word *fluidum* is *fluid* or *liquid* in English, Beijerinck used the expressions 'liquid state' and 'dissolved state' interchangeably in his original Dutch paper to describe the contagium (Kluyver, 1983, p. 119; Bos, 1999, p. 678). His ideas were heterodox for his times, but Beijerinck had experimental and theoretical back-ups for different elements of conception. For instance, he designed a series of experiments to test his hypothesis regarding the solubility of the infectious agent. First, he spread some material (extracts of crushed leaves) from diseased plants on the surface of a thick layer of agar and allowed a diffusion time of about ten days. After washing the surface of the plate, he infected healthy new plants with material extracted from the deeper layers of agar, taking great care to avoid contamination from the upper layers. By his reasoning:

> A virus, consisting of discrete particles, would need remain on the surface of the agar and consequently be in the impossibility of rendering the agar virulent; a virus, really dissolved in water would, on the contrary, be able to penetrate to a certain depth into the agar. (Beijerinck, 1899b, pp. 171-172)

If the material from the deeper layers did indeed produce an infection identical to the original disease when injected into healthy new plants, Beijerinck felt justified in concluding that it contained a soluble, disease-producing agent, i.e. a *contagium fluidum*.

As for the living nature of the agent, Beijerinck was quite clear. To him, the fact that a soluble agent retained its infectivity through serial transfers from a diseased plant to an unaffected one was evidence of multiplication. And, as he responded to a question from the famous botanist Hugo de Vries about the appropriateness of the adjective *vivum* at the Royal Academy meeting, he 'considered the ability to reproduce to be the major characteristic of life' (Beijerinck, 1898a; Bos, 1999, p. 678). In addition, he proposed a completely new mechanism for the multiplication of the disease agent. 'Propagation results only when the virus is connected with the living and growing protoplasm of the host plant,' he reported, noting too that the replication occurred only in young, dividing cells of the tobacco plant:

> The method of reproduction of the virus reminds one in certain ways of that of the amyloplasts and chloroplasts, which also grow only with the growing cell protoplasm, but can also exist and function independently. (Beijerinck, 1942/1898, p. 39)

Given the novelty of his ideas, it was not to be expected that Beijerinck would be allowed to present them uncontested. One of his main opponents was none other than Ivanowski, the first person who had demonstrated the filterability of the tobacco mosaic agent in 1892, but whose interpretation of the results had been quite different. His own conclusion was that the tobacco mosaic disease was 'explained most simply by the assumption of a toxin secreted by the bacteria present, which is dissolved in the filtered sap' (Ivanowski, 1942/1892, p. 30). His ideas were drawn from the example of the French bacteriologists Émile Roux and Alexandre Yersin, who had demonstrated that the major symptoms of diphtheria were caused by a toxin produced by the bacteria, rather than the live bacteria themselves (Roux and Yersin, 1888). Upon reading Beijerinck's reports, Ivanowski was not only understandably piqued that the latter had made no mention of his own earlier discoveries, but also critical of the idea of a soluble contagion. He repeated the agar diffusion experiments and obtained similar results, but extended the studies by testing the infectivity of material from different stages of a fractionated filtration, due to which he maintained his belief that the agent was particulate:

> We see that there is not a single fact which supports the hypothesis on the soluble character of the infectious agent of mosaic disease. On the contrary, the experiment with the diffusion into agar and especially the fractionated filtration clearly indicates that we are dealing with a *contagium fixum*. (Ivanowski, 1903, quoted in Lechevalier, 1972, pp. 140-141)

Ivanowski did not succeed either in isolating or in cultivating a contagium or bacterium that could cause the tobacco mosaic disease and eventually had to concede that the 'question of the artificial cultivation of the mosaic disease microbe remains to be solved by future investigations. But the force of his arguments against the idea of *contagium vivum fluidum* was such that it had persuaded the examiners of his doctoral thesis that he had 'refuted' Beijerinck's hypothesis, which they furthermore deemed as 'a sad chapter in the annals of contemporary science' (Lechevalier, 1972, p. 141).

Meanwhile Beijerinck's ideas were also challenged by a pair of German investigators, Friedrich Löffler and Paul Frosch, former students of the famed Robert Koch, who around the same time published results of their investigations into the causative agent of foot-and-mouth disease in livestock. Although they did not introduce any new labels or even use the term 'virus' in their paper as Beijerinck had, they explicitly came to a similar conclusion about the nature of the agent, namely that it was living and so tiny as to be filterable:

[The] activity of the filtrate is not due to the presence in it of a soluble substance, *but due to the presence of a causal agent capable of reproducing*. This agent must then be obviously so small that the pores of a filter which will hold back the smallest bacterium will still allow it to pass. The smallest bacterium presently known is the influenza bacillus of Pfeiffer. [...] If the supposed causal agent of foot-and-mouth disease was only 1/10 or even 1/5 as large as this, which really does not seem impossible, then this agent would not be resolved in our microscope. [...] This would explain very simply why it has been impossible to see the causal agent in the lymph under the microscope, even after the most extensive search. (Löffler and Frosch, 1961/1898, p. 152; emphasis added)

Contrary to Beijerinck, however, Löffler and Frosch did not believe that the agent was a soluble or fluid entity. Rather, they held that the foot-and-mouth disease was caused by some particulate or corpuscular organism smaller than the limits of visibility even with a microscope, a view that Beijerinck would explicitly dispute in the German version of his talk, where he said in a footnote: 'I cannot agree with the conclusion of Mr. Löffler as regards the corpuscular nature of the virus of the foot-and-mouth disease' (1942/1898, p. 37).

Likely in part due to the lack of the experimental means to further test his hypothesis, and also because he turned his attention to other matters of more pressing concern to him in his academic position, Beijerinck did not attempt to further defend his ideas about the tobacco mosaic virus (TMV) or the *contagium vivum fluidum*. In fact, he himself appears to have only referred to it again in any detail much later in 1913, at yet another address to the Royal Academy, on which occasion he defended his view on the possibility of life existing in liquid or soluble form:

[T]he concept of life – if one considers metabolism and proliferation as its essential characters – is not inseparably linked up with that of structure; the criteria of life, as we find it in its most primitive form, are also compatible with the fluid state. [...] In its most primitive form, life is, therefore, no longer bound to the cell. [...] No, in its primitive form life is like fire, like a flame borne by the living substance; – like a flame which appears in endless diversity and yet has specificity within it; – which can adopt the forms of the organic world [...]; – which does not originate by spontaneous generation, but is propagated by another flame. (Beijerinck, 1913, p. 26, quoted in Kluyver, 1983, pp. 120-121)

The scientific literature of the early decades of the twentieth century, on viruses in general and tobacco mosaic virus more specifically, gives the impression that the *contagium vivum fluidum* had no immediate impact either on the biological sciences or in understanding infectious disease. Indeed, references to Beijerinck in the first couple of decades after he published his findings on TMV were largely negative and display an incomplete or mistaken understanding of his novel ideas and their revolutionary implications. His views were 'not now tenable' said one reviewer (Wolbach, 1912, p. 2), for example, while another claimed that it was too difficult to conclude 'just what Beijerinck wished to convey by these vague and indefinite terms' (Allard, 1914, p. 438).

One notable exception is the microbiologist Felix d'Herelle, who in a 1925 address to the Royal Academy on the occasion of his receipt of its prestigious Van Leeuwenhoek Medal[24] (for achievements that we discuss in the next section) paid the following tribute to Beijerinck and his ideas about viruses, and life:

> [T]here has been much discussion on Beijerinck's conception [of the virus] but I do not think that we have yet understood its true profundity. All of biology was, and indeed is still, based on the fundamental hypothesis that the unit of living matter is the cell. Beijerinck was the first to free himself from this dogma and in fact, proclaim that life is not [solely] the result of cellular organization, but is derived from another phenomenon, which can only reside in the physicochemical composition of a proteinaceous micelle. (D'Herelle, 1925, quoted in Kluyver, 1983, p. 121[25])

With the advantage of hindsight, it is perhaps not surprising that Beijerinck's novel ideas about the nature of life and the possibility of soluble life forms resonated with Felix d'Herelle, another highly original thinker and the originator of a controversy that would have a profound impact on the thinking about the nature of viruses. Beijerinck's idea that an ultramicroscopic entity could cause disease transcended many of then established fundamental biological categories, such as plants and animals. In 1917 D'Herelle stirred

---

24 The van Leeuwenhoek medal was awarded in 1895 to L. Pasteur and in 1905 to M.W. Beijerinck.
25 On a beaucoup discuté la conception de Beijerinck, mais je ne pense pas qu'on en ait saisi toute la profondeur. Toute la biologie reposait, repose encore, sur l'hypothèse fondamentale que l'unité de matière vivante, c'est la cellule. Beijerinck le premier, s'est affranchi de ce dogme, et a proclamé de fait, que la vie n'est pas le résultat d'une organisation cellulaire, mais dérive d'un autre phénomène, qui ne peut dès lors résider que dans la constitution physico-chimique d'une micelle protéique.

the pot even further when, with his discovery of an entity he called the bacteriophage; he claimed that even bacteria could be infected with viruses. His claim was problematic for several reasons, and garnered controversy on at least two distinct but related matters. Before going into these details of the debates, however, a little background might be necessary.

Bacteriophages and the re-definition of viruses

Just as the association of the tobacco mosaic disease with a filterable agent was first reported by Ivanowski rather than Beijerinck, so too was the phenomenon of bacteriophagy first discovered by someone other than D'Herelle. In 1915 a British medical researcher named Frederick Twort first described a phenomenon of a transmissible lysis of micrococci bacteria, in material from which he was attempting to cultivate viruses. He published just one paper about his discovery, in which he made several suggestions as to the possible cause of the phenomenon, which he dubbed as 'glassy transformation' (Duckworth, 1976, p. 794). 'It is clear the transparent material contains an enzyme,' he wrote, on the basis of his observations that the lytic substance could retain its bacteria-dissolving activity for up to six months and was destroyed by heating, but also conceded that 'the possibility of its being an ultra-microscopic virus has not been *definitely* disproved, because we do not know for certain the nature of such a virus' (Twort, 1915, p. 1242, emphasis in original). Partly due to financial considerations and partly because he was called away to serve in World War I, Twort was unable to pursue his work any further and his discovery seemed fated to languish in obscurity (Bull, 1925, p. 95). Two years later, D'Herelle – who was investigating an outbreak of bacterial dysentery in the town of Maisons-Lafitte outside Paris, for the Pasteur Institute – discovered a near identical phenomenon in these bacteria. His first results were presented by Émile Roux to the French Académie des Sciences in September 1917 and published soon thereafter in *Comptes rendus de l'Académie des Sciences* (1917). Unlike Twort, however, D'Herelle never seemed to be in any doubt about the nature of this phenomenon and clearly interpreted his findings one way only. He opened his paper with the declaration that he had isolated an invisible microbe endowed with an antagonistic property against the Shiga bacillus, and in his conclusion, gave this putative agent of lysis a name: 'This microbe [...] is an obligatory bacteriophage' (D'Herelle, 1917, p. 375).[26]

26   Ce microbe [...] est un bactériophage obligatoire.

It is worth offering a word of explanation about D'Herelle's choice of the word 'bacteriophage' here, for it does not appear to mean, as is commonly believed, a neologism for 'bacteria-eater'. Rather, he appears to have used the term in a descriptive sense, as something that lived at the expense of these bacteria in much the same way as the bacteria themselves lived at the expense of their human hosts. As elaborated in his monograph, which D'Herelle published within a few years of his initial discoveries:

> The suffix 'phage' is not used in its strict sense of 'to eat' but in that of 'developing at the expense of', a sense that is frequently used elsewhere in scientific terminology. [...] This is precisely the interpretation to be given the term 'phage' in the word 'bacteriophage'. (D'Herelle, 1926, p. 21)

There was no reference to Twort or his findings in D'Herelle's report and to this day the jury is out among historians and scientists as to whether this oversight was because D'Herelle was unaware of these results or because he did not think them related to his own discovery (Duckworth, 1976, pp. 799-800). Certainly, his reaction was nothing like that of Beijerinck, who had been quick to acknowledge the work's priority 'with pleasure', explaining that he had been unaware of the earlier publications when he delivered his early reports (Bos, 1999, p. 678). In this case, it had been Ivanowski himself who had noticed the omission and remarked in his PhD dissertation:

> [Beijerinck] filtered the sap of diseased plants through a porcelain filter and stated that the sap, sterilized in this fashion, retained its infectivity. The author does not know that I had already established this fact a long time ago. (Ivanowski, 1903, quoted in Lechevalier, 1972, p. 140)

In the case of bacteriophagy, however, Twort appears to have remained as unaware of D'Herelle's initial work as the latter maintained he had been of Twort's 1915 discoveries. Certainly, he made no public comments about it until after his work was brought into the spotlight by the Belgian microbiologist and Nobel laureate Jules Bordet and Mihai Ciucǎ, who at March 1921 meeting of the Belgian Society for Biology announced 'We believe that it is a duty to recognize the incontestable priority of Twort in the study of this question' (as translated and quoted by Duckworth, 1976, p. 797). Unlike Beijerinck though, D'Herelle did not recognize Twort's priority in discovery. In fact, for many years he neither denied nor admitted to having prior knowledge of Twort's 1915 work, but rather would emphasize the difference in their findings, arguing that Twort's description of the phenomenon with micrococci was 'not a question of a real bacterial dissolution, but a transformation of a normal culture on agar into a glassy and transparent one' (D'Herelle, 1922). The dispute on the birthright of the concept bacteriophage should be settled finally by Flu and E. Renaux as umpires (Flu and Renaux, 1932).

The main similarity between Beijerinck and D'Herelle lies in the fact that both men offered explanations for their discoveries that ran completely against the grain of the belief systems about the nature of disease causation and even life at the time. But whereas Beijerinck's ideas about the *contagium vivum fluidum*, as discussed in the previous section, underwent a long eclipse and was not revived for several decades, D'Herelle's work underwent a lull of a mere two years. After that, 'Hundreds of people cited D'Herelle's work, and although he may not have been universally regarded, he was certainly universally acknowledged' (Duckworth, 1976, p. 797).

Although the work of D'Herelle – details of whose background are shrouded in some mystery – cannot be regarded as a Dutch contribution by any means, there is more than one connection to the Netherlands in his story. For one, his mother, Augustine Worms-Mect was a devout Dutch Catholic from near Maastricht, the Netherlands (Summers, 1999, p. 3). More pertinent, to the history of the bacteriophage, is his contact with the Dutch medical researcher Paul Christian Flu, one of the aforementioned 'hundreds', who were intrigued by the phenomenon of bacteriophagy. In 1921 Flu was appointed professor at Leiden University to head the newly formed Laboratory for Tropical Hygiene there. When soon thereafter, D'Herelle 'abruptly left' the Pasteur Institute and embarked on a peripatic career that took him to many places all over the world. His first appointment, thanks to Flu, was at Leiden University. On Flu's recommendation he became associated with the university as conservator of its Institute of Tropical Medicine.

While in Leiden D'Herelle supervised the experiments on bacteriophagy of A.B.F.A. Pondman, a medical doctor who had worked for some years at the Pasteur Institute in the East Indies, where he had been responsible for smallpox vaccine and rabies vaccine production. As it happened Pondman received his doctorate in 1923 – even before his supervisor, for the largely self-educated D'Herelle had never received an academic degree. In fact, it was Flu who proposed his name for an honorary medical degree which Leiden University awarded him in January 1924. Unfortunately, due to financial considerations, D'Herelle could not obtain a long-term position in the Netherlands. Meanwhile, however, his work was also taken up by other Dutch scientists, e.g. at the Laboratory for Hygiene in Amsterdam by S.M. Kropveld, L.K. Wolff and J.W. Janzen (Janzen and Wolff, 1923a and b; Kropveld, 1923), and perhaps most notably by L.E. den Dooren de Jong (see Van Kammen, 2011). Furthermore, as mentioned earlier, in 1925 the Netherlands also honoured D'Herelle for his discovery of the bacteriophage by awarding him with the Van Leeuwenhoek Medal, their foremost prize for a microbiologist (D'Herelle, 1925 and 1928). Surely weighing in on this choice must have been Beijerinck, one of the most eminent of the Dutch microbiologists and a former recipient of the medal,[27] who was enthusiastic about the discovery of bacteriophagy, which he considered a confirmation of his theory of the *contagium vivum fluidum* (Den Dooren de Jong, 1983, p. 43).

Advances in virus research and the rediscovery of Beijerinck's virus concept

In a discussion of the history and legacy of the idea of *contagium vivum fluidum*, the renowned Dutch plant virologist Lute Bos insightfully remarked on 'the striking similarity between Beijerinck's fate in virology and that of Mendel in genetics' (1999, p. 683). Just as there was a gap of some 35 years between the publication of Mendel's famed treatise on his plant hybridization experiments (1865) and the full realization of the import of his work in 1900 – independently by Hugo de Vries, Karl Correns and Eric von Tschermak – so too did the full discovery and final characterization of the of the tobacco mosaic contagium not occur until the 1930s, after Beijerinck's death. But Bos also noted that although 'Beijerinck was 'the Mendel' of virology', unlike the monk who did not live to realize the significance of his work for the discovery of genes, Beijerinck before his death 'had a clear notion already of the close association between virus and host metabolism' (ibid.).

Despite his insights, however, Beijerinck did not pursue his work on *contagium vivum fluidum* for a variety of reasons. The shifting of his interests compounded by the cessation of Dutch commercial tobacco cultivation effectively ended the pursuit of the topic in the Netherlands and Western Europe more broadly (Scholthof et al., 1999). Bibliographic records show that although there was significant progress on understanding different aspects of the tobacco mosaic disease and its agent, much of this work unfolded across the Atlantic. But since this work has little direct bearing either medical virology in the Netherlands or the fate of Beijerinck's concept as such, we will not discuss those advances any further. Instead we take a brief glance at other discoveries – outside the context of TMV (and plant

---

27 Beijerinck was awarded the medal in 1905. Another eminent recipient was Louis Pasteur in 1895.

pathology more broadly) and even foot-and-mouth disease – which also contributed to the idea that there were microscopic disease agents differ-ent from bacteria (or fungi and protozoa). Notable examples include the discoveries of agents of African horse sickness, yellow fever, and rabies, to name but a few (M'Fadyean, 1900; Reed et al., 1900; Remlinger, 1903). In fact, as Creager has observed (2000, p. 29), the publication of a number of reviews on filterable agents of infectious diseases in the first decades of the twentieth century points to an emerging canon about viral diseases (Roux, 1903; M'Fadyean, 1908; Wolbach, 1912). The increasing number of discoveries of diseases caused by filterable viruses, however, was not accompanied by a corresponding progress in understanding the nature of these agents.

By the 1930s, armed with a better picture of the viruses, scientists were in a better position to appreciate Beijerinck's hitherto misunderstood *contagium vivum fluidum*. In contrast to the case of Mendel where the botanist Karl Correns made overt claims about rediscovering his experiment (1950/1900, pp. 39, 48), Beijerinck's re-entry into the history of virology occurred without fanfare, rather matter-of-factly. For example, in 1926, the plant pathologist Louis O. Kunkel and virologist Thomas Rivers would disagree over whether it was Ivanowski or Beijerinck who deserved the label of the founder or 'father' of virology (Benison and Rivers, 1967: pp. 115-116). Neither made any claims about rediscovery, however. And in an address on the nature of viruses to the New York Academy of Sciences, Wendell Stanley opened with a reprise of the investigations of both men, but emphasized the fact that it was Beijerinck 'who first recognized the true significance of the results and the fact that viruses differ from bacteria' (1938, p. 21). But there are two publications that deserve special mention in a discussion of the reawakening of Beijerinck's ideas about viruses: the first, a 1940 biography by three Dutch scholars, G. van Iterson Jr, L.E. den Dooren de Jong and A.J. Kluyver; and the second the journal *Phytopathological Classics* 7 (1942) in which the seminal papers of Mayer, Ivanowski, and Beijerinck were reprinted. In both these publications is a recognition by the author (or in the second case, by the translator) of Beijerinck as a, if not *the*, father of virology. The publication *Martinus Willem Beijerinck: His life and his work*, as the biography is titled, was in fact the final instalment of a much larger project begun in 1920 by Beijerinck's colleagues and successor at Delft on the occasion of his 70th birth anniversary and his retirement after 25 years as professor, to collect his extant publications. Beijerinck, who by the time of his death was internationally respected for his contributions to microbiology, would himself ascribe this fame to these volumes (Van Itallie-van Embden, 1940/1928). The last part of this project, which commenced after his death in 1931, was intended to collect his final (post-retirement) research and included the biography as a sixth and separate volume. Although published in English, the biography had a limited circulation at the time of printing, and only became widely accessible to scholars outside the country when it was reprinted in 1983.[28] It comprises three parts, each undertaken by a different member of the contributing team, of which the third part, dealing exclusively with his microbiological work, was written by Kluyver who was Beijerinck's successor as the head of his laboratory at Delft University. Although just four pages of the nearly 200-page document are devoted to the topic of viruses, there is no equivocation on the Kluyver's part that Beijerinck and his ideas deserved primacy in the founding story of virus research. 'Ample proof is afforded that the contagious agent causing the disease does not belong to the visible microorganisms, but on the contrary is a principle which occurs in the plant juice in a "dissolved state"', he wrote, adding furthermore that, 'anybody reading Ivanowski's 1899 paper will have to acknowledge that this author, even seven years after he made his discovery, was not at all aware of its tremendously far-reaching importance' (Kluyver, 1983/1940, pp. 118-121).

From its inception the *Phytopathological Classics* volume had a more ambitious reach than the biography. The American plant virologist James Johnson, who translated the papers, was a cheerleader for all of the reprinted contributions, but whereas he lauded the importance of Mayer and Ivanowski's discoveries on their individual merits, he attached a much broader disciplinary importance to Beijerinck's discovery. For instance, he claimed that although Beijerinck 'gave only a very small part of his brilliant career to the viruses, the impact of the work was extremely far reaching'. Like other virus researchers of his generation and later, he too noted that Beijerinck's '*vivum fluidum contagium* appears to come very close to the now prevalent concept of a protein molecule as representing the physical structure of a virus' (Johnson, 1942, pp. 5, 31).

In light of such a revival, it is perhaps not surprising that such a leading virologist as Thomas Rivers – who was himself named 'the apostolic father' of the virology of his times by another eminent virologist, John Enders – would accord 'the honor of being the father of virology' to Beijerinck, rather than Ivanowski or Löffler and Frosch. The reason for Rivers's choice, as he later explained to the historian Saul Benison during a series of oral history

---

28   A dozen or so years later the biography was reprinted yet again accompanied by three historical papers read at a symposium held in Delft, The Netherlands, to commemorate the hundredth anniversary of the laboratory started by Beijerinck there (Bos and Theunissen, 1995).

interviews, was that whereas there was no doubt about Ivanowski's priority in the matter of observing the filterability of the tobacco mosaic agent, it was Beijerinck who realized the novelty of the agent and 'put his neck out by calling it a living contagious fluid' (Benison and Rivers, 1967, pp. vii, 115, 119).

The relevance of Beijerinck in the Dutch medical context

Even as Beijerinck's ideas were beginning to make a comeback, it must be admitted that the impact of his virus concept remained low in the medical research circles, at least within the Netherlands. Eventually, however, the science caught up. As one way of gauging this impact, Gerard van Doornum surveyed the contents of the NTvG from 1857 onwards for articles containing the key words 'virus', 'Beijerinck' and names of various diseases (now known to be caused by viruses). He found a total of 85 articles bearing the word 'virus' in their titles were published in this journal during between 1857 and 1950, but as discussed earlier, we must remember that the word had a much broader meaning for most of this period than it does now. In 27 of those 85 articles, for instance, the term 'virus' was used in a wider, less specific sense as simple a source of infectious disease. The more restrictive term 'filterable virus' appeared for the first time in the 1890s and thereafter, about three to five times per decade for two more decades. In the 1930s and 1940s that there were nineteen and eighteen medical articles, respectively, relating specifically to the early virus concept. Remarkably, considering the detrimental effects of World War II on research and publications in general, 1950s saw a steep increase to 89 articles with the word *virus* in the title. Beijerinck's name was hardly mentioned at all: there were two references in 1893 and 1901 in connection with fermentation; and one obituary in 1931. Although the author of the latter, J.J. van Loghem, described Beijerinck's bacteriological achievements in detail, he completely ignored his contributions to virology (1931). The explanation of this omission might be found in an overview entitled 'Het raadsel der vira'[29] in which he wrote that Beijerinck simply repeated the experiments of Ivanowski and confirmed his results, so he believed that the honour of being the father of virology belonged to Ivanowki and not to Beijerinck (Van Loghem, 1944). The single positive reference came from Beijerinck's contemporary, A.P. Fokker, a professor in microbiology in Groningen, who paradoxically supported Beijerinck's views, even though he vigorously opposed the ideas of such leading bacteriologists of the day,

29   'The enigma of viruses'.

such as Pasteur and Koch. For what it was worth, this support came in the form of a tangential reference in an insulting diatribe against a colleague who reported on serum therapy for diphtheria:

> And what was heard about the most important communication of Beijerinck about a *contagium vivum fluidum*, that appeared some months ago, and in more sound times a revolution in science ought to bring? On this issue, to the best of my knowledge, people have remained [...] silent. (Fokker, 1899[30])

Sadly, his words proved all too true, for some decades to come.

One possible explanation for the relatively low early interest in the *contagium vivum fluidum* from the medical circles is that, as suggested by the veteran historian of medicine Bill Bynum, the impact of the science for most of this period was far more striking on diagnosis and the public face of medicine than it was on improving therapeutic measures against various diseases (1994, p. xii). Beijerinck's concept of virus offered neither diagnostic nor therapeutic potential to be tapped into by clinicians and thus they ignored it for many years. We believe that the increased publications on viruses in the NTvG was a reflection of the tremendous growth in knowledge about some fundamental aspects of the virus chemistry and biophysics, such as their composition, structure and multiplication, which had direct ramifications for understanding and treating infectious diseases.

Viruses after the 1930s: New insights in light of technical developments

Although such scientists as D'Herelle would claim that the discovery of the bacteriophage was a step towards solving the mystery of the filterable viruses (1926), there were others – e.g. Jules Bordet (1922, 1923, 1931) – who considered the problem different altogether, and still others who likely thought the phages confounded rather than helped matters (Gratia, 1938, 1945). Looking back at the history of virus research, however, it appears evident to us that one of the main hurdles to understanding the nature of viruses was technical

---

30 En wat heeft men nog gehoord van de allerbelangrijkste mededeling van Beijerinck over een contagium vivum fluidum, die reeds enige maanden oud is en in een meer gezonden tijd een revolutie in de wetenschap zou moeten brengen? Voor zoover ik weet heeft men daarover ... gezwegen.

rather than theoretical, for, as Bos has argued, '*conceptually* virology was conceived in 1898 when Beijerinck's classical paper was published. The development of the new discipline remained embryonic until [...] viruses became subject to isolation and study *in vitro*' (1999, p. 684). Into the 1930s, for instance, Rivers would lament that viruses were still 'characterized by three *negative* properties, namely, *invisibility* by ordinary microscopic methods, *failure* to be retained by filters impervious to well-known bacteria, and the *inability* to propagate themselves in the absence of susceptible cells' (Rivers, 1927; Rivers, 1932, p. 423, emphasis added).

A positive resolution to each of the negatives identified by Rivers would depend on the development of appropriate methods and technologies in the 1930s and 1940s: the development of electron microscopes, as well as X-ray crystallographic techniques to render the invisible viruses visible (Editorial JAMA, 1932; Ruska et al., 1939/1940; Ruska, 1987; Stanley, 1935 and 1938; Bawden and Pirie, 1937); improved instruments, such as the ultracentrifuges that enabled the purification of the ultrafiltrable virus particles (Creager, 2002); and the development of different methods for the cultivation of viruses, e.g. in chick embryos and cultured cell lines (Woodruff and Goodpasture, 1931; Scherer et al., 1953; Temin and Rubin, 1958). Such physicochemical studies of the viruses proved key in triggering the development of molecular biology, which, in combination with the biological information about viruses-host interaction gained from studies on cultivated viruses, provided the further means 'to reveal the true nature of viruses' (Bos, 1999, p. 675). The histories of these various developments are well beyond the scope of this book, and has, furthermore, been described in considerable detail by several distinguished authors to whom we refer interested readers (Waterson and Wilkinson, 1978; Grafe, 1991; Booss and August, 2013; Chastel, 1992; Bos, 1999; Méthot, 2016; Van Kammen, 1999). In the meantime, however, it is worth noting that the medical research community contributed relatively little towards the major advances in learning about the structure, composition and functioning of viruses mentioned in the brief summary of events above. But they were intrigued by the spectacular findings on the threshold of life and reaped the benefits of the new knowledge, as is amply evident from their attendance at various meetings about viruses.

Three symposia held in the Netherlands deserve special mention here, for they provide snapshots of the state-of-the-art in Dutch virus research and also demonstrate the high level of activity and interest in the subject despite very turbulent circumstances. Especially remarkable is the attendance – 20 members and 63 other guests – at the 1940 symposium organized by the learned Society for the Advancement of Science, Medicine and Surgery on

'The Ultravirus Problem' just three weeks before the German invasion of the Netherlands. The two other meetings devoted to viruses were both organized by Netherlands Society for Biochemistry, in 1939 and 1947. Proceedings of these symposia were printed in full in the *Chemisch Weekblad* (1939 and 1947/1948) and the NTvG (1940).

The roster of speakers and topics of the biochemists' symposia bears testimony to the contributions of basic chemistry, physics, and biochemistry towards understanding the nature of viruses. Also evident from these talks is a growing focus among attendees on questions of virus growth and multiplication. For example, H.S. Frenkel, the director of the State Veterinary Research Institute, discussed advances in techniques and new instruments developed in the Netherlands for cultivating animal viruses. Although often overlooked in historical accounts of virology, Frenkel was a pioneer in this area who had developed a method for cultivating the foot-and-mouth disease virus in vitro, which was later used at the French Institut Mérieux for the production of a vaccine (Barteling and Vreeswijk, 1991). His colleague, the colloid-chemist Louis W. Janssen, a virus researcher at the State Veterinary Research Institute, was a prominent presence at all three meetings, where he presented different aspects of his work on virus replication and ideas about biosynthesis. Janssen – whose ideas have attracted very little historical attention, especially from Anglophone scholars, because he hardly published anything internationally – was one of the earliest researchers to suggest a compartmentalization of nucleic acids biosynthesis, i.e. of DNA to the nucleus and RNA to the cytoplasm. He assumed that the thymose-containing machine factories in the nucleus produce ribose-containing machines which are transported to the cytoplasm, where they make in turn the different proteins containing cell products. In the case of a virus-infected cell, the poisoned thymose-containing nuclear machine section is damaged, result-ing in modified machines in the cytoplasm that are no longer capable of producing the normal protein cell products.

Janssen was optimistic that it was up to the present (i.e. his) generation to carry forward the progress of the past 20 years in order to answer the fundamental question of whether life was chemical or physical. Other notable speakers at the 1940 meeting include the above-mentioned Flu, on the nature of viruses as pathogens, and S. Weidinger, a colloid chemist and histologist from Amsterdam who dealt with X-ray spectroscopic studies of viruses and proteins (Flu, 1940; Hermans, 1963; Weidinger, 1940).

The end of the war opened up more opportunities and many senior scientists made research tours to the UK and the USA. One such was the medical researcher J. Mulder from Leiden, whose trip was funded by the

Figure 6   **L.W. Janssen's (1901-1975) hypothetical scheme to interpret biochemical findings: normal situation**

Figure 7   **L.W. Janssen's (1901-1975) hypothetical scheme to interpret biochemical findings: virus infection of a host cell**

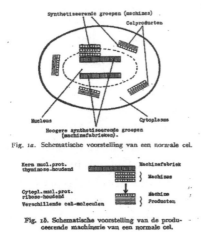

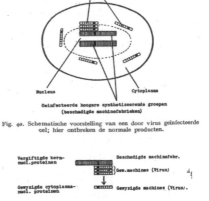

Schematic representation of the producing machineries of the normal cell. He suggested a hypothetical scheme to interpret the biochemical findings regarding virus infecting a host cell. Reproduction by courtesy of NTvG

Schematic representation of the producing machineries of a virus infected cell I. He suggested that a failure in the host cell nucleus led to an aberrant molecular entity which functions as an infectious virus. This mechanical explanation was farfetched at the time, but did forecast the conception of a provirus.
Reproduction by courtesy of NTvG

Rockefeller Foundation and reported in the NTvG (Mulder, 1947). There was also increased travel within the country, e.g. the bacteriophage researcher and former Beijerinck student and colleague, L. Den Dooren de Jong, by then head of the Bacteriology Laboratory for the local hospitals in Rotterdam, was invited in 1954 by the learned Clinical Society Rotterdam to deliver a lecture on 'Viruses and their behaviour in the cell'. The contents of his lecture – primarily focusing on the then current state of the art of biochemical and biophysical virus studies (Den Dooren de Jong, 1954) – is a clear indication of how far different basic and clinical research communities had come in opening up channels of communication amongst themselves.

What we have seen in this chapter then, is the transition in the use of the term 'virus' from a generic label in nineteenth century for the causative agent of any infectious disease to denote a separate category of infectious disease agents with specific distinguishing properties of their own. Because these agents were invisible, they could not be characterized until the development of special instruments and methods to visualize and analyse them. Thus, we see the first tentative steps of the entry of new biological entities into the worlds of biophysics and biochemistry; initiating an interdisciplinary approach that would become so successful after World War II that it would lead to the molecular biology 'revolution'. At the same time this chapter also illuminates two general phenomena about the process of science as it is done in the real world. First, there is the universalism of scientific knowledge. Even in the nineteenth century, when scientific publications were made widely available, researchers worldwide criticized each other and tried to establish and defend their priority in matters of new findings. Beijerinck's interpretations were scrutinized by contemporaries from all parts of the world, from Russia to the US. In other words, a Dutch finding about a filtcrable disease agent had international repercussions. The second phenomenon which is beautifully illustrated in this chapter is the need for scientists to recognize their antecedents and identify with a tradition of practice and thinking. In the specific case of virology, which in the 1930s was beginning to carve out a niche for itself, we saw the new generation of its practitioners create a new order by acknowledging its true forebears. The numerous commemorations of the founding of virology in Russia (Lustig and Levine, 1992; Lvov, 1993), the Netherlands and Germany (Calisher and Horzinek, 1999), are manifestations of this wish to reconstruct the past and, where possible, beat the national drum.

3   On the fringes

The Dutch work on viruses, 1900-1950

's Leven Nevels [*Life's fringes*][31]
– A.J. Kluyver (1937)

The epigraph – a palindrome in its original Dutch – is actually the title of an address by the microbiologist Albert Jan Kluyver to the Dutch Society of Microbiology where he spoke on the status of virus research in the Netherlands at the time. It is fitting from a historical perspective that this topic was addressed by the foremost Dutch bacteriologist of the day and one who was, moreover, the intellectual heir of, and successor, to Martinus Beijerinck (Kamp et al., 1959). It serves to highlight the fact that the origin of virus research was firmly rooted in bacteriology and pathology.

By the middle of the 1870s the basic knowledge about and techniques to work with, bacteria and the diseases they produced (Rosen, 1993/1958) were well in place, with central laboratories for microbiology founded in major European capitals. In 1888 Louis Pasteur had founded Institut Pasteur in Paris; Berlin had the Institut für Infektionskrankheiten with Robert Koch as director; and in London there was the bacteriology laboratory at King's College under E.M. Crookshank, who had worked with Joseph Lister, the third man of the triumvirate that dominated the origin stories of medical microbiology and the germ theory. Pasteur had himself led the development of virology in France with his work on the rabies vaccine – indeed the Pasteur Institute when it opened was dedicated to the treatment of rabies. In contrast, it was not Koch himself but a former student and colleague, Friedrich Loeffler, who pioneered virology in Germany and German-speaking countries (Schmiedebach, 1999). We must recall that Loeffler worked on foot-and-mouth disease in collaboration with Paul Frosch and with Uhlenhuth (Grafe, 1991, p. 99; Loeffler and Frosch, 1898; Löffler and Frosch, 1961/1898) and even now there are virologists who accord him the honour of discovering the first virus over either Beijerinck or Ivanowski (Witz, 1998; Murphy, 2018).

No equivalent to the laboratories of Koch or Pasteur was established in the Netherlands. In Wageningen (1875-1884), for example, Beijerinck had

---

31   's Leven Nevels. Although *'nebulae'* is a closer translation of the Dutch word *'nevels'* than 'fringes', we have kept the translation provided by Kluyver himself (1937).

discussed his plans for a research laboratory to improve the cultivation of
grain with the minister concerned, but the minister did not grasp the import
of Beijerinck's ideas and nothing came of the discussion (Van Itallie-van
Embden, 1940/1928). By the end of the nineteenth century, however, Dutch
bacteriologists with the spirit of enterprise did succeed in establishing a
number of clinical, bacteriology diagnostic laboratories in various cities (Van
Lieburg, 1986; Visser et al., 1986). Meanwhile, existing university laboratories
of hygiene extended the field of investigation to bacteriology as a logical
consequence of these developments. By virtue of the Law on Higher Education of 1875, all four Dutch universities were obliged to establish a chair in
hygiene and medical police and to provide the support for an associated
research laboratory. In addition to these statutory laboratories, private
initiative was taken to establish and fund two specialized laboratories for
tropical hygiene – the first one in Amsterdam in 1917 on the initiative of the
Colonial Institute and the second in Leiden in 1921 by the Society Institute
for Tropical Medicine Rotterdam-Leiden. The latter institute was financed
by rich entrepreneurs (port barons) in Rotterdam who also opened the
Harbour Hospital in Rotterdam. The directors of these laboratories were both
appointed professor at the University of Amsterdam and Leiden University,
respectively. The main stimulus for the specialization in tropical hygiene
was that the Netherlands had deep commercial interests in certain tropical
regions, i.e. the Dutch colonies in the East Indies, the West Indies and
Suriname, where infectious diseases were a real burden both for expatriates
and local inhabitants. The growing interest in tropical disease at the end of
the nineteenth century, which we shall discuss in further detail in Chapter 7,
was also connected with the introduction of the so-called colonial ethical
policy (Beukers, 1989).

In the immediate wake of the first discoveries...

Despite Beijerinck's characterization of the tobacco mosaic virus as a completely different entity from the known bacteria, there was little scope for
fundamental research in virology in the laboratories of hygiene. For one, the
viral diseases of plants, while providing a more convenient experimental
system than infectious diseases of humans and other animals, did not
appear to have much applicability in the latter investigations, at least at
first. After Beijerinck's first investigations at the request of his colleague
Adolf Mayer on the contagious character of tobacco mosaic disease, he left
Wageningen in 1885. His discussions with the Minister of the Interior on the

expansion of his laboratory came to naught, and he accepted the invitation of Jacques van Marken, owner of the Netherlands Yeast and Spirit Works in Delft, where he worked as an industrial microbiologist for ten years (Van Itallie-van Embden, 1940/1928). Then in 1895, after negotiations with the director of the Polytechnic School in Delft and a discussion in the House of Commons over his salary and other terms of employment, Beijerinck was appointed professor of microbiology in Delft (Netherlands Staten-Generaal, 1893). He enjoyed a long and illustrious career as a bacteriologist. Although he never returned to experimental work on viruses after 1899, he would remain interested in the 'invisible' microbes throughout his life; exemplified, for instance, by his enthusiastic reception of the bacteriophage discussed in Chapter 2 (Den Dooren de Jong, 1983, p. 43).

As Dutch microbiologists lacked the state-of-the-art facilities of the more advanced research institutes in their neighbouring countries over the first decades of the twentieth century, they did not engage in cutting-edge virus research themselves. The fact that they closely followed the breakthroughs of their colleagues abroad was indicated, for example, by the proceedings of the Society for the Advancement of Science, Medicine and Surgery (Genootschap ter bevordering van Natuur- Genees- en Heelkunde) in Amsterdam (Delprat and Kummer, 1965; Van Berkel et al., 1991). Another learned society named for Matthias van Geuns[32] in Utrecht met on a monthly basis and the proceedings of their meeting contain reports of epidemiologic and clinical aspects of regularly returning '*morbi epidemici*' or epidemic diseases (Haneveld, 2004; Kühler, 1953; Sypkens Smit, 1953; Utrechts Geneeskundig Gezelschap 'Matthias van Geuns', n.d. a and b). The most frequent communicable diseases around 1900 seem to have been scarlet fever, variola (smallpox), and meningitis. Influenza was mentioned sometimes, but measles, rabies or poliomyelitis hardly at all. In contrast to the meetings of the Amsterdam Society the discussions of this group of Utrecht medical faculty members were oriented chiefly towards clinical problems. The bacteriologist and 1929 Nobel Prize-winning physician Christiaan Eykman whom readers may recall from Chapter 1 for his favourable review of Pasteur's vaccine on pragmatic grounds, was a regular member of this group.

Further evidence that Dutch microbiologists had their finger on the pulse of international research scene at the end of the first half of the twentieth century, and were respected in turn, is to be found in the archives of nominations of the Nobel Prize for Physiology and Medicine. Witness, for example,

---

32   Utrecht Medical Society 'Matthias van Geuns'. Utrechts Geneeskundig Gezelschap 'Matthias van Geuns'.

the fact that Ernest Goodpasture, the American virologist who was the first person to successfully cultivate viruses in the laboratory outside the context of their natural infections (Woodruff and Goodpasture, 1931) was nominated as a candidate for this achievement by no less than four Dutch medical researchers in 1949 (Nobel Foundation, n.d. b). Two of these men also co-nominated Frank Macfarlane Burnet, who developed Goodpasture's methods into an assay technique for the viruses (1936). Since nominations for the Nobel Prize may be made by invitation only (unless the nominator is a former winner), it means that the opinions of the Leiden researchers were held in high esteem in the international community.

One topic that did receive a lot of press – both positive and negative – especially in the NTvG was the anti-rabies vaccine developed by Pasteur and co-workers in 1885. The critiques within the Netherlands closely corresponded to those that Pasteur et al. faced in France and elsewhere as detailed by the historian Gerald Geison. Broadly speaking, these critiques fell under three categories: i) strictly scientific arguments disputing the experimental approaches, ii) clinical concerns, and iii) statistical arguments (Geison, 1995). Reservations notwithstanding, after 1886 it became possible for Dutch patients to travel for treatment against rabies to the Pasteur Institute in Paris, at the expense of the state of the Netherlands (Polak, 1964). Later the travelling time was shortened, when in 1907 the patients were referred to the 'Institut antirabique' of Dr Jules Bordet in Brussels (the self-same Bordet who in 1920 became involved in the dispute with Felix d'Herelle over the nature of bacteriophagy). Because of the lack of the freedom of movement between the Netherlands and Belgium due to the German occupation of Belgium during World War I, Dutch physicians worked to make rabies vaccination possible in the Netherlands itself. In 1915 patients could be referred to the Institute of Pathology of Professor Spronck – the address of which was ironically Pasteurstraat 2, Utrecht – while the vaccine was obtained by diplomatic mail from the Institut für Infektionskrankheiten in Berlin (Ruijsch and Van Asch van Wijck, 1915).

It should also be noted that the Netherlands was not completely devoid of studies related to virus diseases. For example, the 1906 issue of NTvG contains a review by Cornelia de Lange, future professor of paediatrics at the University of Amsterdam, of a thesis by an H. Aldershoff on 'vaccine bodies'. The author, who conducted his experiments in Groningen using corneal tissue cultures inoculated with vaccinia and smallpox viruses, considered these bodies to be products of the cell nucleus enclosed by a shell originating from the protoplasm of the epithelial cell (De Lange, 1906). Another example of an original Dutch contribution is that of the activity of

J.J. van Loghem on the prevention of the possible spread of yellow fever to the Pacific caused by the opening of the Panama Canal in 1914. According to Wickliffe Rose, the chairman of Rockefeller Foundation Yellow Fever Committee, Van Loghem's impressive contribution to the report *Yellow fever: Feasibility of its eradication* highlighted the risk that 'so long as yellow fever exists in America the danger remains for Asia' (Rose, 1914).

It is hardly surprising that the few communications in the NTvG on Dutch research that were related to human virus diseases came from academic laboratories as well laboratories connected with the institutes for tropical hygiene. The involvement of the latter might be explained by the significance in terms of morbidity and mortality of diseases such as yellow fever, dengue, rabies or smallpox in the East and the West Indies, and the importance of the public health measures in combating these diseases due to lack of specific therapeutic possibilities. The progress of medical virology during the first half of the twentieth century in the Netherlands may well be told in terms of the activities at these institutions, and consequently our focus for the bulk of this chapter will be on the work conducted there. Before considering these individual laboratories, however, we will pick up a thread from Chapter 1 and consider the impact of the important outbreaks of viral diseases during this period, beginning with the pandemic that claimed more lives than any other infectious disease outbreak in modern times.

The Spanish influenza pandemic of 1918: Its impact in the Netherlands

On 4 August 1918, near the end of World War I, the *Nieuwe Rotterdamsche Courant* ran an article by P.H. Kramer, an officer of the Dutch Military Health Service (Militair Geneeskundige Dienst), describing a disease outbreak 'of an exceptional epidemic character, which has not honoured the neutral borders of our fatherland, and which has become known to us closely under the name of Spanish flu or Spanish disease'.[33] What Kramer was describing was the beginning of a first wave of a pandemic and which over the next six months would spread over the entire world and kill over 30 million people, which was 'more than three times the number of military casualties suffered'

---

33   een ziekte van een buitengewoon epidemisch karakter, welke ook de neutrale grenzen van ons vaderland niet heeft geëerbiedigd en die ons thans onder den naam van 'Spaansche griep' of 'Spaansche ziekte' van nabij bekend is geworden. (Both the original and the translation quoted in Haalboom, 2014.)

over the entirety of World War I (Patterson and Pyle, 1991). At the time that he wrote this piece, Kramer was as yet unaware of the severity of the problem and under the impression that the influenza epidemic, while spreading quickly, was relatively mild (Haalboom, 2014). But he was very wrong. As medical records show, at its height in the Netherlands during the autumn of 1918, the flu epidemic claimed over 17,000 lives in 1918 and continuing at a lower level until May 1919 with 1,400 deaths. A second outbreak counted 3,700 deaths between January and May 1920 (Quanjer, 1921).

Given its severity, it is probably not surprising to learn that the 1918-1919 pandemic – which, despite its name, most epidemiologists now believe did *not* actually originate in Spain – aroused much more panic within the Netherlands than the previous outbreak of 1889-1890. Both visitations, however, were cause for discussions in the House of Representatives (see Chapter 1 for details about the first incident). During the 1918 outbreak one of the members of the house, W. van Ravesteijn, questioned Minister of Labour P. Aalberse about his awareness of the rumours of a plague outbreak, and further inquired about the preventive measures that the government was intending to take (Van Ravesteijn, 1918-1919). All the minister could offer by way of a response was that bacteriological examination had not revealed the plague bacillus. He also drew attention to the fact the epidemic had begun at the eastern border with Germany, which implied that it might have been introduced by labourers crossing over (Aalberse, 1918-1919). But even with information in hand, we believe that controlling the disease would have been challenging. For one, monitoring the flow of people during the thick of the war would have been virtually impossible. Furthermore, there would have been difficulties posed in identifying infectious individuals who were in the incubation period and therefore asymptomatic. Without any specific information about the disease, the government could take only general measures, which it did by raising the daily allowance of bread to improve the overall health of the population. It also adopted measures to close schools and public places where crowding could be expected. The most detailed – albeit still incomplete – epidemiological report of the epidemic was published in 1921 by the distinguished military physician Major General A.A.J. Quanjer, who was by then inspector of the Military Medical Service (Militair Geneeskundige Dienst). Only incidentally, his report contained information about the respiratory symptoms and airborne transmission of the disease (Quanjer, 1921).

As with many other epidemic diseases, the European encounter with influenza made its way into various works of literature and the arts. The famous Marcel Proust – whose father, the physician-hygienist Adrien Proust, had been involved with the reporting the events of the 1892 flu epidemic – would refer to the Spanish outbreak in his novel *Time regained*. In one scene the narrator is asked at a reception [at the home of] the Princesse de Guermantes, whether he was not afraid of catching influenza of which there was an epidemic at that moment (c. 1918). Overhearing this question, another guest, a well-wisher, interjects with the reassurance, 'Oh no! It's usually only the young who catch it. A man of your age has very little to fear' (Proust, 1981, p. 969; Proust, 1986, p. 328). While we are not sure about the extent of Marcel Proust's medical knowledge, this remark by his character actually represents a rather accurate picture of the demographics of the 1918 outbreak. According to the medical historian Anton Erkoreka, the highest risk groups in Western Europe during the Spanish influenza pandemic were in fact, young people – men and women between the ages of 25 and 34, followed by those between the ages of 15 and 24 (Erkoreka, 2009, 2010). Meanwhile, closer to home, the influenza pandemic also made its appearance in the Dutch literature of the same period with the Dutch author H.W. Gorter writing to one of his lovers: 'Are you also being very careful, my Heart? Gargle again and again, suck, rinse your mouth, swallow, and wash your hands. The latter, especially. I am also being extremely careful' (Frerichs, 2014).[34] His advice reflects the common wisdom regarding precautions against and alleviation of symptoms of the disease, which, in fact persist to the present day.

Given the medical, public health, national, and international importance of the pandemic, it is surprising that it spurred so few virological studies on influenza in the Netherlands. One reason for the lack of progress at this time, not only in the Netherlands but indeed the world over, might well have been the uncertainty over its causative agent. As the prominent American physiologist and bacteriologist Hans Zinsser observed in 1922, the scientific community was 'overwhelmed by the wealth of reported material, but confused at the same time, by its indefiniteness in description of technique and by the frequently defective clinical characterization of the cases studied' (quoted in Gillett, 2009, p. 170). In hindsight, it is clear that one drawback during the 1918 pandemic was that too much effort was expended on finding a bacterial rather than viral agent. Many scientists the world over investigated the bacterial species *Haemophilus influenzae,* isolated by Richard Pfeiffer in 1892 as a possible cause. For instance, as detailed later in this chapter, the earliest studies by L.K. Wolff and J.J.C. van Hoogenhuyze at the Laboratory for Hygiene in Amsterdam were focused precisely on

34   Pas jij ook geweldig op, mijn Hart? Aldoor door gorgelen, zuigen, spoelen, slikken, en handen wasschen. Dit laatste vooral ook. Ik ben ook reusachtig voorzichtig.

finding a bacterial agent (Van Hoogenhuyze, 1919). Another early problem in studying this disease had been the lack of adequate animal models, which hindered scientists in their search for the causative agent. As will be made evident in the sections on virus research in different laboratories, despite the early interest in the 1920s stimulated by the pandemic, it was only in the 1930s that there was any real progress in influenza virus research both at local and global levels.

Dutch progress on rabies, smallpox, polio, and measles, 1900-1950

Compared to influenza, none of the other viral diseases discussed in Chapter 1 had that much of an impact within the Netherlands in the first half of the twentieth century, be it in terms of knowledge about the diseases themselves or virus research more generally. The groundbreaking events around these other diseases were either past or yet lay in the future, and furthermore did not take place within the Netherlands. Rabies research, for instance, had already reached its climax in France with Pasteur's dramatic demonstration of the efficacy of the vaccine in 1885. Whereas his original method remained the method of choice in France and her colonies, modifications to the original method were introduced by others in different parts of the world (Van Rooyen and Rhodes, 1948, p. 854). In the Dutch East Indies, for example, the bacteriologist Maria van Stockum demonstrated the superiority of a formalin-based vaccine over other preparations (Van Stockum, 1935). Her preparation had a longer shelf life, which proved a great advantage in delivering immediate on-site treatment to victims bitten by animals, who did not have to travel to a central facility for treatment.

In the case of smallpox, the World Health Organization (WHO) would triumphantly announce success in its eradication around the globe in 1980, the result of a decades-long campaign initiated in 1959. But this achievement was more a triumph of public health practices than basic virus research, and in any case, not an achievement for which the Dutch could claim any special priority. Between 1900 and 1950, there had been a series of relatively small smallpox outbreaks in the Netherlands, but there was little if any change in the way physicians managed the disease (see Kramer, 1930; Dewhurst, 1955 and 1959). Although there was no shortage of the vaccine, its production in the Netherlands, which was diminished from thirteen to three locations in the 1930s and spread out to Amsterdam, Rotterdam and Groningen, was inefficient, and resources for research were scarce. Despite a recommendation in 1932 and a formal decision in 1938, the Netherlands only centralized its vaccine production in 1955, and reluctantly at that (Van Zon, 1990, p. 278). In the meantime, there were small advances, e.g. on post-vaccination encephalitis, research which had commenced during the 1930s at the Institute for Preventive Medicine in Leiden (Bijl, 1954).

Polio presented a similar pattern of outbreaks as smallpox during the same period, with a series of relatively minor epidemics in different Dutch cities. Certainly nothing compared with the scale of polio epidemics that began in 1918 in the United States, of which Franklin Delano Roosevelt (FDR) was a famous victim in 1921. A member of a prominent and affluent family – he was distantly related to the former president, Theodore Roosevelt, who was also the uncle of his wife, Eleanor – FDR diverted considerable funds towards rehabilitation and basic research on polio, both before and during his presidency.

Meanwhile, although The Hague was home to Karl Landsteiner from 1919 to 1922, the versatile Austrian researcher who had identified the virus causing poliomyelitis (Landsteiner and Popper, 1909), the visit had little impact on polio research in the Netherlands (Haeseker, 2002). Coincidentally, the neurologist F.S. van Bouwdijk Bastiaans, with whom Landsteiner published work on another totally different subject (namely, tuberous sclerosis), would in 1930 publish an overview of the symptoms, diagnostics, prophylaxis, and treatment of polio (Van Bouwdijk Bastiaanse and Landsteiner, 1922). In the absence of any vaccines, Dutch health professionals made use of convalescent immune serum as a treatment against polio. In 1943 a distressing outbreak occurred in Amsterdam, which affected a total of 612 people and claimed 79 lives. The disease spread to the concentration camp in Westerbork, where it killed three out of a total of 58 Dutch Jews afflicted. A detailed report of this epidemic was published in 1946 by neurologist/psychiatrist N. Speijer in the NTvG. It was not until World War II that any Dutch researcher achieved anything of note in polio research. In the second part of the 1940s, D. Verlinde, a microbiologist at the Institute for Preventive Medicine in Leiden, who was interested in infections of the central nervous system, turned his attention to the poliovirus (Versteeg, 1987).

Although A.P. Fokker, a professor of bacteriology in Groningen, optimistically predicted the imminent discovery of a causative agent for measles as early as 1891 (Fokker, 1891). The virus has been grown on chorio-allantois in the 1930s and has been used in human immunization experiments (Van Rooyen and Rhodes, 1948, p. 229; Van Lookeren Campagne, 1943). The communication by Van Lookeren Campagne was published in the NTvG in the middle of World War II, the information came through the Renseignements Scientifiques of the Red Cross. On cell culture the virus was actually grown in 1954 (Enders and Peebles, 1954). In the absence of a known agent, scientists, encouraged by the success of the diphtheria antiserum prepared by the inoculation of animals, adopted similar approaches against measles (De Haan, 1896). The first communication on the application of convalescent serum against measles in the Netherlands was published in 1922 in the NTvG by C.M. Kroes, of the Department of Infectious Diseases of the Wilhelmina Gasthuis in Amsterdam. Working off prior information (Degkwitz, 1920), Kroes prepared the immune serum by drawing blood from recently recovered measles patients about one week after the disappearance of their exanthema, and heating the serum thus obtained at 60°C for one hour, presumably to inactivate the pathogens. In 1925 J.C. Schippers reported on the good results of the application of the convalescence serum for the prevention of serious complications of measles. Later in the 1930s, treatments for measles came within easier reach of the general practitioners as convalescent serum was made available via the National Institute for Public Health at Utrecht (De Ruiter, 1939; Wagenaar, 1938). But this approach posed problems because doctors then needed to depend on the existence of a base of convalescents for their supply. To overcome this problem, they turned to the use of gamma globulin preparations, which were easier to obtain because about 90 per cent of the population contained antibodies against measles virus in their circulating blood (Hüet, 1951). The slight drawback arising from the lesser potency of these preparations – due to lower levels of antibodies in blood as compared to convalescents – was mitigated by the ease of access and collection methods as well as higher volume of available material (Dicke, 1953, pp. 99-100).

The early Dutch centres of activity on virus diseases

In the remainder of the chapter, we describe the progress of virology research at the various centres from the early 1900s through the end of World War II. Most of this work was embedded in laboratories at the four major universities with medical faculties in the Netherlands: the state universities in Leiden, Utrecht, and Groningen, and the municipal University of Amsterdam. Two other sites of considerable activity during this period were the Institute for Tropical Hygiene in Amsterdam and the Institute for Tropical Medicine in Leiden. Although they were funded by private means and had no formal association with the university system, their directors were affiliated with local universities. Due to the overlap of the activities between the universities and tropical institutes, we will treat them as single units in the ensuing

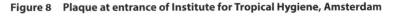

Figure 8   Plaque at entrance of Institute for Tropical Hygiene, Amsterdam

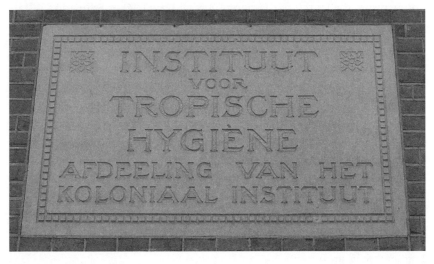

Photo by G. van Doornum

discussion. Finally, we also pay attention to the activities at two institutions that were founded in the 1930s and would later become important for Dutch virology: the State Veterinary Research in Rotterdam, which moved to Amsterdam in 1941, and the Institute for Preventive Medicine, established in Leiden in 1929. As Amsterdam is the capital city, we begin our account with the research activities there.

Amsterdam

Laboratory for Hygiene, University of Amsterdam, and Laboratory of the Department for Tropical Hygiene of the Colonial Institute[35]

The University of Amsterdam as we know it today was originally founded in 1632 by municipal authorities of the city as the 'Athenaeum Illustre' or Illustrious School of Amsterdam. According to the historian P.J. Knegtmans, the school was primarily set up to impart the latest in learning to the city's merchants-to-be and future regents rather more than to teach medicine (2007, p. 20). Over the next two centuries the Athenaeum grew in size and

---

35   Laboratorium voor de Gezondheidsleer, Universiteit van Amsterdam en Laboratorium van de Afdeling Tropische Hygiene van het Koloniaal Instituut.

stature. In 1877 after a long process involving much debate, lobbying efforts and waiting, the Dutch parliament approved the Higher Education Bill in 1876, which granted the city of Amsterdam the right to elevate it to the status of to a full-fledged university the following year. This change in status gave the university the same privileges as national state universities while being funded by the city of Amsterdam (Knegtmans, 2007, p. 133). Although the dramatic rise in costs greatly curtailed the university's growth after WW II, municipal funding continued until 1961, at which point both the funding and the administration of the university were taken over by the national government. When the university was established in 1876 the Higher Education Bill had also stipulated that each university was obliged to teach hygiene, medical police and forensic medicine. Therefore, the university also established a separate Laboratory for Hygiene at the University in 1879. For the bulk of the period covered in this chapter, the laboratory was headed by two bacteriologists, R.H. Saltet (1896-1923), followed by Johannes J. van Loghem (1923-1941).

Meanwhile, in 1910 a number of large private companies had joined forces with the government to found the 'Colonial Institute' – today the Royal Tropical Institute or KIT[36] – specifically to study the tropics and promote trade and industry in the Dutch colonial territories. Two years later, the Colonial Institute founded the Institute for Tropical Hygiene to train medical doctors for future work in the tropics. Van Loghem, who together with his mentor Saltet had drawn up the plans for this institute, was appointed as the first director in 1912. Prior to his appointments in Amsterdam, Van Loghem had served from 1908 to 1909 as a substitute director of a Dutch facility in Sumatra, where together with his wife, he discovered the prevalence of *Aedes aegypti* mosquitoes, the primary hosts of the yellow fever virus, and also played a key role in bringing the threat of yellow fever in South East Asia to the attention of other investigators (Van Loghem and Van der Noordaa, 2000). In 1924, when Van Loghem was appointed professor of hygiene as successor of Saltet, he became head of the university Laboratory for Hygiene. The directorship of the Institute for Tropical Hygiene was taken up by W.A.P. Schüffner, who, in turn, maintained this position in tandem with a professorship at the university until 1937. Originally from Germany, Schüffner had worked in the Dutch East Indies from 1897 until 1929 and afterwards in the Netherlands, he was considered an eminent scientist who ranked among the likes of such respected scientists as Sir Patrick Manson, Ronald Ross, Bernard Nocht and Alphonse Laveran (Dinger, 1950).

36   Dutch name: Koninklijk Instituut voor de Tropen (KIT).

By the time of the Spanish influenza pandemic, the Laboratory for Hygiene was sufficiently established to undertake investigations on different aspects of the problems the pandemic had presented. Investigating the disease at the Laboratory for Hygiene were medical researchers L.K. Wolff and J.J.C. van Hoogenhuyze. Following the conventional wisdom of the times, the two researchers at first attempted to find a causative agent through a bacteriological examination of patients with pneumonia. Van Hoogenhuyze, who performed the actual experiments, tested the blood, sputum and, when available, lymph nodes from the hilum of the lungs, for the presence of bacteria. From 33 of the 37 cases, he was able to detect some small, rather thick organisms, when re-inoculated and grown in sterile serum or saliva appeared to resemble the plague bacilli, although they were soon shown not to be so (Snapper and Wolff, 1919; Van Hoogenhuyze, 1919). Wolff presented the results of this study at a meeting of the Society for the Advancement of Science, Medicine and Surgery in Amsterdam in January 1919, which Van Hoogenhuyze was unable to attend for personal reasons. He also alluded to his own belief – based on a survey of the international literature of the subject – that the primary cause of influenza was probably an as yet unknown, ultrafiltrable virus, and that the bacteria they had detected were responsible for complications due to secondary infection (Wolff, 1919b). In an amusing aside – that is telling of the import of the subject at the time – minutes of the society's meetings reveal that this session had been unusually long and the discussions about influenza had lasted for several hours. In fact, they only ended at 11:15 pm, when the audience was distracted by the entry of an Alsatian dog, sniffing around trying to find its master. As it turned out it has been the head of the laboratory, Saltet, who saw the dog and let him in (Van Riemsdijk, 1928, p. 21).

Influenza was also the main topic of discussion two months later at the March meeting of the society. On this occasion the veterinarian E.C.H.A. Bemelmans presented his views about the causative agent of and therapeutic measures against, influenza. According to him the disease was similar to a contagious equine pleuropneumonia or equine influenza ('besmettelijke borstziekte van het paard') and he advocated the use of Ehrlich's Salvarsan, better known at the time for treating syphilis – to successfully treat both the human and equine influenzas (Bemelmans, 1919; Zwick, 1929). In the discussion following this presentation, Wolff disputed Bemelmans's recommendation. Later, in the face of Bemelmans's opinions that influenza was not transmitted from person to person, Wolff distanced himself even further from the field (1919a).

It must be emphasized that although the possible viral aetiology of influenza was mentioned by Wolff, it was generally accepted that, given the technical and methodological limitations at the time, such agents could not be isolated in any laboratory experiment. Furthermore, to the best of our knowledge there are no indications that Wolff, or other researchers in the Netherlands, actually conducted any experiments to isolate influenza viruses. The 1921 report on the work resulting from 1918 pandemic by the Military Medical Service (Militair Geneeskundige Dienst) inspector, General A.A.J. Quanjer, also confirmed that there were no Dutch publications on attempts to isolate a causative virus (Quanjer, 1921).

Another topic that roused the interest of various members at the Laboratory for Hygiene was the newly described phenomenon of transmissible lysis of bacteria, first by Frederick Twort in 1915 among the micrococci and then more extensively in the bacteriophages of dysentery bacilli by Felix d'Herelle in 1917. It was D'Herelle who, based on his observations of bacterial lysis of a human pathogen, had first speculated about the possible application of the bacteriophages as therapeutic agent against certain bacterial diseases. Then, the Belgian researcher Richard Bruynoghe at Leuven reported the use of staphylococcal bacteriophages in treating furuncles and carbuncles (Lavigne and Robben, 2012). This line of investigation was taken up in Amsterdam first by S.M. Kropveld, a surgeon and later by Wolff as well. Kropveld attempted to isolate and apply bacteriophages obtained from the pus from his own patients, but achieved disappointing results (Kropveld, 1923; Wolff, 1922). Together with D. Herderschêe, who was an internist, Wolff attempted to apply bacteriophage therapy in the treatment of such serious infection as typhoid fever and bacillary dysentery. In consultation with D'Herelle, who supplied the bacteriophage material, they tested the efficacy of two polyvalent typhus phages in treating patients diagnosed with typhoid fever. They reported optimistic results, but they ultimately preferred to treat patients symptomatically (Herderschêe and Wolff, 1924; Janzen and Wolff, 1923a and 1923b).

A team of microbiologists, including J.E. Dinger, W.A.J. Schüffner, E.P. Snijders and N.H. Swellengrebel at the Institute for Tropical Hygiene, carried out a series of remarkable experiments in the 1920s on the transmissibility of the yellow fever virus by mosquitoes. The location of these studies in Amsterdam rather than in the East Indies has an interesting provenance that is worth examining for it shows us the very forward thinking of researchers at the time. Van Loghem first investigated this disease during his 1908/1909 visit to Sumatra and found the prevalence of two species of mosquitoes *Aedes aegypti* and *Aedes albopictus* in the town of Deli as well as aboard the ships of the Royal Paquet Boat Service. These mosquitoes were also found to be abundant in Africa and the Americas where yellow

Figure 9   The staff members of the Laboratory for Tropical Hygiene, Amsterdam

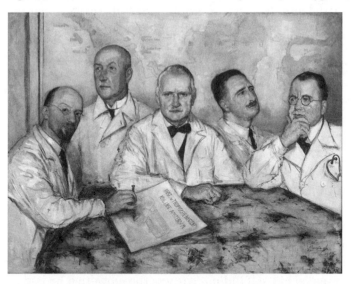

From left to right: J.J. van Loghem, W.A. Kuenen, W.A.P. Schüffner, N.H. Swellengrebel, E.P. Snijders
Painter: Lizzy Ansingh, 1933
Reproduction courtesy of Allard Pierson, University of Amsterdam

fever was prevalent and Van Loghem became convinced of their possible role in carrying yellow fever from the Americas to Asia via the Panama Canal, which was opened in 1914. The work on the canal was significantly delayed by engineering problems and a high mortality among workers due to yellow fever. Since the East Indies had an abundance of the vector but was not plagued by yellow fever, investigators decided against conducting experiments on transmission there so as to minimize the risk of spreading the disease. *Macaca cynomolgus* monkeys from the East Indies were transported to the laboratory in Amsterdam, and the virus was supplied by A. Petit at the Pasteur Institute in Paris. The macaques appeared to be susceptible to the virus – which had originated in West Africa (Dinger et al., 1929a). These results about the susceptibility of, and transmission among, different monkey species raised the spectre of an epidemic outbreak of African yellow fever in Asia, but luckily such an event never came to pass. In a second communication the researchers reported that one of them had accidentally acquired a laboratory infection which was confirmed by the experimental inoculation of a rhesus monkey with the blood of the infected researcher. Luckily, he recovered within four weeks, but the monkey died in agony (Dinger et al., 1929b and 1929c). Work on yellow fever, as well as additional viral infections, such as dengue, lymphogranuloma inguinalis, and psittacosis, continued at the institute during the 1930s. Still later, rickettsial diseases (such as scrub-typhus) also came under the scrutiny of Schüffner and Walch (Dinger, 1951).

The State Veterinary Research Institute[37]

Although strictly speaking beyond the scope of the medical virology per se, the early twentieth century research activities of the State Veterinary Research Institute (SVOI) as described by Verhoef (2005) deserve at least a brief mention. First established in 1930, the institute found accommodation in Rotterdam in 1933, but was transferred to the premises of the Marine Etablissement in Amsterdam in 1941, as originally proposed by the director, H.S. Frenkel. According to Verhoef, who published a richly documented memorial book on the history of the Netherlands Central Veterinary Institute, safety considerations might have prompted this move, as the marine grounds, being military terrain, were guarded. Unfortunately, being of Jewish origin, Frenkel himself did not witness the move that he had so wished for, because in 1940 he was dismissed from the directorship of the institute, in accordance with the laws introduced by the German occupiers. Frenkel and his family were arrested later and deported via Barneveld and Westerbork to the concentration camp Theresiënstadt in Czechoslovakia, from where they were fortunately released in February 1945 and transported to Switzerland (D. Birkenhäger-Frenkel, personal communication, 2012). His problems were somewhat mitigated after the war, for upon his return to Holland in 1945 he was immediately reinstated as the director of the institute.

Upon his return, Frenkel, who was a veterinarian and virologist, resumed his efforts to culture the foot-and-mouth disease virus in epithelial cells of bovine tongues in attempts to produce suitable vaccines against the disease. In March 1948, he was permitted by his superiors to publish the results of his simplified and less expensive methods of vaccine preparation (Verhoef, 2005). Later, in 1950, this method was taken up by the Institut Français de la Fièvre Aphtheuse, in the city of L'Arbresle near the Swiss border, for the large-scale production of the vaccine (Mérieux and Lambichs, 1988). This institute had been founded in 1947 by Charles Mérieux, a French entrepreneur, who had first met Frenkel in 1934 while travelling on business, selling tuberculin. Always on the lookout for new ideas, he re-established ties after learning of the success of Frenkel's method.

---

37   Staatsveeartsenijkundig Onderzoekingsinstituut (SVOI).

Still another noteworthy member of the staff at the State Veterinary Institute was L.W. Janssen, a very competent researcher, interested in such fundamental questions as whether or not viruses were living. Janssen was very well connected with the virus research establishment both at home in the Netherlands and internationally, and throughout his career he maintained contact with such prominent figures as Albert Jan Kluyver in Delft, Hendrik Marinus Quanjer in Wageningen, and Frederik Zernike in Groningen. With the help of a grant from the Rockefeller Foundation, Janssen had worked for several months in 1938 in the laboratory of Norman Pirie in Cambridge, where he learned the techniques for micro-analysis of the viruses. He also worked in the laboratories of the Swedish biochemists Theodoor Svedberg and Arne Tiselius in Uppsala, where he worked on the isolation of the foot-and-mouth disease virus using state-of-the-art techniques of ultracentrifugation and electrophoresis developed there. Based on these experiments he found the phosphorus-containing protein components of these viruses and also determined their nucleoprotein nature (Janssen, 1939, 1940, 1948; Verhoef, 2005, p. 109). But unfortunately, his work failed to garner the attention it deserved (Grafe, 1991). Many years later Kluyver would recall, 'some years before the war, that I was in a rather close contact with Dr Janssen, and that I was more or less fascinated by his theories' (Verhoef, 2005). He also lamented the fact that 'partly owing to the difficulties due to war-conditions, and partly because the author always continued to bring his scheme to perfection', Janssen did not publish his results and ideas in international venues. Had he been able to publish his views, Kluyver added, 'they might well have been a revelation to many biochemists and in any case, they would have acted as valuable stimulant for experimental research' (quoted in Verhoef, 2005, p. 109).

Leiden

Although Amsterdam was and remains the Dutch capital city, the country's oldest university is situated in Leiden, having been founded in 1575 by William, Prince of Orange, as the State University of Leiden (Rijksuniversiteit Leiden, later called Leiden University). Unlike the Illustrious School, the predecessor of the University in Amsterdam, Leiden University was intended, right from its inception, to provide the country and its government a population of men educated in different fields, which included medicine and the biological sciences. The main sites of activity in virus research are described.

Laboratory for Tropical Hygiene, Leiden University

The development of the study of tropical medicine in Leiden has a long history which has been described in detail by H. Beukers (1989) and Van Bergen (2009). Despite some initial difficulties with the Minister of Colonies and the Colonial Institute in Amsterdam, the university was able, at the initiative of the Leiden Society for the Advancement of the Study of Tropical Medicine and financial support from Rotterdam businessmen, to search for candidates for a professorship in tropical hygiene in 1919. But the first person to be offered the position – the above-mentioned W.A. Schüffner, who at that time was working in the East Indies and later served as the director of the Institute for Tropical Hygiene of Colonial Institute in Amsterdam from 1924 to 1937 – did not accept the invitation. Meanwhile, the society was reorganized and in 1920 renamed as the Association Institute for Tropical Medicine Rotterdam-Leiden,[38] whose activities were then divided between two locations: the laboratory in Leiden and a new hospital to be established in Rotterdam. Paul Christiaan Flu, a highly regarded tropical doctor who was intrigued by the possibility that phages might be used to kill bacterial pathogens, was appointed as the first head of this new institute in 1921.

Born and raised in Suriname, Paul Flu began his medical education by taking the classes at the local school for physicians. He finished his studies at the University of Utrecht in 1906 before going on to gain research experience through further studies at the Institut für Schiffs- und Tropenkrankheiten in Hamburg, Germany (Snijders, 1946; Van Thiel, 1946). His experiences working in laboratories in Suriname (1908-1911), the East Indies and Leiden (from 1920 onward) convinced him of the great significance of virus diseases in tropical pathology. This conviction also led to a deep interest in the bacteriophage work of Felix d'Herelle, who was invited by him and two other Leiden professors during the fall of 1921 to move to Leiden and join the new institute. In Leiden D'Herelle worked two years on the 'nature 'of bacteriophages (Summers, 1999, p. 118). One area of bacteriophage research that Flu and others at Leiden pursued long after D'Herelle's departure in 1924 was the investigation of its use in vaccines. Later Flu and colleagues demonstrated that it was possible to immunize rats against plague by injecting them with concentrated suspensions of virulent plague bacteria treated with solutions of bacteriophage antagonistic to these species, but equivalent experiments involving human subjects were never tested (Flu, 1929; Anon., 1948).

38   Vereniging Instituut voor Tropische Geneeskunde Rotterdam-Leiden (VIT). See Anon., 1948.

Figure 10   P.C. Flu (1884-1945)

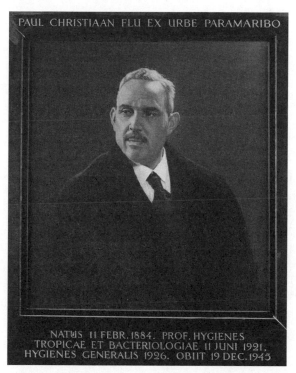

Professor of Tropical Hygiene and Director of the Institute of Tropical Medicine Leiden
Portrait by Jan Rotgans
Courtesy of Leiden University
Bijzondere Collecties Universiteit Leiden, Icones 392

Albert Einstein, who gave an inaugural address in Leiden as special
visiting professor on 27 October 1920, was another famous person with
whom Flu had discussions. Einstein visited Leiden again in November 1921,
May 1922, October 1924, February 1925, and April 1930, although his visiting
professorship was officially terminated on 23 September 1951 (Pais, 1982,
p. 526). Specifically, Flu sought Einstein's help to estimate the diameter of
the pores of bacteriological filters made of earthenware. The procedure
involved using an air pressure test while the filters were immersed in aether
and Einstein helped Flu calculate pore sizes by deriving the equation that
described the relationship between such variables as membrane pore size
(radius) and air pressure when air bubbles begin to appear in the aether
(Einstein and Mühsam, 1923; Flu, 1928; Pais, 1982, p. 489). There is no information as to whether Einstein informed Flu that he had published papers on
this subject together with his Berlin friend Hans Mühsam.

Figure 11   Institute for Tropical Medicine and Laboratory for Tropical Hygiene and Parasitology, Leiden

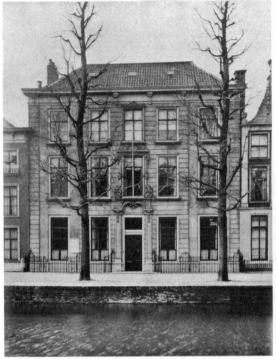

Reproduction courtesy of P.K. Flu and Leiden University

Laboratory for Bacteriology, Leiden University

Although virology departments have traditionally sprung from parent laboratories of bacteriology and microbiology, the bacteriology laboratory at Leiden (established in 1885) did not really publish any work of note on the subject of viruses during the period covered in this chapter. R.P. van Calcar held the position of chair from 1905 until 1935, when financial considerations forced the university to terminate the chair. Following this unfortunate turn of events, individuals in laboratories performing related work, e.g. Paul C. Flu, were requested or otherwise imposed upon to take on teaching duties. One of Calcar's interesting tasks during his chairmanship was to provide in 1910 and 1911 financial support to the then budding artist Piet Mondrian with a commission to make drawings of microscopic observations of preparations on glass slides containing stained bacterial specimens (Entrop, 2003).

Laboratory for Bacteriology and Experimental Pathology of the Netherlands Institute for Preventive Medicine[39]

In 1929, E. Gorter, professor of paediatrics, and J. van der Hoeve, professor of ophthalmology, at Leiden, decided to follow the example of the newly established school of hygiene and public health at the famous Johns Hopkins University in Baltimore, MD, USA. They established the Netherlands Institute for Preventive Medicine, within which was housed the Laboratory for Bacteriology and Experimental Pathology. The paediatrician Gorter was a man with varied talents, who was co-author of a clinical laboratory diagnostics (Gorter and De Graaff, 1915 and next editions). J.P. Bijl of the Central Laboratory of RIV in Utrecht was appointed as the first director in 1933 (Bijl, 1954). Although the original intent was a focus on tuberculosis, post-vaccination encephalitis and smallpox research circumstances deemed otherwise and the earliest work to emerge from the laboratory was on influenza. The person primarily responsible for this output was the German scientist G. Elkeles, who had worked on psittacosis in Berlin but left his country due to problems with national socialism and took up a temporary position at the Institute for Preventive Medicine in Leiden in 1933. Almost immediately he commenced studies on the influenza virus, then very recently isolated by a team of English researchers, W. Smith, C.H. Andrewes, and P.P. Laidlaw, and shown to be amenable to propagation in ferrets (Smith et al., 1933). This crucial breakthrough provided influenza virus researchers with a long-sought animal model. Elkeles was not only able to duplicate results but also successfully demonstrated the transmission of the human influenza virus from humans to ferrets to pigs (Elkeles, 1934; 1971; Rigter, 1996; Tyrrell, 1998). His work was recognized and cited internationally, most notably by the American virus researcher Richard Shope, who would go on to make valuable contributions to understanding the epidemiology of influenza (Shope, 1931 and 1951; Shope and Francis, 1936). In 1934, Elkeles moved away from Leiden to South America, but not before he had secured a place for Leiden in the international influenza research scene.

In 1941 the veterinary virologist J.D. Verlinde was appointed head of the laboratory and following his interests and expertise, the focus shifted to the epidemiology and pathogenesis of various viral infections, including poliomyelitis, arboviruses, rabies, influenza viruses and poxviruses

---

39 Afdeling Bacteriologie en Experimentele Pathologie van het Nederlands Instituut voor Praeventieve Geneeskunde (NIPG).

Figure 12   Entrance of Institute for Preventive Medicine, Leiden

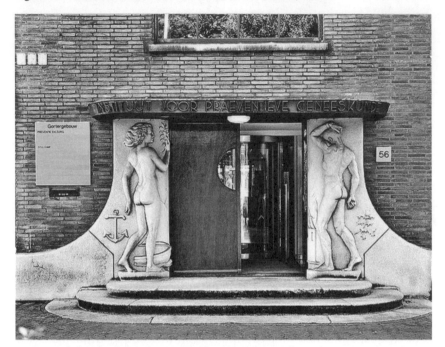

Reproduction courtesy of Rijnlands Architectuur Platform

(Versteeg, 1987). In 1947 he was appointed extraordinary professor of medical microbiology and ordinary professor in 1960; as a consequence, he was also responsible for the medical microbiology department of the academic hospital.

Clinic of Internal Medicine of the Academic Hospital

At the same time of Verlinde's leadership at the NIPG-laboratory, the Academic Hospital also became home in 1946 to J. Mulder, an internist from Groningen, who in the 1930s had begun a program of influenza research there (Van Furth, 2009; Mulder, 1937, 1940, 1941). Mulder was appointed in Leiden as a professor of medicine, where he continued his research on understanding infections of the upper respiratory tract, originally conducted in Groningen in collaboration with the biologist L. Bijlmer, who unfortunately died very young in 1947 due to complications following lung surgery (Bijlmer, 1943; H. Bijlmer, personal communication, 2018; Haex, 1965; Mulder, 1937; Mulder et al., 1940).

Utrecht

Laboratory for Hygiene, State University of Utrecht

The State University in Utrecht was established in 1636, with seven professors
working in four faculties: philosophy, which offered all students an introduc-
tory education, and three higher-level faculties: theology, medicine and law.
As in the other state universities, the laboratory for hygiene was established
in the late nineteenth century in response to the stipulations of the Higher
Education Bill of 1876. The illustrious Dutch researcher Christiaan Eykman,
trained in hygiene and forensic medicine but best known for his work on the
tropical disease of beriberi, was a member of the medical faculty at Utrecht
from 1898 onwards until his death in 1931 (Palm, 1999, pp. 447-449). He held
the position of professor of hygiene and medical police until 1929, when he
was succeeded by Ludwig Karl Wolff, a Swiss-born and Amsterdam-trained
ophthalmologist and bacteriologist who had varied interests in pathology,
epidemiology and pharmacy (Van Loghem, 1938). A clinical lecture delivered
by Wolff in 1932 provides evidence of his interest in the nature of viruses
and bacteriophages. It was in his laboratory that H.S. Frenkel and H.W.
Julius took the first steps towards successfully culturing cells isolated from
various tissues. They were also successful in cultivating vaccinia virus in
cultures of cells from the abdominal cavity from rabbits using the instrument
of De Haan that had been modified by themselves (Wolff, 1932). Another
well-known member of the faculty was Hendrik Aldershoff, he was appointed
in 1924 as an extraordinary professor of serology. He had graduated from
Groningen in 1906 having written a thesis on 'Vaccinelichaampjes' (vaccine
bodies). Although he was a member of the League of Nations Committee on
Smallpox and post-vaccination encephalitis, his interest in virus diseases
did not result in extensive virus research in Utrecht (Aldershoff, 1929; De
Lange, 1906; Josephus Jitta, 1937). Indeed, it would appear as though following
the sudden death of Wolff in 1938, virological research at the university in
Utrecht had to wait until after World War II to flourish again.

National Laboratory of the National Institute of Public Health in Utrecht[40]

Smallpox vaccine and rabies vaccine were produced in the Dutch East Indies
during the first half of the nineteenth century at the central laboratories in

---

40   Centraal Laboratorium van het Rijks Instituut voor de Volksgezondheid.

Figure 13   R. Gispen (1910-2000) and Jacoba G. Kapsenberg

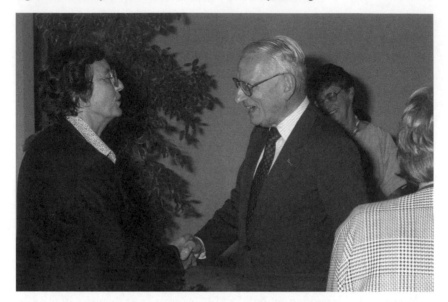

R. Gispen and Jacoba G. Kapsenberg at the farewell reception for Jacoba Kapsenberg in 1989
Reproduction courtesy of RIVM

Java (see Chapter 7). This was not the case at the National Institute of Public Health in the homeland. In 1932, it was advised by the above-mentioned J.P. Bijl to centralize at the Central Laboratory of RIV the Parcs Vaccinogènes, which were located in Amsterdam, The Hague, and Groningen. The decision to centralize was taken in 1938; however, the realization was carried out only in the 1950s when the new accommodations in Bilthoven had been built (Van Zon, 1990, pp. 277-280).

Another virus vaccine, the diluted and glycerine pre-treated rabies vaccine according to the method of Högyes, was available after World War II from Philips Duphar in Weesp as the Hoegyes-Philips vaccine; this was controlled at the Central Laboratory in Utrecht (Gispen et al., 1965). The leading position of RIV in the field of medical virology should come after 1951 with the arrival of R. Gispen and J.G. Kapsenberg and the opening of the Laboratory for Viral and Rickettsial Diseases. The start was in the old building in Utrecht, where a room in a stables was converted for virological research. A year later, more rooms were made available and it was not until 1958 that the laboratory moved to the new buildings in Bilthoven, where one could work according to modern scientific requirements (Van Zon, 1990, p. 251).

Groningen

Laboratory for Hygiene, State University of Groningen

The University in Groningen was founded in 1614. Despite nearly being closed in the 1870s, today it belongs to one of the five largest universities in the Netherlands and has four major faculties. According to the author of *Honderd jaar medische microbiologie in Groningen* (One hundred years of medical microbiology in Groningen), virology did not exist in the university until the arrival of J.B. Wilterdink in 1970 (Westendorp Boerma, 1977) – but we do not know whether the author deliberately overlooked the remarks of A.P. Fokker on the discovery of Beijerinck in 1898 or did not have any knowledge of Aldershoff's 1906 thesis. Although Fokker, the first professor of hygiene and medical police in Groningen (1877-1906), was one of the early scientists to have recognized the significance Beijerinck's hypothesis about viruses, it was a dubious honour for Beijerinck. A prolific albeit sometimes controversial writer, Fokker contributed many reports on various new bacteriological findings to the NTvG throughout his tenure at the university. According to De Knecht-van Eekelen (1984), Fokker supported the doctrine of bacterial heterogenesis, the formation of bacteria from dead organic material. He opposed the 'dogmatic' belief of the 'orthodox' bacteriologists in bacteria as specific elements in disease. Therefore, he mistrusted the value of the treatment of diphtheria with specific antitoxic serum, as was introduced by Behring and by Roux (1894). But at the same time, he was reproachful of bacteriologists. Fokker claimed that bacteriologists had no eye for new achievements such as the discovery of a viral disease, the tobacco mosaic virus disease, by Martinus Willem Beijerinck (1899).

Fokker's successor was A. Klein, who held the chair from 1907 until 1930. Under his directorship there was not much diagnostic microbiology carried out at the university, since he was more committed to research and teaching. A fervent liberal, Klein was politically active and elected to the city council of Groningen in 1923, where he asked critical questions on the bacteriological quality of drinking water. His claims were investigated by G. Kapsenberg, a talented scientist who had successively trained as surgeon, microbiologist, and pathologist. He was the first head of the Laboratory of the Municipal Health Service, established in 1919 (Van Loghem, 1943). Kapsenberg's results contradicted Klein's claims, which had the unfortunate result of angering him so much that he withdrew his council membership, and furthermore, refused any contact with Kapsenberg and the Laboratory of the Municipal Health Service, which provided clinical bacteriology services for the academic hospital. Fate or history, however, had the last laugh for in 1935 after Klein's retirement, Kapsenberg was appointed as his successor. After his nomination Kapsenberg remained head of the laboratory of Municipal Health Service where routine microbiological diagnostics for the academic hospital continued. Although the responsibility for this laboratory was transferred by the municipality to the state university, the location of the laboratories outside the Academic Hospital did not change. In 1943 his immunological and bacteriological work came to a sudden end by his untimely death (Van Loghem, 1943). From the 1950s onward, his daughter, Jacoba G. (Cootje) Kapsenberg played an important role in public health virology and diagnostic virology.

After Kapsenberg's death, his position was taken up in 1946 by A.B.F.A. Pondman, who had been involved in the production of rabies and smallpox vaccine in the Dutch East Indies (Westendorp Boerma, 1960). In 1923 he defended in Leiden his thesis on bacteriophagy which was prepared under the guidance of F. d'Herelle. Before Pondman moved to Groningen, he worked at the National Institute of Public Health (RIV), where he was deputy head of the institute and head of the laboratory for epidemic typhus vaccine production. In 1942, both he and his assistant acquired a *Rickettsia prowazeki* laboratory infection through their experimental work, but both fortunately recovered (Van Zon, 1990, p. 164; Westendorp Boerma, 1960). The bacteriologist who succeeded Pondman as head of the Serologic-Vaccinology Department in 1946 also acquired the same laboratory infection; however, a worse fate struck him – he died of it. In Groningen Pondman's research interests were transferred to serology and immunology and as a consequence research interest in virology was waned at the Laboratory of Medical Microbiology in Groningen.

Also of note among various achievements at Groningen is that J. de Haan of the Laboratory for Physiology, who developed an instrument to culture tissues outside the body using a continuous circulation method (De Haan, 1924). A modification of this instrument was used by Julius and Frenkel in Utrecht as mentioned above.

International developments in techniques

In this chapter we did not discuss systematically the advances in fundamental and applied virus research during the 1930s as the aim of the book is to focus on the development of medical virology in the Netherlands. Nevertheless, the activities of the above-mentioned Janssen (1939), who was a colloid chemist at the State Veterinary Research Institute (Staatsveterinair Onderzoekingsinstituut, SVOI) indicate that the technical advances abroad were followed closely. Therefore, this chapter will be finished with a short summarizing of these technical steps forward. Milestones in the development of virology over the first half of the twentieth century were the colloid membranes as means to determine size and form of virus thanks to colloid chemistry (W.J. Elford, 1931), electron microscopy (E. Ruska,[41] B. von Borries, and H. Ruska, 1932), new methods for physicochemical analysis, such as the ultracentrifuge (T. Svedberg,[42] 1926), electrophoresis (A.W.K. Tiselius,[43] 1930).

The interest in the newest developments in virology is also reflected in the lectures delivered at a symposium organized in Wageningen by the Netherlands Society for Biochemistry in 1939, where among others Janssen was one of the keynote speakers. It must be noted that none of the speakers at the symposium were medical doctors. At the same symposium attention was also paid to the new methods to cultivate viruses. Propagation of human and animal viruses was for a long time dependent of growth in a susceptible animal. Alternative methods as cultivation in tissue cultures were also used to study viruses. P. Rous and J.B. Murphy, for example, used chick embryos in their 1911 study of the Rous sarcoma, the method of cultivation of a virus in fertile eggs (Woodruff and Goodpasture, 1931). Different ways of inoculation can be used: the amniotic route for isolation of clinical specimens, the chorio-allantoic membrane where growth of virus can be observed by production of plaques or pocks (vaccinia, variola, and herpes viruses), the allantoic route for production of large quantities of virus, or the yolk sac route for the isolation of rickettsiae. The discoveries of W. Smith, C.H. Andrewes, and P.P. Laidlaw in 1933 that ferrets and mice were animals in which influenza viruses could be isolated were cases of serendipity (Tyrrell, 1998).

In spite of all these advances, medical virology had to wait until after World War II for the development of easy-to-handle cell culture systems, which heralded a new era in virology. The next chapter depicts the steps forward in the second half of the twentieth century and the accompanying organization of virologists in the Netherlands.

41   Nobel Prize, 1986.
42   Nobel Prize, 1926.
43   Nobel Prize, 1948.

4 From cell culture to the molecular revolution

The rise of medical virology and its organization

> The electronics, radioactive isotopes, and complicated biochemistry of our age
> have threatened to turn medical science into something dangerously resembling
> technology. Now and again we need to be reminded of its fundamental biological
> elements. Against this background we express our admiration of the biological
> common sense, characterizing your approach to important medical problems,
> and of the wonderful simplicity of the solutions you have presented.
> – *Sven Gard* (1954)[44]

The history of science and medicine, especially in virology, has often privi-
leged achievements in research laboratories over all other venues of scientific
enterprise. This narrative slant is not entirely surprising because it is in
these environments that the most dramatic and groundbreaking discoveries
have taken place. It was argued among others by F.M. Burnet that around
the midpoint of the twentieth century virology became an autonomous
discipline based on its concepts, techniques and specific institutes that
were created (1953a and 1953b). Later, historical research underpinned and
reaffirmed this claim of growth to independence for virology (Méthot, 2016;
Van Helvoort, 1993a, 1993b, 1994, 1996). The most useful breakthroughs in
the field of virology that followed the initial spate of discoveries in the 1930s
occurred at university research institutes and laboratories of public health.
As Marguerite Pereira, director of the PHLS Virus Reference Laboratory in
the 1970s and 1980s wrote, 'the history of virological discovery is therefore
largely about technical innovation' (1986). Medical virology in the clinic
hardly benefited from these technical advances until the end of World
War II when easy-to-handle cell culture systems heralded a new era in
virology. The present chapter depicts the steps forward in the second half
of the twentieth century, and the accompanying organization of virologist
networks across the Netherlands.

---

44 Presentation speech at the Nobel Prize Award in Medicine, 1954. The recipients of the prize
were John F. Enders, Thomas H. Weller and Frederick C. Robbins 'for their discovery of the ability
of poliomyelitis viruses to grow in cultures of various types of tissue' (Gard, 1954).

It is not until the last quarter of the century that breakthroughs emerged in larger microbiology laboratories at general hospitals. There, practitioners of the nascent field of medical virology applied the newly discovered techniques and developed networks connecting microbiologists, immunologists and public health workers, so essential to their work (Bradstreet et al., 1964).

Although virology had its origins in bacteriology, diagnostic virology for the most part was not integrated in clinical bacteriology laboratories; the only exceptions arose due to the personal interest of certain heads of these laboratories. An obvious reason for this particular divide is that the activity of a virus-oriented laboratory was not of immediate value to the individual patient (Hawkes, 1979). Another explanation is the lack of technical equipment for and expertise in virology at the average bacteriology laboratory. This problem was solved in the United Kingdom by introducing members of the central PHLS Virus Reference Laboratory into the country's largest bacteriological laboratories in order to set up centres for virology, the so-called regional virus laboratories (Bradstreet et al., 1964).

This policy was not implemented in the Netherlands. Furthermore, because viral infections were not easily treatable until much later in the twentieth century, the initial focus of medical virology was on prophylaxis largely taken care of at public health institutes. For example, during the smallpox epidemic in Tilburg in 1951, only specimens of patients whose clinical diagnosis was not certain were submitted for laboratory diagnosis to the Institute for Preventive Medicine in Leiden, the Virus Laboratory of the National Institute of Public Health in Utrecht and the Laboratory for Hygiene in Amsterdam (Sas, 1954). In addition to common viral diseases of temperate regions, such as influenza, measles, rubella and mumps, a number of viral diseases – smallpox, yellow fever and dengue – were more prevalent in the tropics. Consequently, diagnostics and protective measures against these diseases, especially in the Dutch context, were assigned to the laboratories for tropical hygiene, which underwent significant administrative changes due to the political processes of decolonization after 1945 (see Chapter 7).

The progress of medical virology in the period covered in this chapter may be roughly characterized by three general waves: first, the successful culture of viruses in cell monolayers as described by John F. Enders, Thomas H. Weller and Frederick C. Robbins in 1949; second, the development of new immunology-based techniques, such as immunofluorescence, radioimmune assays and enzyme immune assays as well as negative staining methods in electron microscopy, during the 1960s; and third, an era dominated by biochemistry and molecular biology, especially after the discovery of the polymerase chain

Figure 14   John F. Enders (1897-1985)

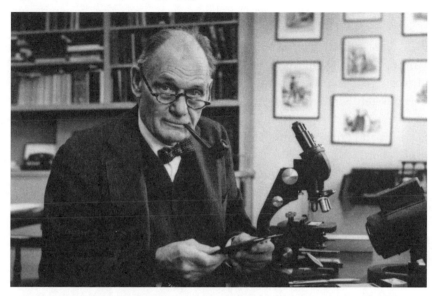

Reproduction courtesy of Harvard Medical School/G.Th. Diamandopulos

reaction by Kary Mullis (1944-2019)[45] in 1983/1985. It should be emphasized that these different techniques did not necessarily compete with one another, of course, and that the advances in any one arena did not immediately replace existing methods. Rather, the developments acted synergistically to expand the investigative scope of the field of virology. It is beyond dispute that advances in fundamental molecular biology – e.g., insights into the structure of nucleic acids, the revelation of the genetic code – and the improved understanding of immunological processes were of tremendous importance for medical virology, but these subjects lie outside the scope of this book.

The first wave: Virus culture

Perhaps the single most significant hurdle in the advance of medical virology in the early part of the twentieth century was the inability to grow viruses in artificial media. Based on their experience from bacteriological research since the 1870s, microbiologists had been well aware of the vital importance of isolating and growing organisms in the laboratory for the advancement of their science. Indeed, in his 1954 presentation speech awarding the Nobel

45   Nobel Prize, 1993.

Prize in Physiology and Medicine to the trio of virologists, John F. Enders, Thomas H. Weller and Frederick C. Robbins, Sven Gard began by comparing the 75-year-old fight against bacterial diseases with the nascent fight against viral diseases with a glowing account of the numerous gains of *bacterial* cultures, pointing out that it was 'not difficult to find the reason why the virologists have failed where the bacteriologists were so successful. They have been severely handicapped by the difficulties connected with the cultivation of viruses' (Gard, 1954). Undoubtedly, the most pivotal breakthrough for isolating and growing animal viruses was the discovery of Enders, Weller, and Robbins, who developed techniques to grow monolayers of cells in continuous and semi-continuous cell lines in which they cultivated the Lansing strain of poliomyelitis virus (Enders et al., 1949).

As with many breakthroughs, serendipity and coincidence played a higher role than any concerted or systematic endeavour, in directing the three men towards their great success. As they recounted their venture upon receiving the Nobel Prize, it was in the course of working with culturing other viruses – mumps and varicella – and having a ready supply of a strain of poliomyelitis virus in storage that 'it suddenly occurred to us that everything had been prepared almost without conscious effort on our part for a new attempt to cultivate the agent' (Enders et al., 1954). Of note, only Robbins, who worked on rickettsia infections, had received training in the field of paediatrics – and hence had some familiarity with polio. Weller, who had been his roommate in medical school, had first specialized in helminthology, and later engaged in the field of virology as a research assistant to Enders, who, although the principal investigator, had originally begun his academic work studying literature (Weller and Robbins, 1991).

At the root of the difficulties that viruses posed for cultivation lay the property that set them apart from all other living creatures – their obligate parasitism in living hosts. Beijerinck had identified this property in his very first report on the tobacco mosaic disease, claiming that 'propagation results only when the virus is connected with the living and growing protoplasm of the host plant' (1942/1898, p. 39). But he could not offer insights into how said connections came about, and the theoretical implications of his observations were not considered for many decades. Meanwhile, however, whether or not they acknowledged or even recognized obligate parasitism, virologists had to accommodate this property in order to make any headway in their studies of viral infections. For many years, the only way scientists had to maintain the unknown and, until the 1930s, invisible agents of the infections of interest had been by repeated passages in susceptible host organisms. Especially in the case of human and animal viruses, this need for live hosts would prove a severe hurdle as animal facilities were expensive to maintain; as P.P. Laidlaw, the famous influenza virus pioneer, wrote with British humour: 'Man is an exceedingly bad experimental animal' (1935). The host specificity of many viruses – for many years the only way to propagate poliomyelitis viruses was in monkeys (see Enders et al., 1954) – meant that an animal facility was needed to keep different species for different studies, which increased costs further.

Although tissue culture had been attempted in non-virology context since the early part of the twentieth century, and the use of the enzyme trypsin to disperse cells from solid tissue had been described in 1916 by F.P. Rous and F.S. Jones, there was a long interval until the first successful inoculations of cell monolayers with viral specimens (Mortimer, 2009). The first successful attempts to culture viruses of multicellular eukaryotic organisms in an assayable manner emerged in the late 1920s and early 1930s. In particular, the discovery that fertilized chicken eggs were a suitable medium for growing animal viruses represents an important stepping stone in the progress of medical virology (Woodruff and Goodpasture, 1931; Burnet, 1936). However, there remained many hurdles to virus cultivation in cell or tissue cultures. Microbial contamination of cultured cells challenged their inoculation with viruses. However, the discovery and use of antibiotics later enabled the maintenance of bacteria-free cultures. In parallel, the belief that tissues that would allow the propagation of viruses had to originate not only from animal species that were susceptible to the disease, but also from the organs targeted by the infection slowed down progress. Such an organotropic presumption was eventually invalidated by Enders, Weller and Robbins as they propagated poliovirus in various human embryonic tissues. From then on, far-reaching applications of the technique were realized at a fast pace. Within ten years of the seminal report, most of the cultivable animal viruses had been isolated in cell monolayers (Huebner, 1957, 1959). In 1948, a mere 20 human viruses had been recognized, of which only nine were established in the laboratory. In 1958, 70 additional human viruses had been established and studied in the laboratory. The culture of virus in cell monolayers also led to the production of a polio vaccine and the large-scale preparation of viral antigens for serological tests, which revolutionized the field of medical virology (see also Enders et al., 1954; Mortimer, 2009).

First wave developments in Dutch clinical virology

A 1953 publication by F. Dekking on the aetiology and laboratory diagnosis of viral diseases offers an overview of the viral diagnostic services offered in the Netherlands around 1950. At the time, Dekking was a virologist-to-be and researcher at the Laboratory for Hygiene in Amsterdam. He was later appointed to a chair in virology at the University of Amsterdam in 1968. In his inaugural lecture he called himself the second professor of virology in the Netherlands and R. Gispen the first as he was appointed in Utrecht in 1960. In comparison Michael Stoker became the first professor of virology at the University of Glasgow in 1958 – which was the first chair of virology to be established at a British university (Thomson, 1957; University of Glasgow, n.d.). Although ten laboratories offered viral diagnostics services in the Netherlands around 1953, Dekking noted that the Dutch were well behind in comparison to the UK and various Scandinavian countries. In particular, the lag in the implementation of cell culture techniques in the Netherlands was remarkable, even though a working group comprising of the NKI-AVL, SVOI and laboratories of histology, hygiene and anatomy at the University of Amsterdam had been set up as early as 1949 for the purpose of developing these technologies (De Bruyn, 1949). Even by 1953, according to Dekking's report, most Dutch laboratories were not equipped with adequate facilities for cell culture and had to rely on monkey inoculations for the isolation and culture of polioviruses. Nevertheless, Dekking expressed his optimism and high expectations over the reorganization of RIV, which entailed the establishment of a new virology laboratory, as well as financial assistance from the Dutch Health Organisation (TNO-NGO)[46] for virus research.

The need for effective liaison and consultation channels between laboratories performing diagnostic tests and the clinicians who were submitting specimens for diagnosis was addressed by Dekking. While he acknowledged that specimens for certain routine diagnoses, e.g. of well-known or common diseases such as smallpox and psittacosis,[47] could be submitted without prior consultation, he instituted a practice of mandatory advance consultation for all other diagnostic requests. Moreover, regardless of the disease, he insisted upon obtaining a résumé of clinical and epidemiological information about the specimens. He divided the diagnostic requests into two main categories: 1) those for the more routine diseases, such as variola, rabies as well as psittacosis and venereal lymphogranuloma, which were categorized as viral diseases at the time; and 2) those requiring more elaborate and specialized examinations. The latter included only about eleven viral diseases to begin with: vaccinia

46 Nederlandse Gezondheids Organisatie TNO (short) or Nederlandse Organisatie voor Toegepast-natuurwetenschappelijk Onderzoek ten behoeve van de Volksgezondheid (in full).
47 Diagnostic procedures for rickettsial and chlamydial infections were performed in viral laboratories because these organisms grow well in eggs and cell culture systems.

Figure 15   F. Dekking (1913-2004)

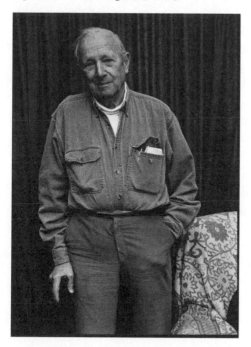

Photo: Henk Thomas, 1996
Reproduction courtesy of Allard Pierson, University of Amsterdam (154.515)

and cowpox, influenza, mumps, Newcastle disease (caused by an avian paramyxovirus),[48] herpes, poliomyelitis, infection with Coxsackieviruses and neurotropic viruses, rickettsioses and Q fever, benign lymphoreticulosis (cat scratch disease), and yellow fever. Diagnostic tests for many viral diseases, such as measles, rubella, varicella, common cold, infectious hepatitis, and serum hepatitis, were not available in the Netherlands at the time of Dekking's report. He also dissuaded laboratories from the overenthusiastic collection of specimens for laboratory diagnosis, only to obtain negative results after many months of labour, and addressed the need for adequate information and collection of two serum specimens with an interval of two weeks to demonstrate a rise of antibody titres in the convalescence sample.

In many respects, viral diagnostics in the Netherlands followed the trends set in the UK a few years earlier. For instance, the isolation of poliovirus using cell cultures had been carried out at the Virus Reference Laboratory of the Public Health Laboratory in London in 1952 and at only a few

---

48   Was considered to cause occasionally human conjunctivitis or meningitis.

laboratories of the Public Health Laboratory Service (PHLS) equipped to carry out such work by 1955 (Williams, 1985, p. 69). In the Netherlands, as indicated in a note in the Annual Report of the Regional Public Health Laboratory in Amsterdam, Dekking had introduced cell culture techniques at the Laboratory for Hygiene in 1955, although not for routine diagnostic purposes. Verlinde introduced cell culture at the laboratory of the Institute for Preventive Medicine in Leiden in 1954 after two years of pioneering (Verlinde and Kret, 1954). B. Hofman had been sent to the USA to gain experience (Versteeg, 1992). In Tilburg, Van der Veen initiated cell culture at the Regional Public Health Laboratory in 1955. The new technique had proved much useful during the polio epidemic the following year (Peeters, 2001). The cell culture media had to be prepared from scratch by suitably trained laboratory personnel, since only some defined components such as Eagle's or Earle's medium were commercially available. Importantly, the use of cells from a wide variety of human and animal organs allowed the discovery of a large variety of hitherto unknown viruses.

The second wave: Immunological and visualization techniques for rapid detection

After virus culture techniques, the developments that had significant impact on viral diagnostics occurred in the discipline of immunology and as technical improvements in visualization techniques. The increased understanding of the nature and specificity of immune reactions – for instance, involving different types of immunoglobulins such as IgG and IgM – enabled scientists to produce and use a range of specific antibodies for various diagnostic purposes. The principle of the fluorescent antibody technique that was introduced in the 1960s was a combination of an antigen-antibody reaction, in which the antibody is bound to its homologous antigen, and of the labelling of the antibody with a fluorescent dye which can be made visible by excitation with an appropriate light wavelength (Gardner and McQuillin, 1980). The application of immunofluorescence for rapid virus diagnosis was meticulously described by Philip Gardner and Joyce McQuillin from Newcastle upon Tyne, UK. Using this technique, the presence of virus could be demonstrated in clinical specimens, for instance, upon respiratory infections. By the use of fixed or unfixed virus-infected cells, specific antibodies could also be detected in serum specimens.

In 1975, Köhler and Millstein were able to create immortal cell lines called hybridomas that could rapidly produce specific single (or monoclonal) antibodies (Köhler and Milstein, 1975). The production of monoclonal antibodies in vitro was a giant step in diagnostics, due to the much-defined specificity of such antibodies for an antigen – in this case, a specific viral component. Monoclonal antibodies could be used in serological assays, for rapid virus detection in cell culture, or for viral antigen detection in clinical specimens.

The 1970s and 1980s were dedicated to the development of the enzyme immunosorbent assay (EIA), also called enzyme-linked immunosorbent assay (ELISA) (see Chapter 6 for the specific role of Dutch contributions in the development of ELISA techniques). The technique built on principles used by radioimmunoassay was developed in the 1960s; here, the reaction between a radiolabelled antigen and a specific antibody was measured by following the competition between radiolabelled and unlabelled antigens. This measurement involved a separation step between bound and free-labelled antigens. Elaborating on this concept, it was found that separation could be increased by immobilizing the antibody or antigen on a solid phase, such as plastic. The use of enzymes instead of radio-isotopes was later exploited as a marker (Kemeny and Challacombe, 1988). A variety of enzymes has been used, such as horseradish peroxidase or alkaline phosphatase. All these techniques dramatically reduced the time needed for individual diagnosis and allowed the instalment of screening programmes.

Electron microscopy became more frequently applied to clinical virol-ogy, when S. Brenner and R.W. Horne described in 1959 the application of the negative staining method as a simple technique for the study of virus particles in suspension. At the same time, methods for embedding tissues for thin sectioning improved. The combination of both techniques revealed excellent information on viral structure (Field, 1986). Uncultivable viruses, such as the noroviruses, Norwalk viruses, and astroviruses, could be detected by this technique. The technique proved also useful in the rapid distinction between smallpox and chickenpox. Possibly due to the barriers posed by the expensive costs of obtaining and maintaining the instruments, however, these methods were not widely used in the routine and rapid isolation of viruses. As a result, S.S. Biel and H.R. Gelderblom, both recognized experts at the Robert Koch Institute in Berlin, had to heave the following sighs: Starting in the 1990s and coincident with the broad introduction of 'modern' diagnostic techniques, the number of electron microscope (EM) diagnostic labs has decreased considerably – in spite of the obvious advantages of this technique (Biel and Gelderblom, 1999). Another passionate plea for electron microscopy in clinical virology was made by S. Biel and D. Madeley during the European Virology Meeting in Glasgow in 2000. Nevertheless, the application of this technique likely will play a greater role in virus research than in routine viral diagnosis (Biel and Madeley, 2001).

Second wave developments in Dutch clinical virology

Perhaps our best source of information about the state of the art in Dutch viral diagnostics during the second wave is a 1975 article by Jacoba G. Kapsenberg published in the NTvG. An internationally recognized expert on enteroviruses who was responsible for viral diagnostics at the National Laboratory of Public Health (1954-1989), she was also later the author of a chapter on enteroviruses in a definitive handbook on infectious disease diagnostics (Lennette et al., 1988). In her 1975 article, Kapsenberg described new immunological and microscopic techniques, with specific details on their application to viral diagnostics. Published some two decades after Dekking's report, Kapsenberg's paper needed much less time and space to enumerate the viruses that could not be propagated in cell culture and therefore, could only be visualized by electron microscopy. The list included molluscum contagiosum, hepatitis A, hepatitis B, epidemic gastroenteritis, and human oncornaviruses. The human parvovirus B19, described in 1975 by Y.E. Cossart as the causal agent of the fifth disease (occurring mostly in children), was not yet included in the list. However, their diagnosis continued to be challenging, because only a handful of laboratories in the Netherlands had their own electron microscopes; multiple laboratories, both within universities and at RIVM, had to share one instrument.

While the serological detection of specific antibodies was performed by immunofluorescence or enzyme immunosorbent assays, older methods, such as complement fixation assay, immunoprecipitation, and hemagglutination inhibition assays, maintained their value during the second wave. In parallel, the propagation of viruses in animals and tissue culture was replaced for the most part by monolayer cell culture using trypsin to disperse cells from tissues and standardized nutrient media with addition of antibiotics. Other technical advances included the improvement of cooling techniques, of the homogenization of tissues, of microscopes, ultracentrifuges, ultrafiltration, and mechanization and the use of micro-instruments for serology. The availability of these new techniques enabled larger hospital-based bacteriological laboratories to perform virological serology testing and direct detection of virus antigen in clinical specimens, for example, the detection of respiratory syncytial virus in nasopharyngeal fluid.

In the intermediate period between the second and third wave, modifications of cell culture techniques were developed that yielded more rapid results. Soon after the publications of Griffiths et al. in the UK on rapid cell culture techniques consisting of a centrifugation step to enhance the contact of the specimen onto the cell monolayer and an early detection of presence of virus amplification by immunofluorescence. These methods were introduced at Groningen, Rotterdam, and at a number of other virology laboratories across the Netherlands (Griffiths et al., 1984; Rothbarth et al., 1987 and 1988; Schirm et al., 1987; Schirm et al., 1992). They became methods of choice for the diagnosis of cytomegalovirus (CMV) and respiratory virus infections because of their high sensitivity, specificity and result-yielding rapidity (Stirk and Griffiths, 1988). The diagnosis of CMV infection in transplant patients could be made much earlier and altered the clinical management of CMV infection in these immunocompromised patients (Griffiths et al., 1984). These methods later became less important when many laboratories downgraded virus isolation methods in favour of molecular techniques around the turn of the twentieth century (Jeffery and Aarons, 2009; Niesters, 2002).

The third wave: The molecular revolution

Without a doubt, the single most dramatic and influential technical advance in molecular biology that occurred in the early 1980s was the development of the polymerase chain reaction (PCR) by the biochemist Kary Mullis (1993). These advances built on the long history of the molecular chemistry of the gene (Booss and August, 2013, p. 294). In the 1970s, hybridization techniques proved to be useful to study viruses that could not be grown in tissue culture (Clewley, 1986). Other methods that were applied in virus research were among others recombinant DNA technology, oligonucleotide fingerprinting of RNA viruses, restriction mapping of double-stranded DNA, electrophoretic migration patterns, Southern, Northern, and Western blotting, and, last but not least, genetic sequencing. Although these techniques had been developed earlier than the PCR, they were not applicable to routine viral diagnostics. The PCR technique broke this barrier because it allowed the rapid and automated amplification of even minute quantities of viral DNA or RNA in a specimen, which could then be detected easily using standard diagnostic techniques, without the need for growing them in culture. Various refinements and improvements of the technique and instruments as well as associated methods, such as digital processing and information technology, accelerated the widespread use of PCR. Despite hurdles posed by problems of cross contamination of specimens and reagents due to the overly rapid generation of large amounts of amplified material, the method quickly became a part of the stock arsenal of both diagnostic and basic research laboratories worldwide. It is no small measure of the success of the technology that just a decade later Mullis was awarded his share of the 1993 Nobel Prize in Chemistry for his invention of the PCR technology.

The rapidly developing nucleic acid-based techniques resulted in a big shift in technical methods used in diagnostic virology laboratories (Persing and Landry, 1989). The presence of human immunodeficiency virus, of hepatitis B virus, of hepatitis C virus (at the beginning of the 1990s) and of other clinically important viruses could be demonstrated in specimens that were negative by the then widely used cell culture techniques. Implementation of the first PCR tests was accompanied by challenging problems of contamination with nucleic acids produced in high numbers by the reaction, resulting in the dire necessity for separate working rooms. An important step forward for diagnostic virology and the management of patients was the development of quantitative molecular assays. Monitoring of viral genome quantities has now become part of most clinical management programs, e.g., to assess the success of antiviral therapy.

Third wave developments in Dutch clinical virology

If there is one area in medicine where virology preceded bacteriology, it would be in the development and implementation of molecular diagnostics. Again, this trend is not surprising, considering that bacteriology relied on tried and tested methods that had been in existence for a long time, compared to virology, which developed alongside molecular biology with the use of molecular assays for the detection of such difficult and non-cultivable viruses as human immunodeficiency virus, hepatitis B and C virus, and human papillomaviruses. Over the late 1980s and in the 1990s, molecular tests were developed and used not only at university diagnostic laboratories or in Groningen at the laboratory of the Municipal Health Service that performed routine clinical diagnostic work in virology for the Academic Hospital, but also at laboratories of RIVM, the Central Laboratory of the Blood Transfusion Service of the Netherlands Red Cross,[49] the laboratory of the Foundation Cooperating Delft Hospitals, and at Organon Technica (see Chapter 6).

49   Centraal Laboratorium van de Bloedtransfusiedienst van het Nederlandse Rode Kruis (CLB), since 1998 Sanquin.

The number of general medical microbiology laboratories with virology diagnostic facilities that used serology and nucleic acid detection assays – based on the wide availability of commercial test kits – had expanded substantially by the turn of the twentieth century. Concurrently, virus isolation by cell culture lost ground in the daily diagnostic practice, but did not disappear altogether, remaining mainly in some university centres as the preferred methodology for propagating viruses for phenotyping and drug susceptibility testing. Application of multiple PCRs for the detection of respiratory viruses replaced rapid viral cell culture tests that were introduced in the 1980s. A financial factor might have also played a role in the rather early introduction of molecular tests in Dutch diagnostic laboratories. In 1996, the COTG,[50] the official body fixing prices in the health sector, approved to charge reasonable tariffs for the refund of these tests.

In parallel, the range of serological tests applied for virological diagnostics changed over the course of the third wave. While in the 1980s, the complement fixation test was carried out at most virological laboratories, a rapid trend towards the use of EIA/ELISA tests and automated instruments could be observed in the last two decades of the twentieth century.

Public health laboratories and medical virology

The involvement of central public health services played a key role in the establishment of diagnostic virology networks worldwide. As noticed by Dekking, the virology laboratory of the National Institute of Public Health (RIV) was central to the development of medical virology in the Netherlands, but in fact, a similar pattern occurred more widely, in other European countries as well as the United States (Bradstreet et al., 1973; Williams, 1985). According to a 1976 summary report by the European Office of the World Health Organization, countries with a federal system of government (Germany, Austria, Switzerland, Yugoslavia) had by this time, some form of a centralized system – for instance, an institute for epidemiology and microbiology – which ordinarily provided reference services, similar to those provided by the PHLS in the UK (Williams, 1985, p. 165). In the Netherlands, the RIV Central Laboratory maintained a policy of contracting out some of its reference services to university or other specialist laboratories. Nevertheless, Dekking made an appropriate remark on the role of RIV with regards to medical virology. In countries such as France, Germany, Italy, and Belgium,

50   Centraal Orgaan Tarieven Gezondheidszorg.

the central institutes had no formal links with the peripheral laboratories apart from the provision of reference services and quality assessment.

The United Kingdom's Public Health Laboratory Service (PHLS) deserves a special mention for its pioneering role in anchoring and shepherding the nascent field of medical virology in its early years. Like many other national public health establishments, its virological work was limited at first to smallpox diagnosis, especially during the early part of the twentieth century. But in 1946, it became one of the first organizations of its kind to establish a dedicated Virus Reference Laboratory (VRL) (Bradstreet et al., 1964; Bradstreet et al., 1973). The VRL was established with a staff of only one qualified virologist and one technician, and expanded by 1950 to a staff of four virologists, who offered diagnostic – mainly serological – services for an array of diseases caused by viruses and similar agents: influenza, psittacosis-lymphogranuloma-venereum group, Q-fever, the pox group, lymphocytic-choriomeningitis virus, mumps virus and primary atypical pneumonia. Cell culture techniques were used from 1954 onward. In 1956, the VRL introduced its members into bacteriological laboratories at its various regional offices, to set up autonomous centres for virology at these locations, thus laying the foundations of a professional network. By 1970, this network had grown to include ten regional laboratories, each with a consultant virologist and nearly 60 so-called area laboratories engaged in virology in addition to bacteriology (Bradstreet et al., 1973). In 1967, J.E. Banatvala and his colleagues at the St Thomas Hospital published a report of their experiences in clinical virology, in which they stressed the importance of laboratories such as their own, which, as an integral part of a research department of a teaching hospital, provided specialized expertise rather than comprehensive services. Meanwhile in her 1986 overview of '40 years of virology in the PHLS', the then-director Marguerite Pereira highlighted the range of immunological techniques that were in routine use for virological diagnostics by the 1970s.

In Germany, medical virology seems to generally be provided in university laboratories rather than in public health laboratories. Klaus Munk published in 1995 a detailed history on the development of virology in Germany in which he stated that nearly all of the listed 37 university virology institutes provided also medical/clinical diagnostic virology services besides their research activities (Munk, 1995). Two out of a total of fifteen non-university centres where virology emerged belonged to pharmaceutical companies, another two were government veterinary laboratories, one was the military virology laboratory, and another one was a primate centre. Among the remaining nine centres were the famous Robert Koch Institute in Berlin, the

Paul Ehrlich Institute in Frankfurt am Main, the Bernard Nocht Institute in Hamburg, the Max Planck Institute in Martinsried, and the Institute for Molecular Virology of the GSF/Research Centre for Environment and Health in Neuherberg. Therefore, from this overview, it may be concluded that in Germany, medical virology and diagnostics occurred in the early years primarily through activities carried out at university laboratories rather than in public health facilities.

In France, medical virology seems to have been omitted from discussions on *historical* overviews of French medicine and medical science. A surprising example of this is Claude Chastel's excellent *Histoire des virus, de la variole au SIDA* (1992), which does *not* provide any specific overview of the development of medical virology in public health or university laboratories in France. In any case, the Institut Pasteur was the stimulating ground for virology in France (Chastel, 1992; Girard, 1988). Nevertheless, six of the eleven authors of the first edition of a French standard work on medical virology entitled *Diagnostic des maladies à virus* came from all over France and were associated with sections of the National Laboratory of Public Health (Sohier, 1964). It may appear as ironic that one of the authors was Chastel himself; his affiliation being the Medical Faculty in Brest, where he was also *biologiste des hôpitaux*.

In the USA, the early years of diagnostic virology were recently described by J. Booss and M.J. August (2013, pp. 158-196). The availability of virology laboratory diagnostics was as limited as in Europe. Epidemiologic studies were conducted by a variety of federal, state, and university-based hospital laboratories. For example, an interesting overview of such studies on virus infections within families is given by J. Fox and C.E. Hall (1980). Diagnostic virology laboratories were located at public health laboratories and university hospitals (Booss and August, 2013, p. 158). In general, virology diagnostics services were provided by hospital-based bacteriology laboratories much later, from 1970 onward, due to the need for highly specialized technical and diagnostic expertise. The techniques that were used consisted of virus isolation and identification techniques, and serological tests revealing the presence of virus-specific antibodies. A lively debate at a 1947 Symposium on Virus Diseases of the Pathology and Physiology section at the 96th annual session of the American Medical Association offers a good snapshot of the status of the field. Stanford University-based Edwin Schultz pointed out that whereas diagnostic procedures had advanced considerably over the preceding decade, they were for the most part highly specialized and out of reach of the ordinary clinical laboratory (1948). The well-known American virologist Edwin Smadel of the Army Department of Virus and Rickettsial

Diseases also warned that the procedures employed in virus diagnostics were still so highly specialized that it required competent research workers to perform the assays in a satisfactory way (Smadel, 1948). He wrote: 'These research procedures are not the physician's to demand for use in routine diagnostic work. Rather they are the physician's to request only, and then in an investigation in which he cooperates with the laboratory worker. If the physician fails to employ these research procedures wisely, he is wasting the common investment in the advancement of medicine' (1948, p. 1079). The laboratory of the Army Medical Department School and that of the National Institute of Health performed regularly all or the great majority of the available tests. The state and municipal laboratories performed some of the diagnostic procedures while a number of laboratories associated with teaching institutions performed but a few of the tests.

The basic and the applied: Separate or joint ways of organization?

Although virology gradually blossomed from the 1950s onwards to become a unique discipline requiring specialized skills and knowledge, it remained within the confines of microbiology. With the growth of the discipline to maturity in the 1960s, workers in the field felt the necessity to meet independently as virologists. At the same time, however, even the field of virology itself was driven by investigators with different interests, such as fundamental virology, plant virology, veterinary and human virology. The endeavours pursued by virologists of these various fields were separate, yet joint at the same time. As the boundaries between these fields were not sharply drawn, it is not surprising that some of the virologists played a role not only in medical virology but also in fundamental or veterinary virology.

Dutch Societies and medical virology

The Netherlands Society for Microbiology

The first Dutch general microbiology organization was the Netherlands Society for Microbiology (NVvM),[51] established in 1911, with Beijerinck as its first chairman. Over the 1960s, members of the NVvM who were interested

---

51   Nederlandse Vereniging voor Microbiologie (NVvM), and since 2011 Koninklijke Nederlandse Vereniging voor Microbiologie (KNVM).

in virology organized informally their own so-called Dutch Virology Day. Unfortunately, the early history of this event remains obscure due to the paucity of archival and oral history records, but some of the early figures involved in convening the 'Virology Days' included well-known representatives from different branches of virology: F. Dekking, R. Gispen, and J. van der Veen in the field of medical virology, J.D. Verlinde in the field of both medical and animal virology, and J. van der Want in the field of plant virology. The first written communication that could be found in the archives of the NVvM is a letter from Verlinde (1969a) dated 18 March 1969 and addressed to the executive committee of the society. It reported on the success of the 'Virology Days', and on the preference of the coordinators to manage their organization independently of the NVvM, because non-members of the society were also regular participants. Verlinde further assured not to intervene with the program of the upcoming autumn meeting of the society.

Around 1970, this group of virologists informally formed the Virology section of the NVvM, to organize the 'Virology Days' as well as symposia on matters of common interest. Eventually, in 1977, after years of discussion on the desirability of sections within the NVvM, the group became one of five official sections of the society, responsible for all subfields in virology, including medical, plant, and veterinary virology. Members of the executive committee of the Virology section were: veterinary virologist M.C. Horzinek, molecular biologist A.J. van der Eb, medical virologist A.C. Hekker, and plant virologist D. Peters. Under the enthusiastic guidance of M. Horzinek, the annual Virology Days were maintained and organized at first by P. van der Marel and after 1983 by H.G.A.M. van der Avoort, both working at RIVM (H.G.A.M. van der Avoort, personal communication, 2017). In 1992, the organization of the 'Virology Days' was turned over to P.J.M. Rottier and R.C. de Groot, at the Veterinary Faculty of the University of Utrecht (P.J.M. Rottier, personal communication, 2018). Under this new management, the 'Virology Days' were renamed 'Dutch Annual Virology Symposium' (DAVS). The format of the meetings included presentations by invited speakers for each of the four disciplines – at least one of these speakers was invited from abroad – and by other participants selected through a review of submitted abstracts. Although the expressed aim of the DAVS was to present research subjects covering all areas of virology, there was a perceptible shift in emphasis to fundamental rather than medical and other applied aspects of virology.

From 1999 to this day, the DAVS has been held at the Royal Netherlands Academy of Arts and Sciences in Amsterdam; the Beijerinck Virology Fund of the Academy allows inviting distinguished foreign keynote speakers;

while the Veterinary Faculty of the University of Utrecht continues to offer secretarial support. The Beijerinck Virology Fund was founded in 1965 by L.E. den Dooren de Jong and his wife, A. den Dooren de Jong-Ris, to honour the memory of Beijerinck, who was his teacher and friend.[52] The fund awards the prestigious Beijerinck Virology Prize every two years to an internationally renowned researcher in the field of virology (Van Kammen, 2011). Certainly, these honours belong to Beijerinck's beneficiaries.

The Netherlands Society for Medical Microbiology

The professional society for medical microbiologists in the Netherlands is the Netherlands Society for Medical Microbiology (NVMM),[53] which was established in 1992 and considered the successor of the pre-existing Netherlands Society of Laboratory Medical Doctors,[54] founded in 1950. This professional society initially regrouped medical doctors engaging into clinical chemistry and clinical microbiology, as well as pathologists until the establishment of their own professional society in 1955. The Science Committee of the NVvM in which each division has a representative, is a link between all divisions, including the medical microbiology division i.e. the NVMM, and it annually organizes a joint scientific meeting on the field of microbiology at large, meant to build bridges between the different communities of microbiology scientists. Over the 1990s a virology session was organized at the joint meeting by the Dutch Working Group for Clinical Virology[55] in collaboration with the Virology section of the NVvM.

The Dutch Working Group for Clinical Virology

A small group comprising an epidemiologist and medical virologists at the National Institute of Public Health (RIV) in Bilthoven was responsible to form the Dutch Working Group for Clinical Virology. The commencement of the working group is not documented on paper and therefore this narrative is mainly based on interviews with Jacoba G. Kapsenberg – known to her intimate colleagues as Cootje. She has vivid memories of those early years. The impetus of the working group was given by epidemiologist M.F. Polak,

---

52   https://www.knaw.nl/nl/prijzen/prijzen/knaw-beijerinck-prijzen-voor-virologie, latest access August 2019.
53   Nederlandse Vereniging voor Medische Microbiologie (NVMM).
54   Vereniging van Laboratorium Artsen (NVLA).
55   Nederlandse Werkgroep Klinische Virologie (NWKV).

who moved in 1960 from the Laboratory for Hygiene in Amsterdam to RIV. In 1964, he took the initiative to collect and analyse monthly data from five virological laboratories (Stenfert Kroese, 1999). Polak invited representatives from each of these laboratories to meet once a month at Bilthoven, to review the summarized compilation of the collected epidemiological data. The laboratories involved were: the Laboratory for Virology at RIV, the virology laboratory of the Netherlands Institute for Preventive Medicine at Leiden University, the Laboratory for Hygiene at the University of Amsterdam, the Regional Public Health Laboratory at the Municipal Health Service of Rotterdam, and the Regional Public HealthLaboratory at the St Elisabeth Hospital in Tilburg. The country's leading virologists – all of those main characters who have already been mentioned – participated in these meetings. J.D. Verlinde from Leiden, F. Dekking from Amsterdam, G.J.P. Schaap from Rotterdam, J. van der Veen from Tilburg/Nijmegen, and, in addition to Polak, R. Gispen and J.G. Kapsenberg from Bilthoven. Not surprisingly, later on four of them were also members of the steering committee of the Virology section of the NVvM. In 1967 and 1970, respectively, N. Masurel from Rotterdam and J.B. Wilterdink from Groningen also joined the meetings. In addition, as the importance of an applied or 'translational' approach to infectious diseases was already well understood, representatives of the Laboratory of Virology at the Veterinary Faculty of the University of Utrecht were also invited (M.C. Horzinek, from 1971 onward). In the 1970s, maybe under the influence of the general democratization of the universities, the meetings became open to non-medical academic staff members of the above-mentioned laboratories.

As indicated, one of the main points on the agenda of the meetings of the working group was to review monthly epidemiologic reports. In addition, items such as technical problems faced by laboratories, the availability of reagents, e.g. antigens and specific antibodies, as well as individual clinical cases, were discussed. Regrettably, however, we were unable to find any records of the meetings over about the first 20 years of the working group.

The system for collecting monthly data on acute virus infections was similar to that instituted at the Public Health Laboratory Service (PHLS) in the United Kingdom. Since the early days of World War II, the UK's public health laboratories, as well as (since 1951) many hospital laboratories outside PHLS, were expected to submit detailed weekly reports on the infectious diseases diagnosed by the laboratory to the central Epidemiological Research Laboratory (ERL) in London (Bradstreet et al., 1964; Bradstreet et al., 1973; Pereira, 1986, p. 10). Based on these reports, the ERL prepared a weekly summary of diagnosed acute infections for wide distribution. The near real-time availability of laboratory results meant that acute virus infections of the respiratory tract or nervous system, in particular influenza and poliomyelitis, were kept under the strictest possible surveillance. The main difference between the British and Dutch systems was that of scale. According to Patricia Bradstreet, in addition to the Central Public Health Laboratory (Colindale, London), where she was appointed director of the Standards Laboratory for serological agents in 1956, nine area laboratories and more than 40 regional laboratories across England and Wales were involved in virology work in 1964. In contrast, in the Netherlands, only the five aforementioned laboratories cooperated in the reportage system. Nonetheless, the small number of virology laboratories in the Netherlands as well as smaller distances between them afforded more opportunities for frequent and personal meetings. Their regular meetings allowed rapid communication among experts as well as prompt deployment of well-conceived public health measures based on international knowledge and individual expertise. All Dutch virologists had international contacts both through personal channels and through more formal institutions such as the World Health Organization (WHO). In the early 1950s, the Netherlands Institute for Preventive Medicine in Leiden was designated as the WHO Influenza Centre for the Netherlands (Bijl, 1954). In 1969, RIV was acknowledged as an 'International reference institute for smallpox vaccine control' of the WHO (Van Zon, 1990).

Expansion of the working group
In the 1970s, the number of general hospital-based microbiology laboratories which provided diagnostic virology laboratory services, increased. As a result, staff members of these laboratories, responsible for viral diagnostics, were invited to take part in the working group. In the early 1980s, residents in medical microbiology were allowed to attend the meetings. After lengthy discussions, the meetings were eventually open to senior technicians as invited guests. By the 1990s, biochemists had gradually made their entry into the diagnostic virology laboratories, initially staffed mainly by medical microbiologists. In 2011, all eight university hospitals, RIVM and fourteen general hospital-based laboratories were represented by medical microbiologists and scientific staff members, mostly of the field of medical molecular biology (the latter discipline indicating that virology had indeed entered its molecular – third – wave).

Working group meetings
By 1980, the meetings of the working group were organized three times a year by a formal steering committee. A scheme rotating the meeting venue

through each of the member laboratories was instituted and remains in place to this day. Meetings typically start with a discussion of routine business and administrative matters, followed by reports of the RIVM liaison officer and since 1997, reports of the liaison officer of the European Society of Clinical Virology (ESCV). Regular items included discussions on the external quality assessment scheme of the Foundation for the Quality Control of Medical Microbiology (SKMM)[56] and later of Quality Control for Molecular Diagnostics (QCMD). Usually, there was a presentation on the research program performed at the hosting laboratory. The agenda for the latter part of the day varied, featuring major as well as more limited virological or technical topics, relevant epidemiological figures, and case reports. The time scheme offered plenty of time for discussions and for the airing of controversial topics. The main themes concerned basic approaches to the diagnosis of viral infections, choices of tests employed, choices of specimen, interpretation of test results, epidemiology, vaccination, and the increasing possibilities of antiviral therapy. Topics of perennial interest – persisting to the present day – include diagnostics of emerging infections, collection and transport procedures for specimens that may contain dangerous pathogens, and the safety of the working environment. As part of permanent education, keynote speakers were invited to deliver lectures on specific subjects. In the 1980s, increasingly more attention was paid to the application of molecular methods in medical virology, such as in situ hybridization and later nucleic acid amplification techniques. In the 1990s, antiviral therapy became of age, enlarging substantially the equipment to fight viral infections. Several sessions of the working group meetings were then devoted to chemotherapy of viral infections caused by human immunodeficiency virus, hepatitis B virus, hepatitis C virus, cytomegalovirus, Epstein-Barr virus, and herpes simplex virus, among others.

Epidemiological reports
According to Jacoba G. Kapsenberg, RIV received in 1979 the WHO's invitation to file monthly epidemiological reports on all laboratory-confirmed cases of viral infections, including such information as virus name, detection methods, confirmation tests, comprehensive clinical anamnesis, and patient age and gender. RIV staff members went to great length to compile the reports from data obtained from all virology laboratories in the Netherlands that were at that time members of the working group (Kapsenberg, 2002). Despite these efforts, the international endeavour proved unsuccessful; there were too many laboratories in too many countries that could not send regular or detailed

---

56   Stichting Kwaliteit Medische Microbiologie.

enough reports. For individual virology laboratories, preparing these reports significantly increased staff workload, due to the need for detailed data and frequent lack of clinical information. This resulted in delays in reporting or even cessation of reporting on a monthly basis, by the contributing Dutch virology laboratories. Obviously, this trend also occurred elsewhere. By the beginning of the 1980s, only the United Kingdom, Israel and the Netherlands sent consolidated monthly reports to WHO (J.G. Kapsenberg, personal communication, 2015). RIV continued to maintain the reporting system to support the field of medical virology with all new information on viral diseases that could be generated by the community of Dutch clinical virologists and clinicians.

In 1985, J.M. Ossewaarde at RIVM initiated the design and development of a computer programme to facilitate input and maintenance of the epidemiological data. Data had to be sent on a floppy disk to RIVM as the internet was not yet in existence. But the programme proved to be premature for the majority of laboratories. In 1989, A.M. van Loon, then head of the RIVM Laboratory for Virology, proposed and organized a change from monthly to weekly epidemiological reports that included much less clinical information. Following a series of lengthy discussions, a new system of weekly reports containing nothing but laboratory results was introduced in the mid-1990s. Reports were faxed to RIVM, where they were further processed using a computer programme designed by P.M. Schrijnemakers. The system evolved from fax- to internet-based, and was communicated in the form of spreadsheets. Nowadays all virology diagnostic laboratories submit weekly epidemiological reports to RIVM. The received data is analysed and compiled into the electronic report *Weekly Reviews of Infectious Diseases Signals*,[57] which is available to all Dutch professionals working in the field of infectious diseases. The number of epidemiological reports has not ceased to increase, probably due to increases in the number of specimens examined and/or due to the use of more sensitive techniques. This reporting system has nevertheless some limitations, for example, because laboratories only report positive specimens. As a result, only the numerator and not the denominator of reported viral infections are known. However, the aggregated data from 23 nationwide laboratories are sufficiently reliable to rapidly show epidemiological trends in viral infections. Despite the absence of detailed clinical and epidemiological information, outbreaks of viral diseases can be assessed. If detailed information is required, special surveys are prepared and performed. Since the establishment of the National Coordination Structure for Infectious Diseases (LCI),[58] which provides guidelines on how to

57 Wekelijks overzicht van infectieziektesignalen (Signaleringsoverleg).
58 Landelijke Coördinatiestructuur Infectieziekten (LCI).

record data during suspected epidemics using standardized formats, in 1994, results of the surveys are made available to all health professionals, including clinicians and laboratory and public health workers.

Professionalization
Although Polak had initiated the meetings in 1964, it was not until 26 September 1989 that the status of the working group was formalized as the Dutch Working Group for Clinical Virology with the introduction of a set of regulations. A.M. Dingemans-Dumas was appointed chairperson at this time. The stated aims of the working group were the promotion of virus diagnostics and of the study and management of viral infections in humans, including epidemiology and immunology. The regulations were modified in 2001 in order to integrate the working group within the Netherlands Society of Medical Microbiology, which necessitated the revision of the by-laws of the latter since until that time the society had no provisions for including working parties. By 2011, the working group meetings had representatives from all eight university hospitals in the Netherlands as well the RIVM and fourteen general hospital-based laboratories.

Standardization and external quality control

In 1981, virology diagnostic laboratories in the Netherlands began to participate in a national external quality assessment scheme led by the Foundation for the Quality Control of Medical Microbiology (SKMM).[59] This foundation had been established the same year by medical microbiologists convinced of the value and necessity of such a system. In 2005, the SKMM merged with the Foundation for the Quality Control of Medical Laboratory Diagnostics[60] (SKML), a Dutch consortium including participants from laboratories of clinical chemistry, medical microbiology, pathology, haematology as well as clinical pharmacy.

Meanwhile a similar initiative for an external quality scheme for molecular tests was undertaken at the European level. One of the founders of the Quality Control for Molecular Diagnostics (QCMD) organization was A.M. van Loon, a prominent member of the working group (QCMD, n.d.). This organization was established by the European Society of Clinical Virology (ESCV) in cooperation with the European Society of Clinical Microbiology and Infectious Diseases (ESCMID) and supported by the European Union Concerted Action on Virus Meningitis and Encephalitis, initiated by the British virologist G.M. Cleator of Manchester, UK. Nowadays, the QCMD operates as

59 Stichting Kwaliteit Medische Microbiologie (SKMM).
60 Stichting Kwaliteitsbewaking Medische Laboratoriumdiagnostiek (SKML).

an independent International External Quality Assessment (EQA)/Proficiency Testing (PT) organization, providing wide-ranging quality assessment services, especially for diagnostic molecular testing for infectious diseases, to over 2,000 participants in over a hundred countries. A relatively large number of Dutch virologists played an important role in QCMD as part of the executive board or as scientific experts; among them were A.M. van Loon (chair, 2001-2016), J. Schirm, H.M.G. Niesters, Gerda T. Noordhoek and R. Schuurman.

The Working Group for Molecular Diagnostics of Infectious Diseases (WMDI)

The increasing applications of PCR and other molecular techniques in diagnostic virology led to the formation of a spin-off working group in 1997. Van Loon and Schuurman from UMC Utrecht, Niesters from Erasmus MC Rotterdam, and Gerda Noordhoek from the Regional Public Health Laboratory in Leeuwarden were the founders of the Working Group for Molecular Diagnosis of Infectious Diseases (WMDI)[61] in the Netherlands. This new group had broader ambition than the mere detection of viruses, and aimed at the widespread application of molecular techniques across all branches of medical microbiology, including bacteriology and parasitology. There is a major crossover between this working group and the above-mentioned Dutch Working Group for Clinical Virology, as many individuals are members of both networks and joint annual meetings are organized.

European societies and Dutch medical virology

At the European and international level, the following societies served Dutch clinical virologists as meeting venues for the exchange of knowledge and expertise

European Group for Rapid Viral Diagnosis

The rise of rapid virus diagnostic techniques occurred worldwide, urging international initiatives to collaborate. Among others, P.S. (Philip) Gardner (UK), M. (Monica) Grandien (Sweden), C.M.V.P. Halonen (Finland), U. Krech (Switzerland), P. Leinikki (Finland), H. Schmitz (Germany), and J. van der Veen (the Netherlands) founded the European Group for Rapid Viral

61   Werkgroep Moleculaire Diagnostiek van Infectieziekten (WMDI).

Diagnosis (EGRVD) in 1975. According to Gardner, even the WHO had an increasing involvement in rapid viral diagnosis (Gardner and McQuillin, 1980). In 1977, Gardner was invited to act as an adviser for the Provisional American Group for Rapid Viral Diagnosis, established by M. Chernesky, E. Lennette, K. McIntosh, S. Plotkin, C. Wilfert, and others. In 1978, its name changed to the Pan American Group for Rapid Viral Diagnosis (PAGRVD) to accommodate individual requests for membership originating from Mexico, Central America and South America (Chernesky, 2000). The first congress of the European Group took place at Amsterdam in 1977 and was organized together with the European Association against Virus Diseases (Gardner, 1978). J. van der Veen from Nijmegen was member of the organizing committee. This and subsequent meetings offered ample opportunity for international contact.

European Association against Virus Diseases

ESAVD was officially established on 19 May 1951 in Geneva, Switzerland, initially as the European Association against Poliomyelitis and Allied Other Virus Diseases (Union of International Associations, n.d.). It seems that the association was already active before its official establishment and organized the following conferences: 1946, Brussels; 1949, Paris; 1950, Amsterdam. In 1974, the name changed to European Association against Virus Diseases, or Association Européenne contre les maladies à virus.

European Society for Clinical Virology

The European Society for Clinical Virology (ESCV) is the successor of the aforementioned European Group for Rapid Viral Diagnosis and European Association against Virus Diseases, which merged into ESCV on 1 January 1997. ESCV is open to anyone interested in viruses as causes of disease in humans and animals, either as a (general) physician, paediatrician, veterinarian, infectious diseases specialist, (clinical) virologist or microbiologists, pure or applied, or just out of curiosity. Dutch members of the ESCV council were both from Groningen: J. Schirm (1998 to 2007, including president from 2001 to 2004), and Sytske Welling-Wester (1997 to 2005 as meetings secretary).

European Society for Virology

The European Society for Virology (ESV) is a non-profit organization officially founded on 30 October 2008. The need for such a society had already been felt much earlier, during the organization of the European Virology 2000 Congress that was held in Glasgow, Scotland, UK. A total of 25 national organizations collaborated for the organization of this meeting. Its success prompted the decision to organize a joint meeting covering all fields of virology every four years. Since 2008, ESV has provided a forum for scientists active in all aspects of virology, and organizes the quadrennial congresses in collaboration with ESCV. The stated aim of the society is to promote and stimulate the exchange of information and collaboration among individual scientists as well as among national and international associations of virology throughout Europe. To achieve these goals, ESV also organizes meetings and courses, offers fellowships and promotes education in virology at all levels. It represents the science, art and profession of virology to governmental and regulatory institutions of the European Union, the media and the general public.

Waves of development and organization of clinical and fundamental virology

In the beginning of the 1950s, the main first-wave advance in clinical virology occurred rather slowly, with the refinement of cell culture techniques. The realm of clinical virology appeared to lay at public health, preventive medicine, and university laboratories. Since the 1970s, and during the second wave, virology diagnostics, with new automated immunological assays and visualization techniques, expanded to general hospitals. University laboratories, the Central Laboratory of the Netherlands Blood Transfusion Service,[62] and the laboratory of the Foundation of Cooperating Delft Hospitals (SSDZ)[63] played a pioneering role in the advent of nucleic acid amplification techniques, resulting in a third wave of expansion of molecular virology diagnostics in general hospitals in the 1990s. In conclusion, the three technical waves drove medical virology into existence, as well as important medical services as a profession with numerous networks for discussion, education, training and exchange.

Concomitantly, in the 1960s, virologists active in clinical as well as fundamental research, in the Netherlands and worldwide, felt the increasing need for independent meetings in their field. A working group for clinical

---

62 Centraal Laboratorium van de Bloedtransfusiedienst van het Nederlandse Rode Kruis (CLB), since 1998 Sanquin.
63 Stichting Samenwerkende Delftse Ziekenhuizen (SSDZ).

virology as well as a rather independent Virology section within the General Microbiology Society was established in the Netherlands. The Clinical Virology Working Group also joined the Society of Medical Microbiology, an independent medical section of the General Microbiology Society. Although it seems that fundamental and clinical virologists engage sometimes into different or separate endeavours, their paths remain connected not only through their organizations and societies, but all the more by fruitful personal contacts and research collaborations.

In conclusion, we are compelled to highlight that, unlike in most other European countries, Dutch fundamental virology and medical virology remain joined through common organizations and societies. These two fields tend to function rather independently within the General Microbiology Society and the Society for Medical Microbiology, respectively. Although medical virologists may be outnumbered by bacteriologists in the NVMM or by fundamental researchers in the Virology section of the Royal Netherlands Society for Microbiology (KNVM), there are ample opportunities to meet and network through these organizations. Furthermore, judging by the number of Dutch virologists present in the executive boards or advisory councils of ESCV and ESV, we should be pleased with the excellent representation of Dutch clinical virology in international virology societies.

5 Medical virology in the Netherlands after 1950

Laboratories and institutes

> I hope to have made it clear that virus diagnostics must be performed completely
> with isolation and serology in fully equipped laboratories, and that a correct
> application of the available techniques together with the interpretation of the
> obtained results require such a professional knowledge and attention that this
> demands full attention of the virologist.[64]
>
> – *Anton Hekker (1982)*

As seen in the previous chapter, medical virology in the Netherlands underwent a diagnostic turn in the last half of the twentieth century. This turn went hand-in-hand with a great expansion in the number of laboratories offering virus diagnostic services, not only at such institutions as universities, or public health centres, but also in general hospitals. During this period, private pharmaceutical companies and the emerging biotechnology industry also turned to virus research and development of laboratory techniques. The number of universities with medical faculties doubled; in addition to the universities in Amsterdam, Leiden, Utrecht, and Groningen that were discussed in Chapter 3, two new medical faculties were founded at existing universities in Amsterdam and Nijmegen, while two new universities with medical faculties were established in Rotterdam and Maastricht. The 1951 establishment of a Laboratory for Viral and Rickettsial Diseases at the National Institute of Public Health (RIV) in Utrecht also had tremendous consequences for the availability of reference laboratory services in the country. In this chapter we provide a survey of the virological work in these laboratories.

---

64 Ik hoop duidelijk te hebben gemaakt dat virus diagnostiek volledig dient te geschieden dus mèt isolatie en serologie in volledig geoutilleerde en geëquipeerde laboratoria en dat een juiste uitvoering van de beschikbare technieken samen met de interpretatie van de verkregen resultaten een zodanige vakkennis en aandacht vereisen dat dit de viroloog volledig opeist.

The impact of the AIDS pandemic on Dutch virology

Just as the 1918-1919 Spanish influenza pandemic left an indelible mark on the history of virology in the early twentieth century, so too did the outbreak of a new virus disease in the 1980s – what eventually came to be known as the Acquired Immunodeficiency Syndrome or AIDS. Perhaps more than any other pandemic in the twentieth century, AIDS exercised a profound and lasting impact on multiple aspects of life. Although this book is not the right venue for a detailed discussion, we would be remiss if we did not mention in passing at least, that the human experience with the disease brought to the fore myriads of issues; not only related to medical research and public health, but also such social matters as sexual mores, discrimination and social identity, to name but a few.

Unlike influenza, AIDS, when it first appeared, was entirely new to the human experience. Indeed, although acronyms such as HIV[65] and AZT[66] and of course AIDS itself are now commonplace and recognized by people from different walks of life, these terms were not even coined until after the 1980s. It was first recognized as a disease in the late 1970s and early 1980s – and at first thought to be confined to the male homosexual community, haemophiliacs, and injecting drug users. But very quickly the disease was recognized all over the world, affecting both sexes with equal ferocity, notably in Africa and Asia. The causative agent for the pandemic remained elusive until 1983, until a team of French virologists isolated the virus we now know as HIV in 1983, although R. Gallo claimed that this virus was independently isolated in his laboratory (Barré-Sinoussi et al., 1983; Gallo et al., 1983).

The first Dutch AIDS patient was diagnosed in Amsterdam in 1981 and the first official cases reported the following year (Van Wijngaarden, 1984; Houweling et al., 1994). Much later, however, tests on serum samples collected from patients in a previous hepatitis B vaccine study revealed that HIV has already been introduced in homosexual men in Amsterdam in the late 1970s (ACS, 1996). Meanwhile, in 1984 J. van der Noordaa, professor of virology at the Academic Medical Center initiated a series of multidisciplinary studies into various aspects of disease encompassing epidemiology, social science, virology, immunology and clinical medicine. Because multiple research groups and laboratories from different institutions were involved in addressing the crisis, we have devoted a separate subsection under the discussion of laboratories in Amsterdam on the Dutch work on HIV/AIDS.

65   HIV (human immunodeficiency virus).
66   AZT (azidothymidine).

Amsterdam

University of Amsterdam[67] and the Academic Medical Center (AMC)

Virology at the University of Amsterdam expanded greatly after the end of World War II spreading well beyond the confines of the Laboratory for Hygiene where it was first established. In 1940, the university appointed microbiologist Charlotte Ruys as extraordinary professor to teach medical microbiology, although she retained her existing position as head of the Regional Public Health Laboratory of the Municipal Health Service. Ruys had broad interests in virology and public health. After Van Loghem's retirement in 1948 she was promoted as professor of bacteriology, immunology and hygiene, and she was appointed head of the Laboratory for Hygiene, a position she maintained until she retired in 1969. After she retired, the chair was split into two separate positions: one in bacteriology and epidemiology, and the other in virology. Meanwhile, in 1954, the virus researcher F. Dekking, who since 1949 had held the position of conservator at the Laboratory for Hygiene, was tasked with creating a separate dedicated unit of virus research within the Laboratory for Hygiene. Later in 1968 Dekking was appointed professor of virology and in his inaugural lecture he identified himself as the second professor of virology in the Netherlands, the honour of the first having gone to R. Gispen, who had already been appointed to his position at the University of Utrecht in 1960 (Dekking, 1968). Dekking's research focused on psittacosis, lymphogranuloma venereum, and the poxviruses. In the course of the 1960s another virologist, K.W. Slaterus, was given the responsibility for viral diagnostics at the university hospitals. The diagnostic laboratory remained housed in the building of the Laboratory for Hygiene, although it was planned in the Academic Wilhelmina Hospital.

Dekking was succeeded after his retirement in 1979 as the head of the laboratory by Jan van der Noordaa, who had first come to the University of Amsterdam's Laboratory for Hygiene in 1960 as part of his compulsory military training after completing his medical studies at Leiden University. While there he worked on the development of a smallpox vaccine using an attenuated strain of vaccinia virus. Reminiscing about this period, Van der Noordaa remarked that in light of the current concerns about workplace safety, it seemed a wonder that there were no cases (at least reported cases) of laboratory-acquired infections during the entire time that he worked on vaccinia viruses in a safety cabinet under the stairs in the hall of the

67　Universiteit van Amsterdam, Academisch Medisch Centrum.

laboratory (J. van der Noordaa, personal communication to G. van Doornum, 2014). After defending his doctoral thesis on the subject of adult vaccinations (mainly conscripts) of vaccinia virus in 1964, he spent 1965 in John Enders's laboratory at Harvard Medical School, where he worked on the herpes simplex virus and the process of cellular transformation by a simian virus – SV40 – before returning to Amsterdam. With regard to this period, it is a pity that George Miller, another postdoc of Enders, did not carry out a plan to write a short piece about the 'early days of viral oncology in the Enders lab', as he wrote to Van der Noordaa in a personal letter of May 1986. After his return he introduced studies on oncogenic viruses and initiated the formation of an active research group studying DNA tumour viruses based on the SV40 model. This line of research was started in the early days of the molecularization of cancer aetiology with rather rudimentary methods when compared with the present technology, such as deep sequencing. The laboratory also investigated many other viruses, including the herpes simplex, varicella zoster, cytomegalovirus and Epstein-Barr virus. The cutting-edge technologies of restriction enzyme analysis were used to construct the first maps of two different orientations of the varicella-zoster virus genome (Dumas et al., 1981).

Well informed about developments in other fields, Van der Noordaa astutely recognized the primary importance of the developments in molecular biology for guiding studies of oncogenic viruses. Consequently, by 1975 he brought in molecular biologists J. ter Schegget and C.J. Sol as members of the staff of the virus research unit. Influenced by the ideas of Van der Noordaa's friend, the virologist Harald zur Hausen – later the 2008 Nobel Prize recipient for his discovery of the cervical cancer-causing papilloma viruses – the focus of the virus lab was redirected to human papilloma work, under the leadership of Ter Schegget.

The Laboratory for Hygiene moved in 1984 to the new building of the AMC (Academic Medical Center) that was founded in 1983 through a merger of the Academic Hospitals at the University of Amsterdam (Wilhelmina Gasthuis and Binnen Gasthuis) and the Medical Faculty of the University of Amsterdam. Soon after the emergence of the AIDS epidemic a Department of Retrovirology was established within the AMC headed by J. Goudsmit (for more, see below under Amsterdam Cohort Studies). When Van der Noordaa delivered his farewell lecture in 1995, he expressed the wish that his position should not remain vacant for long. He had to wait twelve years until in 2007 M. de Jong was appointed at his chair to teach clinical virology. The research line was already covered by appointments of B. Berkhout and H. Schuitemaker (for more, see below).

State Veterinary Research Institute[68]

The virologist H.S. Frenkel, who had been instrumental in getting State Veterinary Research Institute off the ground in the 1930s – and who, despite many years of Nazi persecution, was able to return as its director in 1945 (see Chapter 3) – maintained his position at the helm of the institute until his retirement in 1959. He continued to play an important role in medical virology in the Netherlands during this period, not only with his own achievements but also because the students that he supervised at his laboratory during their training and research for their thesis would go on to become the country's well-known virologist and infectious disease specialist, notably J.G. Kapsenberg (1955), and J. Huisman (1956), respectively. After his retirement from bench work, Frenkel turned to philosophical speculation about whether or not viruses were living. He took a Spinozian approach to the question; like the Dutch philosopher, he believed that all earthly material was God's creation and composed of the same substance, which was animated, albeit to different degrees in different creatures (Frenkel, 1963).[69] Among the people with whom Frenkel discussed these philosophical views on viruses was the virologist Albert Sabin (Frenkel, 1961). For a more detailed account of the history of this institute, readers are referred to *Strenge wetenschappelijkheid en practische zin*[70] by Peter Verhoef (2005).

Regional Public Health Laboratory of the Municipal Health Service of Amsterdam[71]

Although it was established as early as 1896 and from 1929 on, was headed by Charlotte Ruys, who was known to have broad interests in virology, the Municipal Health Service in Amsterdam did not commence viral diagnostic work until after 1950. As late as 1956, according to the annual reports of the Municipal Health Service, cerebrospinal fluid specimens from patients suspected of having meningitis serosa were still sent for laboratory diagnostics to Dekking's lab at the University for laboratory diagnosis (GGD Amsterdam, Archief, 1956). The earliest independent virological studies – on the epidemiology of poliomyelitis and rubella – began in 1956, but it was not until 1959 that

68   Staats Veeartsenijkundig Onderzoekings Instituut.
69   omnia, quamvis diversis gradibus tamen animata sunt (translation by G. van Doornum).
70   *Strict science and practical senses.*
71   Streeklaboratorium van de Gemeentelijke Geneeskundige en Gezondheids Dienst.

the laboratory began to culture viruses in its own premises. The cell culture system was started under the guidance of medical researcher G.J.P. Schaap, who had been associated with the laboratory since 1953, but who moved to Rotterdam in 1962. In 1965, a culture of rubella virus was introduced by M. Wabeke, who had defended a thesis on this subject in 1964, just two years after the first successful attempts to propagate rubellavirus in cell culture (GGD Amsterdam, Archief, 1965; Wabeke, 1964). In the 1970s the laboratory extended its reach to the hepatitis B virus. In the face of various infectious outbreaks during the 1970s and 1980s, the Regional Laboratory was compelled to expand their capacity for tissue culture, specifically for the cultivation of respiratory viruses as well as *Chlamydia trachomatis*, a bacterial species that, like viruses, has a requirement for living cells for its growth. During this time, other cutting-edge techniques, including ELISA-based assays and immunoblotting assays, were introduced. The modernization of the laboratory with automation, an information system, and a quality control system, resulted in the designation of the Regional Laboratory as a reference laboratory for virology by RIVM.[72] The 1990s saw a shift in the focus of the clinical virology at regional laboratories to the epidemiology and improvement of detection of sexually transmitted viral diseases such as AIDS; hepatitis A, B and C; and genital warts (caused by human papillomaviruses) as well as *Chlamydia trachomatis*. Also evident in this period was an upsurge in the development of new diagnostic methods based on molecular biology, often in cooperation with commercial companies (Van Doornum, 1990, passim). In 1999 a new staff member, Sylvia Bruisten, was recruited to strengthen the molecular section; she came from the CLB, where she had acquired expertise in HIV detection.

Central Laboratory of the Netherlands Red Cross Blood Transfusion Service (CLB)[73] and Red Cross Blood Bank of Amsterdam[74]

The Netherlands Red Cross was originally founded in 1867 and its Central Laboratory of the Blood Transfusion Service, which performed research for all regional blood banks, established in Amsterdam sometime in 1939. Facilities for culturing HIV became operational in 1984 around the time that the CLB became a participant in the Amsterdam Cohort Studies (ACS, see details below). The unit was formally established as the Department

---

72   Bijzonder Instituut voor de Virologie.
73   Centraal Laboratorium van de Bloedtransfusiedienst van het Nederlands Rode Kruis (CLB), since 1998 Sanquin.
74   Rode Kruis Bloedbank Amsterdam.

of Clinical Viro-Immunology in 1992, headed by the immunologist Frank Miedema. The Department of Clinical Viro-Immunology and the Laboratory for Retrovirology of the AMC were international leaders in trashing out the immunology and the virology of HIV/AIDS through their work within the ACS.

The regional Red Cross Blood Bank of Amsterdam that was housed in the same building as the CLB was responsible for the screening of donor blood for the prior exposure to, or presence of various infectious agents. The growing risks posed by viruses such as hepatitis B virus, HIV, and later by 1989 hepatitis C virus, intensified research efforts at the blood bank together with the CLB, not only to develop methods to efficiently screen donor blood and blood products for possible viral contamination, but also to identify the specific viral contaminants. Over the years the Amsterdam Blood Bank and CLB became proficient in testing for a large number of viral diseases, including hepatitis A, B, C, D and E, cytomegalovirus (CMV), Epstein-Barr virus (EBV), and human retroviruses such as HIV, HTLV-1, HTLV-2, and human parvovirus B19, using a large number of serologic and molecular assays.

Since the discovery of the hepatitis B virus by S. Blumberg in 1963 and the availability of tests for screening of hepatitis B surface antigen (HBsAg) donor blood was screened for the presence of HBsAg. Since in the middle of 1985 screening for HIV antibody was performed at all blood banks in the Netherlands. The names of a number of people who work in the 1980s and 1990s on hepatitis B, hepatitis C and HIV screening might be mentioned here: the medical doctors H.W. Reesink, C.L. van der Poel, and H.L. Zaaijer, as well as H.T.M. Cuypers, H. Huisman and P.N. Lelie on the laboratory side. With regard to testing donor blood on possible transmission of virus infections, Van der Poel defended his thesis on the transmission of hepatitis C virus and Zaaijer evaluated serological and nucleic acid assays detecting presence of HIV-1, HIV-2, HTLV-I, HBV, and HCV. In 1995 he defended his PhD thesis: *Confirmatory testing of blood-borne viral infections*.

VU University Medical Center Amsterdam (VUmc)[75]

The Free University of Amsterdam was founded in 1880, but its medical faculty was slow to gain momentum. A first step was the appointment of L. Bouman as professor of psychiatry in 1907 (Van Deursen, 2005, p. 110), but a full-fledged medical faculty was not established until 1950. At that time, only bachelor-level courses were introduced, but masters-level courses and clinical training facilities soon followed. The first person to graduate

---

75   Vrije Universiteit Amsterdam. VU Medisch Centrum (VUmc).

with a medical degree from the Medical Faculty at VU was Miss S.W. van Duinen, who passed her examination in 1957 (Van Deursen, 2005, p. 246).

In 1959 the veterinarian H.A.E. van Tongeren, who had trained with Verlinde in Leiden, was recruited to teach medical microbiology and was appointed as ordinary professor of microbiology in 1963. He held this position until 1978, at which time the position was given to D.M. MacLaren, a bacteriologist, while Van Tongeren himself was given a chair in medical virology, due to his main research interests. Unfortunately, however, over the 1960s and 1970s the institute was too small to make an impact in either diagnostic or research virology. It was not until the twenty-first century, after the appointment of a molecular biologist, P.H.M. Savelkoul, who was also given charge of viral diagnostics, that molecular tests for the diagnosis of viral diseases were introduced properly at VUmc. However, at the Department of Pathology the molecular biologist J.M.M. Walboomers was appointed head of the Molecular Pathology unit in 1987. From then onwards the Free University began an internationally successful program in human papilloma virus research under the leadership of pathologist C.J.L.M. Meijer and Walboomers, together with their doctoral student students A.J. van den Brule and P.J. Snijders (Van den Brule et al., 1992).

Amsterdam Cohort Studies (ACS)

Although it cannot be pinpointed to a single laboratory or university, the activities of the Amsterdam Cohort Studies are worth discussing separately because of the group's high visibility and output in the wake of the AIDS pandemic of the 1980s. The cohort was the result of Jan van der Noordaa's efforts to initiate a multidisciplinary attack on AIDS encompassing approaches from virology, immunology, epidemiology and public health. Multiple laboratories and departments from four different institutions in Amsterdam joined forces in 1984 with the express purpose of addressing the various problems posed by the AIDS epidemic. They included the Academic Medical Center, the CLB, the University of Amsterdam, the Department of Public Health and the Environment of the Municipal Health Service of Amsterdam. Two additional participants, the Departments of Gay and Lesbian Studies and of Social and Organisational Psychology of the University of Utrecht, were also involved in the ACS right from the beginning. Van der Noordaa remained as its coordinator until 1995, after which R.A. Coutinho of the Municipal Health Service took over (ACS, 1996; ACS, 2001). The ACS also spurred the creation of AIDS research units in participating institutions. Coutinho, for instance, set up a dedicated department of AIDS research at the Municipal

Health Service in 1984. Three different facilities at the Academic Medical Center were set up, starting with the Department of Human Retrovirology, headed by J. Goudsmit. In the hospital an AIDS unit headed by S.A. Danner was established in the Department of Internal Medicine, while J.M.A. Lange was responsible for the AIDS outpatient clinic activities; he also became head of the trial centre called the National Antiviral Therapy Evaluation Centre (NATEC). It was during this period also that the CLB set up its Department of Clinical Viro-Immunology (headed by Frank Miedema) in cooperation with the Laboratory for Experimental and Clinical Immunology of the University of Amsterdam. Later, all of them were successively appointed professor at the University of Amsterdam. In the twentieth-first century researchers of the first generation would be appointed, such as B. Berkhout (in 2002) and H. Schuitemaker (in 2004).

The extensive activities of the ACS participants are evident from its prodigious output: between 1988 and 1995, various members of the ACS published some 188 reports and 24 academic theses in addition to numerous summaries. Studies dealt with a variety of practical concerns, such as prevalence and incidence of infections, risk factors for transmission, sexual behaviour in affected and at-risk populations, the natural history of HIV-1 infections and interventions to limit the disease. It became apparent that the presence of a low-circulating CD4+ number predicts the development of AIDS. Another key area of concern for the cohort was vaccine development and extensive studies were undertaken to find the antibody-eliciting components of the viral envelope. To date one of the most challenging hurdles in this arena has been the antigenic variation in certain envelope proteins.

The epidemiological data collected in the ACS studies gave insights into the prevalence, incidence and risk factors for HIV infections and AIDS. The cohort study among homosexual men started in 1984 and one year later the longitudinal study among injecting drug users followed. Anal-receptive sexual practices were found to be the most important risk factor for transmission among the study participants, most of whom were homosexual men. These and other epidemiological data on transmission were not only important scientifically but also were instrumental in shaping prevention for the HIV/AIDS risk groups. The samples collected from the periodic examinations of AIDS patients, in combination with clinical data and questionnaires that they answered, enabled the ACS to make a systematic study of factors related both to primary infections as well as the natural history of the disease. The biology of HIV – for example, its predilection or specificity for different cell types and affinity for different types of receptors on the surface of various immune cells appeared to have a prognostic relevance. For instance, the cellular tropism of different HIV variants could be explained by their capacity to induce the formation of syncytia in the cells they infected. The infection of cells with HIV depends on the recognition of a combination of molecules or receptors on the cell surface which bind to the virus. A surface antigen called CD4 is necessary, but not sufficient, for HIV to bind to the cell surface; additional co-receptors appeared later to be required for facilitating the fusion of the viral envelope to the cell membrane. These co-receptors also arbitrate the binding-specificity of the virus to different cell types, such as T-cells or macrophages. Whereas SI variants that could induce syncytia were tropic for T-cells, the biologic properties of the non-syncytium (NSI) HIV-1 variants revealed an enhanced tropism for monocytes. The discovery of syncytium-inducing variants proved useful as an independent predictor in the progression to AIDS. In 1988 the first article on the relevance of the HIV-1 phenotype was published and many others should follow (Tersmette et al., 1988; Schuitemaker et al., 1991). The most rapid progression to AIDS was observed in individuals with high-replicating SI HIV-1 isolates; most individuals with low-replicating NSI isolates remained asymptomatic during the study period. Thereupon, studies have been performed to explain the observed differences in cell tropism. In 1995, it was discovered that the coreceptor for T-cell line-tropic SI variants and some macrophage-tropic NSI variants was the α-chemokine cell-surface receptor CXCR4. Studies on the coreceptor usage of NSI variants obtained from progressors in the ACS studies showed that these HIV variants use CCR5 as coreceptor (ACS, 2001, p. 23; Cocchi et al., 1995; Deng et al., 1996; Dragic et al., 1996; Feng et al., 1996; Van Rij et al., 2000). When Tersmette moved to clinical microbiology in the second half of the 1990s, Hanneke Schuitemaker took over his leading role in this part of the ACS.

A turning point in the antiretroviral therapy occurred in 1995 when the use of protease inhibitors was approved. The dual therapy of one protease inhibitor and two reverse transcriptase inhibitors appeared to be a successful combination. The efficacy of the therapy could now be monitored by determination of the HIV-1 RNA plasma viral load (ACS, 2001, p. 34).

A 2013 publication by Antoinette C. van der Kuyl, a senior staff member, offers an overview of the activities of Laboratory of Human Retrovirology (headed since 2002 by B. Berkhout and renamed in 2006 as the Laboratory of Experimental Virology), from 1983 until 2013. The report mentions among others protocols for novel diagnostic assays for detecting HIV superinfections and for measuring amounts of intracellular virus. Other topics covered in the report include studies of drug-resistant mutants, HIV evolution, and

Figure 16   Collaborators of the Amsterdam Cohort Studies on HIV infection and AIDS (1998)

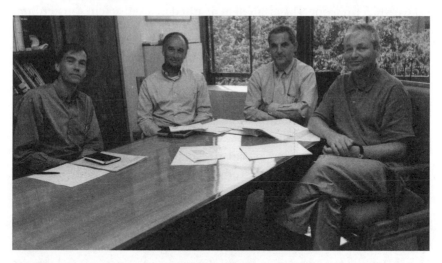

Access to Patients Is Key to the Success of the Dutch Quartet. From left to right: immunologist F. Miedema, public health expert R.A. Couthinho, clinician J. Lange, virologist J. Goudsmit. In the corridors this team was also known as the Amsterdam Politburo.
Reproduction courtesy of R. Coutinho, *Science*, NKI-AVL and Sanquin, Amsterdam

the changing epidemiology of HIV infections linked to immigration from HIV-endemic areas.

The so-called Buck-Goudsmit affair that attracted considerable publicity in the Netherlands in 1990 is worth recounting here, in part because it draws attention to the dangers of pronouncing clinical judgements during the very early stages of basic research (Eijgenraam, 1991). In 1990, a research team headed by H. Buck, a respected organic chemist from Eindhoven Technical University, published what seemed to be a very promising method for interrupting the replication of HIV in the journal *Science*. He synthesized methylated oligonucleotides complementary to portions of the cellular genome integrated HIV DNA, which were supposed to bind to their complements in the integrated virus DNA and thereby prevent the replication of that specific DNA and predicted that his method would lead very quickly to a successful treatment (Buck et al., 1990). Unfortunately, however, his claims that the oligonucleotides blocked virus infectivity could not be substantiated fully when his samples were tested at Goudsmit's laboratory in Amsterdam (Moody et al., 1990; Maddox, 1990). The investigation committee suggested that Goudsmit's 'heavy workload' prevented him from properly supervising his co-workers. Furthermore, Buck's samples were not merely impure; it subsequently appeared that they contained no detectable modified DNA at all. The paper had to be retracted and the disgraced Buck was forced to take early retirement. The affair also resulted in a setback in Amsterdam, but luckily Goudsmit was able to continue his research with the help of new senior staff members and the Laboratory of Human Retrovirology recovered and flourished again.

In 1990 the Academic Medical Center (AMC) was founded separate from yet interwoven with the National AIDS Therapy Evaluation Centre (NATEC) for the purposes of coordinating clinical trials of different anti-HIV therapies with Joep Lange as director. Lange was trained in internal medicine and in 1987 defended a thesis on serological markers in HIV infection. Rather early he had published the results of a study evaluating the dosing and toxicity of the drug AZT among a population of symptom-free HIV-positive patients who were considered to be at high risk for fast progression to full-blown AIDS due to the presence of certain HIV-related antigens in their blood. In 1992, soon after his appointment at NATEC, Lange was also appointed at the World Health Organization's Clinical Research and Product Development branch of the Global Programme on AIDS. He held this position from 1992 to 1995 and played a pivotal role in many international studies on HIV/AIDS, being a strong advocate for improving the access to antiretroviral drugs in low-income countries (Hankins et al., 2014). Tragically Lange was a passenger on the ill-fated Malaysia Airlines Flight 17 from Amsterdam to Kuala Lumpur, which was shot down by a missile on 17 July 2014, leaving no survivors. It is especially poignant in the context of this book, that when he died, Lange was travelling to attend the International AIDS Conference in Melbourne.

Leiden

Leiden University Medical Centre[76]

The Leiden University Medical Centre was officially created in 1996, the result of cooperation between the Faculty of Medicine and the Academic Hospital of the old university. At this time all the laboratories on or near the premises – both those discussed in Chapter 3 and new ones that were established after World War II – came under the common jurisdiction of the University Medical Centre.

76 Leids Universitair Medisch Centrum (LUMC).

Laboratory of Bacteriology and Experimental Pathology and Central Clinical Virology Laboratory

As discussed in Chapter 3, this laboratory was first set up in the 1920s within the Netherlands Institute for Preventive Medicine[77] at Leiden University. NIPG was administratively reorganized in 1960 to become part of the Dutch Health Organisation (TNO-NGO) that was established in 1949 within the Netherlands Organisation for Applied Scientific Research (TNO),[78] a non-profit company focusing on applied science. The laboratory was split off and was transferred to the Medical Faculty and was renamed as Laboratory for Microbiology, however, it did not change location and remained housed in the same building near the Academic Hospital. Much later, in 1980, the laboratory was split into two separate branches: the Central Clinical Bacteriology and Parasitology Laboratory and the Central Clinical Virology Laboratory (Versteeg, 1987).

The veterinary microbiologist J.D. Verlinde, who had been appointed as the head of the Laboratory of Bacteriology and Experimental Pathology in 1941, was promoted to the position of extraordinary professor in 1947 and full professor in 1960; he served in this capacity until 1976. Firmly believing in the mutual benefits between bench science and daily medical practice, he made sure, right from the start, that the laboratory undertook the routine examination of specimens from patients of the neighbouring Academic Hospital. He created an enduring tradition of research on many different infectious viruses, including viruses infecting the central nervous system, enteroviruses, polioviruses, and arboviruses, evidenced by the many publications to emerge from the laboratories during the 1960s and 1970s. His far-reaching influence is also reflected in the appointment of six of his former trainees as professors of virology in different institutions in the country. Verlinde died in 1987, and his former student J. Versteeg was appointed, first as professor of virology in 1978 and then in 1980, as the head of the Central Clinical Virology Laboratory. Among his best-known personal accomplishments is the authorship of *A colour atlas of virology*, published in 1985.

In the early 1950s, the NIPG was designated as a World Health Organization Influenza Centre for the Netherlands. Interestingly, the Netherlands had already played a role in the establishment of such centres. According to a report from the WHO, the impetus for the first WHO World Influenza Centre, set up in 1947 at the National Institute for Medical Research under the direction of Sir Christopher Andrewes in London, 'came from a proposal by

77 Nederlands Instituut voor Preventieve Geneeskunde (NIPG).
78 Nederlandse Organisatie voor toegepast-natuurwetenschappelijk onderzoek (TNO).

the Delegate of the Netherlands who stressed the international importance of influenza and the need to have early information on epidemics wherever in the world they emerged' (Cockburn, 1964, 1973:162). Regrettably, we could not retrieve the identity of the Dutch delegate, but the timing of the event leads us to guess that it must have been one of the three Dutch persons mentioned: NIPG's director J.P. Bijl, J.D. Verlinde or J. Mulder.

During the 1980s the clinical virological laboratory gained recognition for work that resulted in the development of diagnostic tests for the human parvoviruses at Leiden (Brown et al., 1990). The circumstances leading to this development were serendipitous to some extent. In 1986 H.T. Weiland, a senior staff member of the clinical virology laboratory, was requested to consult on the case of a pregnant woman who had acquired an exanthematous disease. Weiland consulted a colleague, the British virologist Mary Anderson, who was involved in a study on the clinical symptoms of human parvovirus B19 infection (Weiland et al., 1987). Following this collaboration, the laboratory began research on parvoviruses, and was successful in producing high quantities of the viral antigens necessary for developing the diagnostic kits.

The arrival of W.J.M. Spaan, who was appointed in 1991 as successor of Versteeg, shifted the focus of the laboratory from applied to basic research on questions about the structure and function of different RNA viruses, such as coronaviruses and hepatitis C virus. At the turn of the twentieth century E.J.H.J. Wiertz was appointed professor in experimental microbiology. A trained veterinarian, Wiertz defended a thesis on T-cell recognition of *Neisseria meningitidis* outer membrane proteins. He became interested in the immune evasion by human cytomegalovirus during a stay as an EMBO[79] fellow at the laboratory of Hidde Ploegh at MIT. In 2009 he moved to the UMC Utrecht, where he continues his research where virology meets immunology and cell biology. After Spaan turned his ambition to governing hospitals, E.J. Snijder, whose research focuses on molecular biology of +RNA (Baltimore classification) virus replication, was appointed professor in 2007. Clinical virology regained its importance at Leiden with the appointment of clinical virologist A.C.M. Kroes as professor in 2003.

Department of Clinical Respiratory Virology

The Department of Clinical Respiratory Virology was created within the Department of Internal Medicine at the Academic Hospital in Leiden not long after the arrival of the internist and virologist J. Mulder from Groningen

---

79   European Molecular Biology Organization (EMBO).

1946 (see Chapter 3). Together with his colleagues J.F.P. Hers and N. Masurel, Mulder conducted internationally recognized investigations on different aspects of the clinical pathology of influenza (Mulder and Masurel, 1958; Hers and Mulder, 1961). Especially remarkable was the discovery by Masurel pinpointing the specific causative agents of pandemics past. During the influenza epidemic of 1956-1957, for example, these investigators noticed that many elderly people – normally at high risk for such infections – remained healthy. The discovery that this age group already had a high level of antibodies to the specific strain of the influenza A virus – called H2N2 – in their serum, which led to the realization that they had been exposed to the virus during the earlier pandemic of 1889/1890 (Mulder and Masurel, 1958). Similar strategies during a 1968 outbreak revealed a common denominator with the 1900 pandemic – the H3N2 strain, also of the influenza A virus (Masurel, 1969). Around the reorganization of the NIPG in 1960 the laboratory of Mulder was recognized by the WHO as National Influenza Centre in the Netherlands instead of the NIPG laboratory. Unfortunately, this laboratory at the Department of Internal Medicine closed operations towards the end of the 1960s, unable to survive the double blows of Mulder's sudden death in 1965 and Masurel's departure to a new medical faculty in Rotterdam in 1969. Its legacy endured, however, because Masurel's new laboratory in Rotterdam was recognized as a WHO centre in 1971 (Masurel, 1971).

Laboratory for Tropical Hygiene

We include here a short note on the fate of the Laboratory for Tropical Hygiene, which was headed by Paul Flu until his death in 1946. After the appointment of J.E. Dinger as professor of tropical hygiene in 1947 this laboratory remained housed at Rapenburg in the centre of the city. After the proclamation of the Republic of Indonesia in 1946 and the transfer of Dutch New Guinea to Indonesia in 1963 it was difficult for Dutch tropical doctors to find employment elsewhere in the tropics. This caused changes in the Dutch tropical medicine teaching and research programmes (Beukers, 1989). When Dinger retired in 1962, the Minister of Education, Arts and Sciences decided that the chair of tropical hygiene had to be abolished; from then onwards the laboratory shifted in focus primarily to parasitology (Beukers, 1989). Virology, however, remained a secondary interest as evidenced by the fact that H.L. Wolff continued to publish work on virology into the early 1980s (Croon and Wolff, 1980). As mentioned above, the laboratory was transferred in 1981 to premises of the Medical Faculty and in 1996 in the LUMC.

Utrecht/Bilthoven

National Institute of Public Health and Environment Bilthoven

The National Institute for Public Health (RIV)[80] had been set up in Utrecht in 1934 by merging the pre-existing Central Laboratory for the Public Health and the State Serologic Institute, already located in the city. In 1951, the Laboratory for Viral and Rickettsial Diseases was set up within RIV under somewhat questionable circumstances as a diagnostic laboratory operating out of an old stable (Van Zon, 1990, p. 251). For many years it functioned as research laboratory as well as the primary provider of viral diagnostic services not only for the nearby Academic Hospital but also many other hospitals and laboratories in the country; reports were conveyed via the postal service, and by telephone when needed. Fortunately, before any major mishaps occurred, it moved in 1958 to a new facility in Bilthoven, where it is headquartered to this day, although the diagnostic services were transferred to the UMC Utrecht in 1993. The institute underwent further organizational changes when in 1984 it was expanded by merging with the National Institute for Drinking Water Supply and Institute for Waste Research and renamed as the National Institute for Public Health and the Environment (RIVM) to represent its broadened scope.[81]

R. Gispen was appointed as the first director of the Laboratory for Viral and Rickettsial Diseases (later called the Laboratory for Virology). Trained by Van Loghem in medical microbiology and tropical hygiene at Amsterdam, Gispen had left to work at the Queen Wilhelmina Institute for Hygiene and Bacteriology in Batavia in the Dutch East Indies soon after completing his thesis in 1927 (Cohen and Kampelmacher, 2001). In 1951 he returned to the Netherlands and became director Fundamental Scientific Research at the National Institute of Public Health, in this function he initiated already the start of the virology laboratory. He was involved in the new housing development of the institute in Bilthoven that was funded by the European Recovery Program initiated by the US Secretary of State George Marshall in 1947.

Jacoba G. Kapsenberg, daughter of the late G. Kapsenberg from Groningen, joined the Laboratory for Virology in 1956 and thanks to her efforts the

---

80   Rijksinstituut voor de Volksgezondheid (RIV).
81   Rijksinstituut voor de Drinkwatervoorziening; Instituut voor Afvalstoffenonderzoek en Rijksinstituut voor Volksgezondheid en Milieu, respectively.

laboratory functioned in the capacity of the national virological reference laboratory. Different functions of the laboratory were, to a large extent, similar to those of the Virus Reference Laboratory of the PHLS in London. Common tasks, for example, included investigation of less common viral agents as smallpox and rabies. Furthermore, the laboratory served as reference for typing of viruses isolated but not identified in other laboratories, such as enteroviruses (polioviruses) and respiratory viruses; studying and developing techniques which might be of value in other virus laboratories was another task (Bradstreet et al., 1964). In its original remit, the laboratory was also intended to provide diagnostic serves and scientific support for the production of vaccines against smallpox and poliomyelitis, but, as mentioned earlier, this function ceased after 1991.

The RIV Laboratory for Virology turned out to be pivotal in the development of clinical virology in the Netherlands, as it faced and met with one epidemic challenge after another. In 1951, very soon after it was set up, the Laboratory for Viral and Rickettsial Diseases was confronted with an outbreak of smallpox in Tilburg. Luckily, Gispen had acquired experience with control measures and laboratory investigation of smallpox while in the East Indies and under his leadership the lab successfully met the challenges posed by this outbreak. Two serious epidemics of poliomyelitis followed in 1953 and again in 1956, resulting in a governmental decision in 1957 to offer mass immunization on a voluntary basis (see Chapter 9). Free inactivated vaccinations against polio (of the type originally developed by Jonas Salk) were offered to children up to fourteen years of age all over the country (Lindner and Blume, 2006). In the meantime, the 1956 influenza epidemic intensified the activity in the field of the respiratory viruses. The 1962 outbreak of rabies in Amsterdam also brought the diagnosis of this disease under the purview of RIV. This incident offered an opportunity for testing a vaccine developed in-house, which appeared to have fewer side effects than the then available vaccines (Gispen et al., 1965).

As a result of their work on so many different viruses, the RIV Laboratory for Virology also established a considerable reputation as a repository of meticulously typed strains, especially of enteric and respiratory viruses. Typing was based on eliciting in horses large quantities of specific antibodies to known viruses by hyperimmunization. Unknown viruses could be typed by testing their reactivity against a panel of such antibodies to known viruses (Kapsenberg, 1988b). This approach allowed for the rapid typing of a large number of viruses through micro-neutralization. In 1968, for example, the laboratory had produced equine antisera against some 20 echovirus serotypes and Coxsackievirus A9; by the 1980s the range for these typing pools had expanded considerably and the repertoire broadened to include separate pools for typing polioviruses and Coxsackie B.

As indicated in Chapter 3, discussions about the centralization of production of smallpox vaccines had begun as early as 1934 and the production was restricted to three institutes in Amsterdam, Rotterdam and Groningen. Twenty years later, in 1954, all production was centralized at the RIV laboratory in Bilthoven, using a Danish strain from the Statens Serum Institute in Copenhagen, because of its low rate of post-vaccinial encephalitis. The 1964 demonstration that the side effects of another strain called Elstree were less frequent and less serious than the Copenhagen strain prompted a switch to the use of the latter in vaccine production (Polak et al., 1964). Meanwhile, the newer virus cultivation methods, using embryonated chicken eggs and cell cultures, replaced the use of live animals, which greatly increased the efficiency of vaccine production. From 1958 onward, vaccines could be lyophilized, which greatly extended their durability over time (Van Zon, 1990, pp. 211, 251, 283).

In 1966 RIV became a participant in the WHO's smallpox-eradication programme, where the capacity of its production line and the advisory role of the virologist/epidemiologist M.F. Polak were significant elements. The very next year the institute was recognized as an International Reference Centre for Smallpox Vaccine in 1967 (Arita, 1988, p. 547). The eradication programme ended with the 1979 declaration by WHO certifying the global eradication of smallpox. In 1981, escorted by police, A.C. Hekker, then the head of the virology laboratory, personally transported the last remaining smallpox viruses from the Netherlands to the repository at the Centers for Disease Control in Atlanta in the USA (Van Zon, p. 279). Other members of the RIV Laboratory for Virology who played important roles in propagating the vaccinia virus for the production of vaccines included B. Hofman and L.M. Brans, who came to RIV from Leiden in 1957, and A.L. van Wezel, who arrived in 1967 (Brans, 1959; Polak and Brans, 1962; Polak et al., 1964).

Vaccination against polio was introduced in 1957 in the Netherlands and as mentioned earlier, the inactivated vaccine was used right from the start. Although over 95 per cent of the general population of one year of age received vaccinations, the occurrence of local epidemics of poliomyelitis persisted into the 1960s and 1970s. The largest of these outbreaks occurred in 1978 with 110 cases reported in that part of the population which had not received any vaccinations (Bijkerk et al., 1979). The Laboratory for Virology was intensively involved in the diagnostics and preventive measures related to this outbreak. Similar outbreaks occurred again in 1992/1993 when poliovirus type 3 infections were introduced into a large, socially clustered community that had refused vaccination for religious reasons (Oostvogel et. al., 1994; Van der Avoort et al., 1998). Thus, the important international work on public health and disease prevention started by RIV scientists Gispen, Kapsenberg and Van Wezel was continued by the likes of Van Loon and Van der Avoort.

Other virus laboratories in the Netherlands also took advantage of Van Wezel's improvements to methods for the production of viruses to use in vaccines, particularly his technique for dispersal of monkey kidney cells and growing them at high density on microbeads (Plotkin and Vidor, 2008: p. 605; Van Wezel, 1967). His method used tertiary (cynomolgus) monkey kidney cells that were excellent for the propagation of enteroviruses and respiratory viruses. Because these cells were readily available at all diagnostic virus laboratories, the adoption of Van Wezel's method greatly reduced the number of monkeys needed for vaccine production and diagnostics.

Gispen retired as head of the Laboratory for Virology in 1975 and was succeeded by A.C. Hekker, who had studied medicine in Leiden where he had been inspired by Verlinde to specialize in vaccinology (Kapsenberg, 1988a). In 1957 he began an investigation into the inactivated polio vaccine produced at RIV, which culminated in a PhD dissertation on the subject (Hekker, 1962; Kapsenberg, 1988). From polio he turned to smallpox and played a prominent role in RIV's participation in the WHO smallpox-eradication programme in the 1960s. Upon his promotion as the head of the laboratory, Hekker turned to more basic problems in medical virology. In particular, he became interested in specific IgM serological tests. After the advent of AIDS in the 1980s he also took a leading role in ensuring that various materials became readily available in the Netherlands for the diagnostic virology laboratories. For example, in 1985, when Western blot assays were not yet commercially available in the Netherlands, Hekker made arrangement for the necessary HIV-antigen to be purchased from the Americans and distributed among five Dutch laboratories recognized as HIV-confirmatory facilities (A.M. van Loon, personal communication, 2017).

A.M. van Loon succeeded Hekker as the head of the Virology Laboratory. He came from the Virology Department of Radboud University in Nijmegen. He aimed to stimulate more scientific research in and publications from the laboratory besides the regular reports of the virology laboratory in RIVM's annual reports. In 1989, under Van Loon's leadership, the virology laboratory became involved in the Global Polio Eradication Initiative as well as the Global Polio Laboratory Network (GPLN) of the WHO. One of the main responsibilities of the GPLN was to distinguish between polio and other causes of acute flaccid paralysis (AFP). In December 1989 Van Loon and Oostvogel organized a workshop on laboratory methods for the diagnosis of poliomyelitis at Bilthoven. The impetus for this workshop was a decision by the WHO to establish the cell culture techniques for isolation and identification of polioviruses developed by Cootje Kapsenberg and Anton van Wezel as the standard for nearly all 150 laboratories in its Global Polio Network. The appearance of laboratory scientist H.G.A.M. van der Avoort as Santa Claus distributing chocolate letters caused much hilarity and is still vividly remembered by the participants of the workshop. The outcome of this workshop was the designation of the Virology Department as a WHO Collaborating Centre for Reference and Research on Poliomyelitis the following year. To the present day, the laboratory serves as a member of the WHO Polio Laboratory Network specially tasked with the preparation and distribution of standardized reagents and cell lines, not only within the Netherlands but also throughout Europe and globally. Meanwhile, Van Loon and Van der Avoort continued to play an important role in the Global Polio Eradication Initiative of the WHO and dozens of Technology Transfer workshops organized from RIVM have followed in years since the first workshop.

Over the years, the question of whether or not RIVM was obliged to perform clinical diagnostic facilities for hospitals and general practitioners had become a matter under consideration within the institute. In 1991 the directorate decided that such routine functions did not fall under the core duties of RIVM so the diagnostic unit was moved to the Academic Hospital of the University of Utrecht (UMC Utrecht) in 1993. Van Loon was appointed head of this laboratory and for a time pulled double duty between the new position and his older function as head at Bilthoven. In 1995 T.G. Kimman was appointed head of the research laboratory. His arrival occurred at a time when the focus of the epidemiologic research at RIVM varied, depending on either public health needs or on technical developments. Whereas, for instance, the epidemiology of bacterial causes of gastrointestinal diseases was important during the 1970s when such infections posed serious public health problems, the possibilities opened up by the invention of the polymerase chain reaction based and associated techniques in the 1990s caused a shift in priorities to studies of such viral pathogens as rotavirus and norovirus (Lodder et al., 1999; Van der Heide et al., 2005; Vinjé and Koopmans, 1996). Kimman was succeeded in 2002 by Marion P.G. Koopmans, a distinguished veterinary scientist who studied the interface between human and animal virus infection; she initiated research on gastrointestinal infections caused by viruses, such as Norwalk-like viruses, rotaviruses, and norovirus. Koopmans maintained this position until 2014, when she moved to Rotterdam in 2014 as A.D.M.E. Osterhaus's successor as head of the Viroscience Department at Erasmus MC. In 2006, she had already been appointed professor in Rotterdam to teach in public health and virus infections.

Another figure who deserves recognition is the late J.C. de Jong, probably best known for his work on influenza. Between joining RIVM in 1973 and retiring in 1998, he played an important role in identifying adenoviruses types 40 and 41 as causative agents of viral gastroenteritis and identifying two others – adenovirus types 50 and 51 – in stool specimens of immunosuppressed patients (De Jong et al., 1983 and 1999). Although his research was not sufficiently appreciated by the management, who had a different vision for the future of the institute in public health, De Jong was not deterred, and in fact, conducted some of his most significant work after his retirement in 1998. After taking early retirement he moved to the Department of Virology of the Medical Faculty in Rotterdam in 1997 (Van Doornum and Osterhaus, 2017).

Laboratory for Medical Microbiology, UMC Utrecht

As described above, diagnostic virology for the Academic Hospital of the Utrecht University was carried out for a long time at the Laboratory for Virology of the National Institute of Public Health (RIV). When in the 1990s the decision was taken that clinical virology was not a main task of RIVM, the diagnostic unit was moved in 1992-1993 from RIVM to the University Medical Centre of the University of Utrecht (UMC Utrecht) that was now located in a new building at the Uithof since the mid-1980s. As mentioned above A.M van Loon held the same position in the UMC Utrecht from 1992 until 2013. He continued research on enteroviruses within European Concerted Action programs and collaborated in the Global Polio Eradication Initiative of the WHO, applying newly developed molecular diagnostic tools. Clinical studies were performed in cooperation with clinicians of UMC Utrecht on respiratory viruses and on herpesvirus infections in transplant patients and neonates. HIV antiviral drug resistance studies were set up by C.A.B. Boucher and R. Schuurman, who had moved in 1995 from the AMC in Amsterdam to Utrecht.

University of Utrecht, Veterinary Faculty

Officially established in 1925, University of Utrecht boasted such significant pioneers of virology as Frenkel and Verlinde among its students, well before it established its Institute for Veterinary Virology in 1955. Lest readers think there is a spelling error in the name of the institute, we assure you that there is no mistake – the faculty made the deliberate choice to use the etymologically correct term 'virulogy' instead of the more common 'virology'. Jac. Jansen, who until then was the chair of infectious diseases, became the head of the new laboratory. Even before taking over in this capacity, he had made waves with his recommendation that Utrecht University award Richard Shope, a virologist trained as a physician, with an honorary degree in veterinary medicine for his achievements in research on rabbit papillomas, Aujesky disease and the aetiology of swine influenza (Tyrrell, 1998). Jansen had to defend his proposal before a rather important group within the university's Senate, who considered the nomination of a non-veterinarian as a *testimonium paupertatis*[82] of veterinary researchers (Haalboom, 2017, p. 91; Jansen, 1951). Evidently, he was successful in his arguments, for the university did make the award in 1951, but the episode points to the somewhat strained relationship between veterinarians and medical doctors at that time.

Another member of the veterinary faculty who merits a mention is M. Horzinek, who brought youthful enthusiasm and optimism to the Institute of Virology, which needed some fresh blood at the time of his appointment in 1971. Friends, colleagues and former students, including H. Lutz, M.P.G. Koopmans, A.D.M.E. Osterhaus and P.J.M. Rottier would describe him as the 'founding father' of veterinary virology in the Netherlands (Lutz et al., 2016). Many of his 'scientific offspring' have become professors in leading positions within and outside country and his legacy continues to contribute to the highly productive field of virology research in the Netherlands. His students and colleagues W.J.M. Spaan, A.D.M.E. Osterhaus, M.P.G. Koopmans, B.A.M. van der Zeijst, P.J.M. Rottier, R.H. Meloen, and H.G.M. Niesters were appointed to positions in Leiden, Rotterdam, Utrecht, and Groningen.

Groningen

UMC Groningen[83] and Virology Unit of the Regional Public Health Laboratory of the Municipal Health Service

Despite the long and illustrious history of its medical faculty, the University of Groningen did not enjoy an equivalent reputation in virology. The subject

82 Proof of indigence (translated by G. van Doornum using Pinkster, 2003).
83 University Medical Centre Groningen.

remained fallow through the 1960s, until recognizing the lacuna, the university appointed virologist J.B. Wilterdink as a professor of microbiology in 1970, specifically tasking him with building virology up (Westendorp Boerma, 1977). With the exception of a short period from 1946 to 1952, it was the Regional Public Health Laboratory of the Municipal Health Service that performed routine clinical diagnostic work in virology. Clinical virology tests were introduced at the Virology unit of the Regional Laboratory that was housed within the UMC Groningen by F.P. Schröder and later also by J. Schirm, while Wilterdink served as stimulating advisor (Schröder, 1992). They successfully established a modern virology diagnostic unit within a few years. Jurjen Schirm's nomination as president of the European Society of Clinical Virology (2001-2004) reflects the widespread recognition of his work in Groningen.

Although he had performed research on enteroviruses under Verlinde in Leiden, Wilterdink's interests shifted after his appointment in Groningen, and after close consultation with his collaborators, he decided to shift his research focus to persistent rather than acute virus infections (Westendorp Boerma, 1977). He became especially interested in the possible association of herpes viruses with cancer, a topic very much in keeping with the ascendance of cancer virus studies in general. Under his enthusiastic leadership as an editor, the first edition of the Dutch textbook *Medische virologie* (Medical virology) for students was published in 1976 (Wilterdink et al., 1976). After his retirement in 1992 the medical virology chair remained vacant for fifteen years, although the appointment of cell biologist J. Wilschut in 1999 maintained at least some continuity on the basic virology front. Clinical virology at UMC Groningen resumed with the appointment of H.G.M. Niesters, a molecular biologist from Rotterdam, to the virology chair and the founding of a diagnostic virology laboratory in 2007.

Nijmegen/Tilburg

Radboud University Nijmegen

Situated in one of the oldest cities in the Netherlands, Radboud University was established in 1923 as the Catholic University of Nijmegen. Its medical faculty was founded in 1951 and J. van der Veen was appointed as the professor of hygiene, bacteriology and virology in 1954.

Van der Veen came to the position with experience in both academic and industrial settings. After studying medicine in Utrecht, he obtained research experience during his military service working on influenza with J. Mulder in Leiden in 1947-1948. Thereafter he started training in bacteriology with Charlotte Ruys in Amsterdam. During this time, he also headed the medical department of the Weesp-based pharmaceutical company Philips Duphar, which produced vaccines against influenza and whooping cough. In 1951, following a short stint in New York, Van der Veen moved to Tilburg as the head of the Laboratory of Bacteriology of the St Elisabeth Hospital there. When he was appointed professor of hygiene, bacteriology and virology in Nijmegen in 1954, he accepted only on the express condition that he would continue his work in Tilburg even though it was 70 km away. Former students and colleagues, such as M.F. Peeters, who would later become his successor in Tilburg, remember Van der Veen's dedication; every week he would personally transport both colleagues and laboratory materials from Tilburg to Nijmegen to conduct practical classes in microbiology and virology for medical students (Brabers, 2009, p. 113; Peeters, 2001; M.F. Peeters, personal communication to G. van Doornum, 2005).

Van der Veen did not actually move to Nijmegen until 1960 after the research laboratory facilities were built properly, but meanwhile, for financial reasons, he remained affiliated as a consultant with the hospital laboratory in Tilburg (Brabers, 2009, p. 114). His main research focused on the respiratory viruses, particularly adenovirus infections, and he undertook a series of investigations on the interactions between viruses and white blood cells (Van der Veen and Kok, 1957; Pereira et al., 1963; Van der Logt et al., 1982). In 1976, upon the request of his clinician colleagues at the academic hospital, his laboratory also began to provide clinical diagnostic services in virology. Under his leadership, scientists A.M. van Loon and J.T.M. van der Logt developed new ELISA protocols, notably a haemadsorption immunosorbent technique for the detection of immunoglobulin M against the parainfluenza virus types 1, 2, and 3 (Van der Logt et al., 1982a and 1982b). He retired in 1986 but his chair remained vacant until 1991, when J.A.A. (Mieke) Hoogkamp-Korstanje was appointed professor of medical microbiology, but she was more concentrated on bacteriology. Van Loon served as interim head of the virology branch for a time during this period, but ceased to do so after his move to RIVM in 1988.

Since the 1990s, the medical microbiology department has made great strides in the adoption of cutting-edge techniques of molecular biology, especially in the study of enteroviruses and human papillomaviruses, developed by the like of W.J. Melchers, J. Zoll and F.J. van Kuppeveld. These new methods have been applied with great profit for diagnostic procedures, epidemiology and research not only in virology, but also in bacteriology and mycology. But despite such advances, the authorities delayed making a decision about establishing a separate chair in virology and it was not until February 2001 that the medical virologist J.D.M. Galama delivered his inaugural lecture. His research was focused on the virology and immunology of measles and enterovirus infections (Galama, 2001). In 2004 Van Kuppeveld was honoured with the Beijerinck Premium for his excellent virus research; in 2012 he moved to Utrecht where he was appointed professor at the Faculty of Veterinary Medicine for his research on virus-host interactions, antiviral drugs, and vaccine development.

St Elisabeth Hospital, Tilburg

As described above, Van der Veen was appointed head of the Laboratory of Bacteriology and Serology in 1951. His arrival was marked by the confirmation – by Verlinde's lab in Leiden – of a smallpox outbreak in Tilburg; as it happens, the last such incident in the Netherlands. Control measures were instituted with the help of RIV, headed at the time by Gispen. According to G.J. Sas, who covered the episode in his thesis (1954), the outbreak likely began with the infection of an animal-dealer, the index patient, through contact with a vulture that he had imported from India. As Sas reported, the good vaccination status in the city and vicinity meant that the epidemic did not spread extensively – a total of 51 people contracted the disease and there were only two deaths.

It was Van der Veen who initiated diagnostic virological techniques in the laboratory. Cell culture techniques, which were introduced in 1955, proved especially useful during the poliomyelitis epidemic that struck the following year. The work on the diagnosis of respiratory infections resulted in a thesis, *Infectious respiratory diseases by adenoviruses among military recruits using the cell culture technique*, defended by G.J.P.M. Kok in 1957. After Van der Veen's final departure from Tilburg in 1982, M.F. Peeters, who had trained in biology, medicine and medical microbiology in Nijmegen, became responsible for the clinical virology. He took advantage of the facilities to culture cells and was also involved in the establishment of an in vitro fertilization unit in cooperation with the hospital's gynaecology and obstetrics department. In 1990, he introduced molecular biology into the clinical microbiology laboratory, and in 1996 expanded the team with two molecular biologists, although the activities of the newer arrivals focused more on the detection of bacteria.

Rotterdam

Regional Public Health Laboratory of the Municipal Health Service of Rotterdam

In the early part of the twentieth century, the medical needs of the people of Rotterdam were served primarily by Coolsingel Hospital, which was established between 1839 and 1848. Although the hospital building was destroyed during the 1940 bombing of Rotterdam, it was not replaced for nearly two decades until the Municipal Dijkzigt Hospital opened its doors in 1961. It was at this time that clinical virology began in Rotterdam. H. Esseveld, a bacteriologist who followed a training programme on mycology, parasitology and virology in the USA after World War II, was involved in drawing up plans for the new hospital that was to be built on the premises of the Hoboken complex (Bänffer et al., 1979). But in 1950, he incorporated into the designs, a combined bacteriology and virology unit within the central microbiology laboratory of the future Dijkzigt Hospital. M.S.M. Daniels-Bosman was made responsible for the virology unit when it opened in 1961, and worked at first with the help of two technicians on cell cultures and the serological tests. Although a municipal hospital, the tests conducted at this facility were considered as research rather than diagnostics, largely because reimbursement for virology tests was not regulated properly.

One of the earliest studies emerging from this laboratory that was published in the NTvG was an investigation of a case of congenital cytomegaly, using material from urine samples to grow viruses in a cell culture (Daniels-Bosman and De Villeneuve, 1963). In 1963 G.J.P Schaap, who came from Amsterdam, took over the responsibility for the virology. The cells that were used in the 1960s were primary monkey kidney cells derived from adult monkey tissue obtained from the Leiden University Hospital, T-cells (derived from human kidney cells) from Tilburg, courtesy of Van der Veen, and human foetal lung fibroblasts as a semi-continuous cell line. Later continuous cell lines, such as Vero cells, LLC-MK2 and RK-13 cells, were used. Schaap displayed ingenuity and ability to devise and maintain instruments. He looked like a fully qualified serviceman when the 'The Super Paljas', an ingenious cell culture instrument, had to be started up or sterilized (R. Woudenberg, personal communication, 1985).

The Dijkzigt Hospital underwent further renovations and was converted into a university hospital following a 1966 decision to add a medical faculty – the seventh in the Netherlands – to the University in Rotterdam. The virology laboratory expanded under the capable leadership of Schaap and extended its scope to studies on CMV infections in pregnancy and the presence of antibodies against the varicella zoster virus. From 1970 the laboratory, which remained in its Dijkzigt Hospital location, became responsible for providing diagnostic services for the Municipal Health Service. In 1973 it moved to twentieth floor of the new building of the Medical Faculty. Meanwhile, however, the Municipal Health Service felt the need to have its own autonomous laboratory on the spot, and in 1977 moved the epidemiological virology unit and part of clinical virology to a new building of the Municipal Health Service at the Schiedamsedijk. Designing this Virology Laboratory of the Regional Laboratory of the Rotterdam Municipal Health Service required a great effort of Schaap. Equipment and facilities at the new location comprised autoclaves, deep freezers for the storage of virus stocks, fluorescence microscopes, an electron microscope and in the attic a facility for housing small laboratory animals, such as mice, hamsters, guinea pigs, and pigeons.

In 1978 the Netherlands was confronted by a poliovirus epidemic that demanded much of the time of the personnel of the laboratory. Other topics pursued included diagnostics of imported viral diseases, Q-fever, respiratory viruses, rubella, enterovirus typing, and rotavirus typing. The viruses that were needed for the preparation of viral antigens employed for serological diagnosis of imported viral diseases as dengue, O'nyong-nyong, Chikungunya, infections caused by Sindbis virus, West Nile virus, Rift Valley virus, and Ross River virus were obtained from Van Tongeren when he retired from the VUmc in Amsterdam. Molecular biological assays were introduced in 1981 when Johannes Buitenwerf, a molecular biologist, joined the laboratory; he started rotavirus diagnostics using electrophoresis, as well as the polymerase chain reaction technique within some years.

After Schaap's retirement in 1983, A.M. Dingemans-Dumas took over the responsibility as head of the clinical virology laboratory. Her rise through the ranks is worthy of special notice because she had commenced her career as a technician in the laboratory in 1965. With the establishment of the medical faculty in Rotterdam, she completed a bachelor's and a master's degree in medicine besides her laboratory work, and later had a traineeship in medical microbiology. She became a staff member in 1977 and maintained the position until 1995, when the laboratory was transferred to the Zuiderziekenhuis, a hospital in the south of Rotterdam. At that time Dingemans-Dumas moved to the Department Infectious Diseases of the Municipal Health Service, because of the decision by the municipal authorities of Rotterdam that a Regional Public Health Laboratory was not the city's responsibility. The authorities no longer considered diagnostic virology (including the laboratory diagnosis of imported viral diseases) to be their public health responsibility, but as the task of general or academic hospitals. Such policies, which were pursued by the municipality of Rotterdam as well as by the directorate of the National Institute of Public Health, diverged from those pursued before the 1990s.

Erasmus MC

The medical faculty and the academic hospital in Rotterdam were relatively young. In 1966 a bill attempting to temporarily restrict the number of medical students was rejected in the House of Representatives. But after the interpellation of the minister, a motion to promote a medical faculty in Rotterdam was immediately proposed and passed the House of Representatives, in recognition of the need to extend the training facilities for medical doctors (Van Raalte, 1977, p. 207). The Dijkzigt Hospital that was renovated to meet the standards of an academic hospital and the medical faculty was established in 1966, merging with the existing Foundation of Higher Clinical Training. Andries Querido, a professor of internal medicine from Leiden, who had worked with André Lwoff at the Pasteur Institute in 1938, was the founder of the Medical Faculty (Mandema, 2010; Querido, 1971, p. 262; Querido, 1990, pp. 60-79, 191-212).

In 1971 the Sophia Children's Hospital located on other premises joined forces with the Dijkzigt Hospital to form the Academic Hospital Rotterdam. At that time N. Masurel was recruited as the head of the virology department, he too came from Leiden, where he worked on influenza with Mulder and Hers at the Unit for Respiratory Virology of the Department of Internal Medicine. He continued to focus his research on influenza and, under his leadership, the WHO National Influenza Centre for the Netherlands also moved from Leiden to Rotterdam, officially on 1 May 1971 (Masurel, 1971). Administratively, Masurel had to expend considerable efforts on organizing the geography of different functions of the laboratory: the basic research laboratory was housed in a new building of the Faculty of Medicine, while the clinical virology services were divided between two locations: one in the renovated Dijkzigt Hospital at the Hoboken complex and the other in the Sophia Children's Hospital, which until 1993 was housed elsewhere at the Gordelweg in Rotterdam. In 1977 the virological epidemiology unit, headed by Schaap, and also part of the clinical diagnostic unit, where tests for other hospitals in the region and local general practitioners were performed, was split off and transferred from the academic hospital to the municipal health service. It lasted until 1993 when the children's hospital at the Gordelweg was closed and then moved to a new

Figure 17   Collaborators of the Erasmus MC Department of Virology (2019)
a: A.D.M.E. Osterhaus; b: R.A.M. Fouchier; c: G.F. Rimmelzwaan

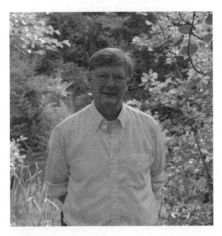

A.D.M.E. Osterhaus. The Research Center for Emerging Infections and Zoonosis (RIZ) of the University of Veterinary Medicine Hannover (TiHo) is a 'one health' research center embedded in the University of Veterinary Medicine in Hannover. The Dutch scientist in virology, Prof. A.D.M.E. Osterhaus, PhD, DVM, is scientific head of RIZ.
Reproduction courtesy of Lourens Gengler (photo) and TiHo Hannover

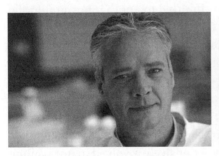
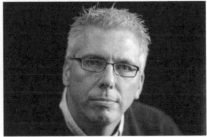

R.A.M. Fouchier, expert in molecular virology and virus evolution
Reproduction courtesy of Erasmus MC, Rotterdam, and L. Willemse (photo)

G.F. Rimmelzwaan, viroimmunologist
Reproduction courtesy of Erasmus MC, Rotterdam and TiHo, Hannover, and L. Willemse (photo)

building at the Hoboken complex where the medical faculty and the Academic Hospital were situated. Besides these organizational duties he continued the study of the drift and shifts of the influenza viruses and immunization of groups at risk (Masurel and Anker, 1978; Masurel, 1979)

The Department of Virology of Erasmus MC Rotterdam underwent a rapid expansion in clinical virology and research after 1990. Masurel retired in 1991 and A.D.M.E. Osterhaus was appointed as professor in virology in 1993. He was trained as a veterinarian in Utrecht, where he received his virology education in the laboratory of M. Horzinek. As head of the Immunobiology Department of RIVM, he described the first phocid herpes virus and the first phocid distemper virus in 1985 and 1988, respectively (Osterhaus et al., 1985; Osterhaus et al., 1988). When he arrived in Rotterdam, the bulk of his research group at RIVM moved to Rotterdam, where their work on measles, HIV, herpes viruses, and exotic virus infections continued. Research on influenza viruses was broadened to respiratory viruses in general. A vivid and vigorous personality with a passion for travelling, Osterhaus may be compared to the principal character in Ludovico Ariosto's *Orlando furioso*,[84] who travelled all over the world from Frisia and Selandia in Holland to the volcano Mount Etna on Sicily and to the River Ganges in India (Van Dooren, 1999, pp. 227-235). With Osterhaus as head, the department expanded its staff and broadened its research interests, and thus acquired an international reputation for excellence. His interest in virus infections in wild life did not diminish after his nomination at the Erasmus University, and he established a unit where specimens could be submitted for the diagnosis of exotic virus infections. In the 1990s, the laboratory also took over the task of the diagnostics of imported viral diseases, which had been given up by RIVM. A notable success in this area was the successful diagnosis of rabies in a Moroccan patient who had first been admitted to another hospital in the Netherlands (Groen et al., 1998). Under Osterhaus, the laboratory also became a WHO Reference and Research Centre for ARBO viruses and haemorrhagic fever virus infections. Furthermore, it received accreditation by the WHO as Measles and Rubella National Reference Laboratory.

In 1988 the Dijkzigt Hospital was confronted with iatrogenic hepatitis B among patients of the in vitro fertilization program and later in 1995 also among heart transplant patients (Alberda et al., 1989; Osterhaus et al., 1998). The Department of Virology was extensively involved in unravelling and resolving this problem. In 1997 the department was able to identify the avian influenza A H5N1 virus that was isolated in Hong Kong from humans, thanks largely to J.C. de Jong, who had moved to Rotterdam after his retirement from RIVM in 1998. In 1997 while yet in Utrecht, De Jong had been consulted by W.L. Lim, an overseas colleague at the government Virus Unit in Queen Mary Hospital, Hong Kong, who had isolated a 'new' non-typable strain of an avian influenza. Under little pressure from Osterhaus, by then head of the department, De Jong went in person to Hong Kong to exclude laboratory contamination as cause of an avian influenza virus which had proven lethal for a three-year-old boy. This strain was typed as

84 *Razende Roeland.*

an avian influenza virus H5N1. The virus identification was important as it was the first documented isolation of influenza A virus of this subtype from humans (De Jong et al., 1997). E.C. Claas and G.F. Rimmelzwaan were important participants in the laboratory work back in Rotterdam (Claas et al., 1998). Other newer landmark achievements of this laboratory include the identification of human metapneumovirus (2000), SARS coronavirus (2003), and avian influenza A H7N7 virus (2003), performed by researchers, such as R.A. Fouchier, T. Kuiken, and G.F. Rimmelzwaan (Fouchier et al., 2005). All three researchers would be appointed to chairs in molecular virology (2007), immunovirology (2010) and pathology (2009), respectively. J. de Jong was also instrumental in the discovery of both HMPV and coronavirus NL63. In addition, at the clinical virology side chairs were instituted in 2007 on which G.J.J. van Doornum and C.A. Boucher were appointed.

Maastricht

Maastricht UMC

As in Rotterdam, the medical faculty in Maastricht owes its existence to the growing need for training opportunities for medical students after the 1960s. Although the national shortage of training facilities was already being addressed, the university in Maastricht established its medical faculty, started more or less unlawfully, a year before official permission was granted in 1975. Two distinguishing features of the medical faculty established there included a problem-based learning system of education and a mandate to link medical research to primary care. With the arrival of Cathrien Bruggeman as head of the Department of Medical Microbiology in 1994, virology received more attention, particularly in the areas of cytomegalovirus infections (basic research) and in-patient care.

General hospitals

From the 1970s onwards an increasing number of laboratories in top clinical training hospitals began to offer viral diagnostics services, rather than relying on outside laboratories to provide such services. With the availability of techniques such as enzyme-linked immunosorbent assays and the growing automation and integration of instruments, more and more hospital laboratories were able to perform serological assays. In addition, they also began to include cell culture facilities for cultivating viruses. By 1990, 23 university and general hospital laboratories participated in a national external quality assessment scheme for virus culture and serology (SKMS, 1990). Molecular methods entered the diagnostic routine in general hospitals in the course of the 1990s. This transition was facilitated by the change of the reimbursement system in 1996, under which these assays qualified for refunds.

Military Medical Service

After World War II, when he played an important role in the Resistance against the German occupants, B.J.W. Beunders was re-conscripted to military service and nominated as the head of the Preventive Military Medicine section. He deserves special mention because of the role he played in selecting medical doctors who were drafted for military service and trained at the Military School of Hygiene and Preventive Medicine. He offered these enthusiastic and talented young doctors research positions via the Inspectorate of Military Medical Service. Besides an interest in tuberculosis control, Beunders's major concern was the prevention of post-vaccination encephalitis due to the fact that the army administered a total of 120,000 primo-vaccinations between 1945 and 1950. Also noteworthy is that at least seven persons obtained their doctorates under his guidance: J. Huisman (1960), M. Bleiker (1960), W. Nanning (1961), J. Driessen (1963), J. van der Noordaa (1964), A.J. van der Eb (1968), and C. Walig (1970).

Commercial companies

The recent history of medical virology in the Netherlands, and for that matter any medical discipline anywhere in the world, would be incomplete without a mention of commercial concerns – namely, pharmaceutical companies and, increasingly in the latter half of the twentieth century, biotechnology firms – that are responsible for the manufacture of various medicines, vaccines, and therapies, as well as diagnostic kits for any number of diseases. The advent of AIDS and various emerging and re-emerging infections, in particular, spurred a growth in these industries after the 1990s. Here we focus our attention on the links between the medical virology laboratories at various medical and academic institutions, and laboratories at some Dutch companies. Compared to commercial laboratories for vaccine production and clinical services (see below), national or foreign companies offering viral diagnostics services to hospitals are relatively uncommon in the Netherlands. Although some foreign companies located along the Dutch-German border expanded their microbiologic and clinical chemistry activities to Dutch hospitals and local public health services in the 1990s, such laboratories fall outside the scope of our discussion.

Philips Duphar

It might seem odd that Philips – and yes, it is the very same Philips – known worldwide as an electronic company, became involved in medical virology. Unsurprisingly enough, this arm of the company has its origins in the development of an electronic device, the sunlamp, for therapy against rachitis. In 1927, A. van Wijk and E.H. Reerink, two scientists based in the Philips laboratory in Eindhoven, discovered that the UV radiations produced by the sunlamps transformed provitamin ergosterol into vitamin D2 (De Groot, 1951). This led to the cooperation with the chocolate producer, Van Houten in Weesp, in the manufacture of vitamin D-supplemented chocolate pastilles (under the joint label Philips van Houten). Then in 1936, Van Houten withdrew from the joint venture and Philips became the sole owner of Philips van Houten as well as acquired a number of other smaller companies and consolidated all into the formation of the Philips Duphar branch of Philips Industries, a multifaceted industry engaged in the production of a number of pharmaceutical and chemical products, including insulin, liver extracts, plant hormones, insecticides, and weedkillers. Soon after World War II, anti-viral vaccines also joined that list. An enthusiastic 1951 report by Klein and Hertzberger, virologists hired to develop vaccines, offers some sense of the company's reasons for investing resources in this direction: The production of virus vaccines, a peculiar form of mass production taking place partly in some large egg hatcheries and promising to be of great importance, not only for the Netherlands but also far beyond its frontiers (for a more detailed discussion of this subject, see Chapter 9 and Bosgra and Roerink, 1967). To this day, the Weesp-based laboratories, now under the ownership of Abbott Biologicals BV, a subsidiary of Abbott Laboratories, are engaged in the commercial production of human influenza vaccines.

Organon Teknika

Organon Teknika was founded in 1972 as subsidiary of the pharmaceutical company Organon, then officially a business unit of AKZO after the 1969 merger between Koninklijke Zwanenberg-Organon (KZO, Royal

Zwanenberg-Organon) and AKU (Algemene Kunstzijde Unie), an artificial silk fibres company. Its main task was to develop tests and instruments for hospitals and medical laboratories, and for a time it was the leader in developing innovative enzyme-immuno-assays and NASBA[85] technique-based test for detection of virus nucleic acids (Tausk, 1978; Warmerdam et al., 1998, p. 78). In 1994 AKZO and Nobel Industries merged into AKZO Nobel. In a wave of divestments Organon Teknika was sold to BioMérieux in 2002. In light of the closure of this subsidiary in 2009, it is bitterly ironical to look back at the press release issued at the time, which optimistically predicted that the new leadership under BioMérieux would provide a solid basis for the future of the business and its employees. The importance of their research in the field of virology will be discussed further in Chapter 6.

Crucell

A biotechnology firm specializing in vaccines and biopharmaceutical technologies, Crucell has its roots in the universities at both Leiden (IntroGene BV, 1993) and Utrecht (U-BiSys BV, 1996). According to a press release dated 20 June 2000, both companies merged under the new name Crucell that year (Pharmaletter, 2000). In 2006 Crucell acquired two more vaccine companies: the Swiss Berna Biotech and the Swedish SBL Vaccines, to expand its capacities (Crucell, 2006; PharmaTimes, 2006). Subsequently a collaboration begun in 2009 with Johnson and Johnson for the production of an influenza vaccine, soon led to the complete takeover in 2011 (BioPharm, 2011). Today, the company – renamed as Janssen Vaccines, remains a subsidiary of Johnson and Johnson, still headquartered in Leiden. The major contributions of this company were in the fields of the adenovirus vectored AIDS vaccine program and adenovirus vectored Ebola vaccine programme. The company was a pioneer in deploying the high capacity PER C6 cell line for the production of these vaccines (for a more detailed description, see Havenga et al., 2006). The development of influenza vaccines based on the universal recognition site of the broadly protective antibody CR9114 in the HA stem remains its most intense focus; one of the problems that need resolution is the development of suitable models to test the protective responses in serum samples to replace the hemagglutination-inhibition techniques, which were for the first time used in the 1940s and still remain the officially accepted technique for measuring the levels of protective antibody elicited by a vaccine.

85   NASBA: Nucleic acid sequence-based amplification.

Delft Diagnostic Laboratory (DDL)

DDL started in 1985 as part of the regional diagnostic centre SSDZ[86] in Delft; it became a legal entity in 1994 as a joint venture between the Molecular Biology Department of the Reinier de Graaf Hospital in Delft and Innogenetics N.V. (now Fujirebio Europe N.V.), a Belgian diagnostics company headquartered in Ghent (W.G.V. Quint, personal communication, 2018). Since 2003 DDL has been independent of its original shareholders due to a management buyout. It offers research and clinical trial support services – in epidemiology, screening, diagnostics, and vaccine development – in working with human papillomavirus (see, for example, Wheeler et al., 2016).[87]

The initiator was J. Lindeman, pathologist at the regional diagnostic centre of the joined general hospitals in Delft, who established the formation of a Laboratory for Molecular Biology in the early 1980s. From 1985 onwards, molecular diagnostic assays were performed in collaboration with the departments of Microbiology, Clinical Chemistry and Pathology. W.G.V. Quint became head of the Molecular Biology laboratory in 1986. Quint trained at Radboud University in Nijmegen, where he defended his doctoral thesis on endogenous murine leukaemia viruses: germline transmission and involvement in generation of recombinant viruses in 1984. Both Lindeman and Quint were keen to perform scientific research besides daily diagnostics for the clinic. Their research program was intended to develop novel molecular assays and encompassed studies on human papillomavirus. Since 1989, there also was an active collaboration between the laboratory and Innogenetics N.V (Ghent, Belgium) in the field of diagnostics for infectious diseases. This resulted in the founding of Delft Diagnostic Laboratory (DDL), which participated in phase II and III clinical trials, in particular related to HPV screening and development of HPV vaccines and hepatitis C virus. In December 2003, the DDL became independent by a management buy-out.

Viroclinics Biosciences BV

Viroclinics was founded in 2001 as a commercial spin-out of the Viroscience Laboratory at the Erasmus Centre in Rotterdam.[88] It has since grown into a company exceeding 130 FTE of dedicated scientists and technical experts,

---

86 Stichting Samenwerkende Delftse Ziekenhuizen (SSDZ).
87 https://www.ddl.nl, latest access July 2018.
88 https://www.viroclinics.eu, latest access January 2019.

and operates within a network of key opinion leaders as consultants. In 2013 the private capital fund Gilde Healthcare obtained a majority interest in Viroclinics Biosciences. Since 9 August 2017 the company has been fully owned by Parcom Capital.

As we did not want to transgress the time limit of the year 2000, we dealt only very summarily with the activities of the above-mentioned commercial companies in the twenty-first century.

6   Techniques and instruments

Their introduction in the Netherlands and the main
contributions of the Dutch

> The future belongs to science.
> – *Sir William Osler (quoted in Vallery-Radot, 1901, p. xvi)*

> Admittedly the most spectacular advances have concerned molecules rather
> than patients, but it is the molecules which cause the diseases and in the long
> run, papers in the *Journal of Molecular Biology* may contribute as much to
> medicine as those in *The Lancet*.
> – *Michael Stoker (1967)*

We started this book arguing that the first elements of medical virology
rose in the late nineteenth century. For many infectious diseases, bacteria
or fungi could be delineated as aetiological agents, especially because they
could be isolated and cultured by in vitro methods. However, there was a
category of diseases for which no aetiological elements could be isolated nor
observed by microscopic techniques and/or propagated on solid, semisolid,
or in liquid media. The agents of diseases like smallpox, poliomyelitis, rabies,
and influenza escaped the techniques of the bacteriological paradigm.
This made the laboratory a crucial tool in human and veterinary medicine.
Even in the early twentieth century, these diseases could only be studied
at the clinical and epidemiological level and epidemics were countered
principally by hygienic measures. The only exception was the possibility
of immunization against smallpox and rabies to interfere with the natural
course of the disease. The preparation of vaccines rested on the modification
of an invisible viral agent, which was presumed to be present and to be
responsible for the disease.

In this chapter, we specifically address the laboratory techniques that
were in use in the Netherlands for diagnostic virology and medical virology in
a broad sense. We also aim at presenting examples of techniques developed
by Dutch researchers, and that contributed to the field of virology. As one
enters a laboratory, now or in the past alike, instruments were and still
are very prominent. Nowadays, white freezer-like boxes hide benchtop
centrifuges which can readily rotate at a speed of 10,000 rounds per minute
(rpm). Larger ultracentrifuges, typically installed in separate rooms with

strengthened walls, can spin up to 100,000 rpm, offering forces up to 802,000 x g, and capable of separating molecules, membranes, viruses, and other microscopic constituents of cells. Nucleic acid and protein sequencers used to be large instruments with an array of blinking lights while now newspapers are filled with the spectacular news that the human genome can be sequenced by an instrument no larger than a mobile phone connected by a USB port to a laptop. In short, instruments are the fundamental tools by which scientific claims have been and continue to be generated.

We have seen that a first categorical recognition of the inconsistency of viral diseases with the bacteriological paradigm was made by Beijerinck. Based on the technical tools at his disposal, he reached a somewhat farfetched conclusion, namely that the infectious agent he was studying in tobacco plants was at the same time living – shown by its multiplication for which it needed living cells – and 'fluid', or, better said, 'soluble', which was shown by its movement through solid agar (Beijerinck, 1899b). After the discovery of Beijerinck, it took three decades before physicochemical properties of viruses could be studied effectively, when techniques and instruments such as ultracentrifugation, filtration through collodion membranes of known porosity, electrophoresis, and electron microscopy became available. These new techniques showed that viruses were very small indeed but nevertheless in a certain sense corpuscular, but not cellular as bacteria.

The small size of viruses and the failure to culture them in the absence of living cells were the main causes of the technical problems that had to be solved to study viruses. In the first decades of the twentieth century, filtration experiments yielded only information on the maximum size of viruses (Boycott, 1928). At that time, propagation of viruses could only be performed by animal inoculation. For instance, the agent of poliomyelitis could be cultured in monkeys. On the other hand, experiments in horses, cows, pigs, rats, cats, and rabbits by S. Flexner and P.A. Lewis, or in rabbits, guinea pigs, sheep, and dog pups by K. Landsteiner and C. Levaditi, remained negative (Levaditi, 1922, p. 35). Interestingly, Levaditi showed in 1914 that he could propagate fragments of spinal ganglia obtained from infected monkeys in so-called bottles of Gabritschewky in the presence of monkey plasma during at least 21 days (Levaditi, 1922, p. 58), predating the rise of tissue and cell cultures.

From 1931 onwards, the use of embryonated chicken eggs replaced the inoculation of appropriate laboratory animals for the propagation of viruses. Tissue and cell culture techniques were introduced in medical virology around 1950, when recognition of specific cytopathogenic patterns became evident. Inclusion of the recently discovered antibiotics in the medium avoided bacterial contamination, and suspensions of tissue cells could be prepared using treatment with trypsin. Decades later, viruses were 'transformed' into 'laboratory tools' themselves in order to study cellular biological processes in the first place. This way of experimenting led to new insights in the field of tumour virology and the molecularizing of cell biology and cancer causation, in particular. Together with breakthroughs in immunology over the twentieth century, the twenty-first century is now on the brink of promising new diagnostics and drugs that are based on previous key achievements brought by these technical tools to medical virology.

In the study of human viral diseases, principles of serological techniques as applied to bacteria were demonstrated to be useful, but only after minor modifications. As pointed out by Van Rooyen and Rhodes, a principal difficulty involved the preparation of suitable antigens (1948, p. 95). We do not intend to give an overview of all common cell culture or serological techniques that have been used in Dutch virology laboratories, but will highlight the main techniques that paved the way to modern (molecular) virology, highlighting those developed by Dutch researchers. In the 1970s, the development of the enzyme immunoassay turned out to be an important Dutch contribution to medical virology.

To honour the simple instruments that were used in so much pioneer work on viruses, we will start with the filters which were used to remove bacteria from solutions.

Four types of filters

In the first days of virology, filters were the only tools available to differentiate between bacteria and smaller viruses. The nature of the materials from which filters were made included the following: diatomaceous earth or *Kieselguhr*, unglazed porcelain, asbestos, or glass. The Berkenfeld filter made of diatomaceous earth was originally made in Germany; a British-type Berkenfeld filter later appeared and was constructed differently from the German type. The porcelain Pasteur-Chamberland filter was made in France (Van Rooyen and Rhodes, 1948). Beijerinck applied in his pioneer work on tobacco mosaic virus the Pasteur-Chamberland filter that was developed by Charles Chamberland in the laboratory of Pasteur to obtain 'physiologically pure water' (Beijerinck, 1899c; Bos, 1999). He also used the simple, yet effective method of diffusion in agar to study the solubility of the virus. From about 1930 onwards, these filters were superseded by the collodion membrane filters developed by W.J. Elford (Barnard and Elford, 1931; Elford, 1933; Van Rooyen and Rhodes, 1948, pp. 34-47).

The average pore diameter of the filter is one of the physical characteristics that determine the ability of a particle to traverse a filter. P.C. Flu of Leiden University reported that Albert Einstein acquainted him of a method to experimentally assess the permeability of filters, as previously used methods were crude (Flu, 1928, p. 4773). Einstein and Flu might have met each other in November 1921, May 1922, May 1923, October 1924, or February 1925, when Einstein spent a few weeks at Leiden University as a visiting professor (Pais, 1982, p. 526). In fact, Einstein did not produce the formula off the cuff; together with Hans Mühsam, a physician and friend of Einstein in Berlin, Einstein developed and tested the method called the bubble-point measurement that has been widely used since then (Illy, 2012, pp. 94-95; Pais, 1982, pp. 488-489). Mühsam presented the method at a meeting of the German Microbiological Association and they published the paper in 1923 (Einstein and Mühsam, 1923).

Light microscopy

Light microscopy could not give any information on the size or nature of viruses, because it was generally not powerful enough to magnify individual viral particles. However, the detection of elementary bodies in human or animal cells was key to the recognition of certain viral diseases, such as vaccinia and variola (Van Rooyen and Rhodes, 1948, p. 1). Elementary bodies can be described as clumps of viruses that are visible as stained particles under the ordinary light microscope. The limit of visibility attainable with the ordinary microscope is about 67 mμ (Van Rooyen and Rhodes, 1948, p. 74). In 1892, G. Guarneri observed by light microscopy, vaccine bodies or cell inclusions, which he named *cytoryctes variolae et vaccinae*, and which he considered living smallpox virus. About a decade later, at the State University of Groningen, where he defended his thesis in 1906, H. Aldershoff studied these elementary bodies in rabbit cornea after inoculation with vaccinia fluid. Based on his experiments, he rightfully concluded that the elementary bodies were specific products of the vaccinia or smallpox virus and at the same time products of the cell nucleus (chromatin) surrounded with a border originating from the protoplasm (De Lange, 1906).

Tissue culture – early days

The challenge posed by the in vitro culture of viruses was interrelated with the development of tissue culture itself (Waterson and Wilkinson,

1978, pp. 71 and 183). Tissue culture techniques were developed in the first decades of the nineteenth century as a method of morphogenetic study, and became a mainstay of biomedical research. Alexis Carrel, who left France for the United States in 1904, used tissue culture for his work on vascular sutures and transplantation of blood vessels and organs. Carrel, who joined the Rockefeller Institute of Medical Research in New York in 1906, was the first scientist working in the USA to receive the Nobel Prize (in 1911). The publications of Carrel, who had built his work on that of Ross Harrison among others, attracted much attention (Carrel, 1912; De Haan, 1924).

However, as described in Chapter 4, there was a long hiatus between the first communications on tissue culture and multiplication of viruses in tissue or cell culture. An important reason was the belief that viruses would only grow in the cells of the relevant diseased organ of their target species and such cells were often very hard to keep alive outside the body (Mortimer, 2009). This view was held by Alexis Carrel for decades. If interest in tissue culture in the Netherlands was present in the first decades of the twentieth century, this is not reflected by a great number of articles in the NTvG through 1900 to 1950.

Based on his experiments at the Laboratory for Hygiene in Groningen in the years before 1906, the above-mentioned H. Aldershoff might be considered as one of the first researchers who applied a primitive form of in situ tissue culture in the Netherlands. In his experiments studying the development of vaccine bodies, he inoculated rabbit corneae with vaccinia virus or varicella virus, removed them after inoculation, and incubated them at $37°C$ suspended in rabbit serum or physiological saline solution (De Lange, 1906).

Also affiliated at the University of Groningen (Laboratory of Physiology), J. de Haan published on culturing tissues using a continuous perfusion method in 1924 (De Haan, 1924). At the meetings of the Biology section of the Society for the Advancement of Science, Medicine and Surgery,[89] presentations on tissue cultures were given in 1924, 1926 and 1928 by De Haan, H.C. Voorhoeve and J.P.M. Vogelaar, respectively. Both last researchers performed their experiments at the laboratory of Histology and Microscopical Anatomy of S.T. Bok at Leiden University (GNGH, 1924, 1926, 1928). In 1930, several presentations were given by P.J. Gaillard; he came also from the laboratory of Bok in Leiden. Later in 1947, Gaillard was appointed professor in Leiden, where he delivered his inaugural lecture entitled 'Tissue culture and the clinic'. His research was focused on the feasibility of transplantation of thyroid tissue (Galjaard, 1977; Gezondheids Organisatie TNO, 1952, p. 58).

---

89 Genootschap ter bevordering van Natuur-, Genees- en Heelkunde (GNGH).

Except from the work of Aldershoff, all the previously mentioned experiments by De Haan, Vogelaar, Voorhoeve, and Gaillard were nonetheless not used to study and culture viruses. Of note though, the aim of the experiments of De Haan was to study migrating cells which were present upon infection (De Haan, 1924).

At a joint meeting of the Internal Medicine and Microbiology sections of the GNGH in 1931, Albert Fischer from Berlin was an invited speaker; the title of his presentation was 'Proliferation und Differenzierung der Gewebezellen in vitro'.[90] The meeting was enlivened by the showing of a film and attracted a large audience. As Fisher moved from Berlin to Copenhagen in Denmark, he had in 1931 no laboratory room at his disposal. As a result, a co-worker of his, Mrs A. Hollmann, was invited to work at the NKI in Amsterdam to pass on knowledge and tricks related to tissue culture techniques to researchers of the institute for the whole year of 1931 (GNGH, 1931; NKI-AVL Annual Reports (A), 1931).

Another source of information on the use of tissue culture for propagation of viruses in the Netherlands is the dissertation of G. Stoel. He defended his thesis *Weefselcultuur in vitro als hulpmiddel in de bacteriologie*[91] at the University of Amsterdam in 1931 (Stoel, 1931). The experiments were not executed in Amsterdam but performed at the famous laboratory of Levaditi of the Institut Pasteur in Paris. Neither in the overview of the literature on cytotropic viruses in tissue culture, nor in the thesis chapter describing an overview of experiments with cytotropic viruses, was any Dutch experiment referred to. This suggests that there was little research activity on tissue or cell culture in relation to the culture of viruses in the Netherlands until 1930.

In the third decade of the twentieth century, H.S. Frenkel, who was a veterinarian, and H.W. Julius, a medical doctor, investigated in Utrecht at the Central Laboratory for Public Health, the culture of the vaccine virus in the 'flowing-through apparatus' of Julius that was a variant of the instrument of De Haan (Frenkel and Julius, 1932). They actually succeeded growing the vaccine virus in the instrument with continuous perfusion; however, the instrument was not practical in use and susceptible to bacterial contamination. In 1930, Frenkel was appointed head of the newly founded State Veterinary Research Institute[92] in Rotterdam, where he continued experiments to propagate foot-and-mouth disease virus using a modified De Haan's instrument (Frenkel and Van Waveren, 1935; Verhoef, 2005, pp. 107-108).

90   Proliferation and differentiation of tissue cells in vitro.
91   Tissue culture in vitro as tool in bacteriology.
92   Staatsveeartsenijkundig Onderzoekingsinstituut (SVOI).

After World War II, Frenkel was very successful with the development of a specific type of culture method. He used explanted epithelial tissue from normal bovine tongue mucosa for the preparation of foot-and-mouth disease vaccine (Verhoef, 2005, pp. 113-120). The 'Frenkel vaccine' was sold from 1950 onwards by the Institut Français de la Fièvre Aphteuse that was founded by Charles Mérieux in 1947. Frenkel and Mérieux had met each other for the first time in 1934, when Frenkel disclosed to him the idea to propagate foot-and-mouth disease virus on the epithelium of bovine tongues, obtained after slaughter (Mérieux and Lambrichs, 1988, p. 47).

In 1954, Frenkel and Jacoba G. Kapsenberg published a new method to obtain a vaccine against smallpox by culturing vaccinia virus in explanted foetal bovine and ovine skin tissue in a liquid medium. After experiments on animals and revaccination of human volunteers, a number of children under the age of two years were vaccinated successfully with virus of the 30th passage (Frenkel and Kapsenberg, 1954). Frenkel published in 1957 a variant method using the deep layers of the bovine tongue epithelium to increase the titres of infectious virus present in the culture fluid (1957). Although the titres could reach high values, it seems that this method has never been actually applied for the production of vaccinia vaccine.

Amidst war circumstances, P.H.H. de Bruyn of the Institute for Preventive Medicine in Leiden reported in 1942 on the state of the art of the culture of filterable viruses in vitro. In his conclusion, he stated that 'cultivation of viruses in vitro is otherwise significant for theoretical research than the cultivation of bacteria' (De Bruyn, 1942). Furthermore, tissue culture might be an easy and inexpensive method for obtaining a highly concentrated substance for vaccination or for obtaining modifications of virus suitable for vaccination. Although this overview was clear and insightful, further virology research has not been subsequently published by this author.

Tissue culture and cell monolayers

It was mentioned previously (Chapter 1), that Eykman paid much attention to the crusade of anti-vivisectionists against the Pasteur's rabies vaccine (Eykman, 1900). At that time, the Netherlands Association for the Protection of Animals[93] had published a pamphlet that was recommended by the polemical medical doctor G. Luchtmans. Eykman successively retorted the doubts related to the scientific foundation of the Pasteur

---

93   Nederlandsche Vereeniging tot Bescherming van Dieren.

experiments, the execution of the vaccine preparation, and the statistics of the results. Eykman refuted all assertions and allegations put forward by the anti-vivisectionists.

Recently, Duncan Wilson depicted the public awareness and the incredible sensationalism when he examined the early history of tissue culture in Britain (Wilson, 2005). It is beyond the scope of this chapter to examine whether in the Netherlands advocates of tissue culture also tapped into popular sentiment to overstress its potential and raised the same rhetoric and public engagements as in the UK. Judging by the paucity of articles on tissue culture that appeared in the NTvG in the same period, it seems that tissue culture did not meet fantastical speculation or popular repugnance at the use of human or animal material. On the other hand, during the interbellum, a special commission of the Health Council was installed and concluded that medical experiments using animals did not entail any abuse. However, a proposal of a bill designed by the Health Council and regulating the conditions of such experiments was declined by the Minister of Health in 1934 (Rigter, 1992, pp. 136 and 313). In fact, the reason to request advice from the Health Council was a complaint by the Anti-Vivisection Association against the Paediatric Clinic of Leiden University Hospital because of experiments with the Bacillus Calmette-Guérin vaccine against tuberculosis on children and not on animals.

Until the discovery and implementation of cell monolayer culture by Enders, Weller and Robbins in 1949, one may draw the conclusion that tissue culture or cell culture techniques were mainly used in anatomy and physiol-ogy research laboratories in the Netherlands but not in virus diagnostics. The situation in the Netherlands was not different from that in the United Kingdom. P. Mortimer described that when the first public health virology laboratory in England and Wales opened in 1947, its workbook referred merely to the isolation of pox viruses on the chorio-allantoic membranes of eggs, inoculation of specimens into mouse brains, and complement fixation tests using egg- and brain-grown antigens (Mortimer, 2009). Within a decade from the publication of Enders, Weller and Robbins, the use of cell monolayers had become routine. The authors had shown that neurotropic poliomyelitis virus could be propagated in human embryonic cells that were of non-neural origin. In any case, with regard to the use of human embryonic cells Mortimer wrote: 'Whether, *de novo*, such uses of foetal tissue would receive ethical approval today is debatable; but if ends ever justified means, then here was an example of it.' It must be noted that poliovirus replicate after entry via the mouth in the gastrointestinal tract in cells lining this tract, tonsils, and associated lymph nodes, with occasional spread to neuronal cells. In 1952, Moscona, among others, such as Dulbecco and Vogt, improved the method of growing viruses on cell monolayers by applying enzymatic digestion of tissue to establish monolayer cell cultures that facilitate recognition of virus-induced cytopathic effects (Moscona, 1952; Dulbecco and Vogt, 1954).

Immediately after the publication of Enders et al., the Study Group for Tissue Culture was established in Amsterdam by members of five different research disciplines: cancer research (W.M. de Bruyn, R. Korteweg), histology (G.C. Heringa), anatomy (M.W. Woerdeman), medical microbiology (A.C. Ruys) and veterinary research (H.S. Frenkel) as announced in the NTvG (Sluiter, 1949). Unfortunately, proceedings of this study group could not be found. Nonetheless, in the 1963 annual report of the NKI-AVL, De Bruyn mentioned a course of the Foundation Institute for Tissue Culture Amsterdam that she organized. This foundation seems to be the legal entity of the above-mentioned study group; after the retirement of De Bruyn in 1964, the foundation was likely dissolved.

Cell culture techniques were introduced in diagnostics laboratories in the course of the 1950s (see Chapter 4). In Amsterdam, F. Dekking introduced cell culture techniques at the Laboratory for Hygiene somewhere between 1953 and 1955, and G.J.P. Schaap did so at the diagnostic Regional Laboratory of the Municipal Health Service in 1959 (GGD Amsterdam, Archief, 1959). In Leiden, cell cultures were applied gradually, with B. Hofman first sent to the USA to gain experience. Cell culture (without inoculation of specimens) was performed in non-aired cabinets with a glass front panel. Later, from about 1950 onwards, culture of inoculated cells was performed on the insistence of Wilterdink in closed glass cabins with a well-closing door and equipped with a workbench (Verlinde and Kret, 1954; Versteeg, 1992). For protection of the worker, air circulation was applied with airflow over the table ascending to the ceiling. Information on air exhaust or filters could not be found. Precautions were taken because of the dangerous nature of a virus like the poliovirus. As such, this seems to be a prototype of a safety cabinet. In other laboratories, the handling of cells and viruses was carried out under a glass hood without any further protection. It might be questioned to what extent such a glass hood actually achieved any protection of laboratory workers. In fact, the glass hood gave a false impression of protection as aerosols could spread around the device and be inhaled by the worker.

At RIV, cell culture was performed in the new building in Bilthoven in 1958, yet it is not clear when this new technique had been previously introduced in the old building in Utrecht. During the smallpox epidemic of 1951, laboratory diagnosis of smallpox was performed in Leiden (NIPG),

Amsterdam (Laboratory for Hygiene), and Utrecht (RIV) using the chorio-allantoic membrane culture.

In the laboratory of the Elisabeth Hospital in Tilburg that was affiliated with the Medical Faculty of the Catholic University of Nijmegen, cell culture was initiated in 1955 (Peeters, 2001). This was in sharp contrast with the development of the medical microbiology laboratory at the University of Groningen. According to F. Westendorp Boerma, virological studies were not executed in Groningen until the arrival of Jan Wilterdink in 1971 (Westendorp Boerma, 1977). This statement might be true for the diagnostic unit of the Laboratory for Medical Microbiology; however, virus research and diagnostic virus serology were being performed in Groningen before 1971. For instance, in 1939 and 1940, J. Mulder and L. Bijlmer examined in the laboratory of the Clinic of Internal Medicine the antigenic structure of an influenza virus strain that was isolated from a patient in Groningen in 1939 (Mulder et al., 1941). Nonetheless, they isolated the strain in ferrets and performed mouse-protection experiments without using tissue, cell cultures or embryonated eggs.

The 1950s and 1960s were characterized by the refinement of tissue culture methods in cell monolayers (Pereira, 1986). The presence of viruses was detected by morphological changes in the infected cells of the monolayer: the cytopathic effect (CPE), which may range from a rapid and extensive rounding of cells, causing detachment from the surface, to a slowly progressing CPE with discrete foci of infected cells. The changes can be found in the cytoplasm, in the nucleus, or in both, and are indicative of the nature of the virus.

Because cell culture techniques provide much more satisfactory host cell systems for the isolation of viruses, they have obviated to a considerable extent the need for use of experimental animals (Schmidt, 1979). Before the introduction of cell culture, the laboratory diagnosis of one case of poliomyelitis was made by intracerebral inoculation of each specimen in one or two monkeys (Versteeg, 1992). Using cell culture, about 400 tubes with monkey kidney cells could be made from each kidney of one sacrificed monkey. Instead of requiring one or two monkeys for the diagnosis of a single suspected case of poliomyelitis, only four tubes were now needed. Furthermore, in order to type by neutralization an isolated strain, at least six or preferably twelve monkeys were typically needed (the monkeys had to be euthanized for pathological examination). The introduction of cell culture reduced considerably the number of monkeys the poliovirus laboratory needed to use for propagation and neutralization tests for typing the isolated strains.

Figure 18   Equipment for purification of a poliovirus by means of gel filtration

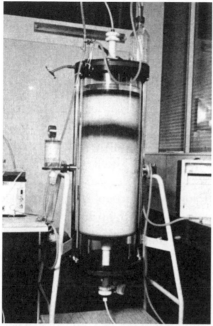

In the dark band, impurities, such as medium and serum components, are separated from the virus
fraction, which then undergoes further purification via an ion exchanger.
Reproduction courtesy of RIVM and Natuur en Techniek

Cell culture and vaccine production

The work on tissue culture of A.L. van Wezel at the National Institute of
Health in Bilthoven deserves a special mention. Van Wezel and his co-
workers developed new approaches for the production of concentrated and
purified inactivated polio and rabies cell culture vaccines (Van Hemert
et al., 1969; Van Wezel, 1967; Van Wezel et al., 1973; Van Wezel et al., 1978;
Van Wezel, 1985). They worked out a highly efficient system to produce
vaccines according to a process that comprised trypsinization of animal
kidney cells by the perfusion method, cell and virus culture in microcarrier
culture, and concentration and purification of the virus suspension. The
advantage of such an approach for clinical virology laboratories was the
availability of the so-called tertiary monkey kidney cells that were produced
by trypsinization of monkey kidneys by the perfusion method. These cells
were most suitable for the detection of enteroviruses and respiratory viruses,
including influenza viruses.

Phase-contrast microscopy

The phase-contrast microscopy that was described by the Dutchman F. Zernike offered opportunities for the study of unstained biological material (Zernike, 1935). In the second edition of 1948, Van Rooyen and Rhodes wrote: 'Since Zernike (1935) described this method, further research by Bennett et al. (1946) has revealed its possibilities for the examination of unstained biological material. The value of the phase-contrast technique in the study of virus elementary bodies is yet unexplored' (Van Rooyen and Rhodes, 1948, p. 7). The answer to the question whether this technique would find relevant applications in diagnostic virology might be found three decades later in Lennette and Schmidt (eds), *Diagnostic procedures for viral, rickettsial and chlamydial infections* (1979). In this virology cookery book, phase-contrast microscopy was not even mentioned. Eventually, the principle of phase contrast was successfully integrated with the electron microscope, for the examination of biologic relevant macromolecules, including viruses (Matijević, 2011). Viruses and the principal cellular macromolecules – DNA, RNA and proteins – are composed of these weak-phase objects mainly consisting of elements with low atomic numbers, such as carbon, oxygen, nitrogen, hydrogen, phosphorus, and sulphur (C, O, N, H, P, and S), that can be easily viewed under phase contrast.

Electron microscopy

The use of the *ordinary* microscope in virology was at first of considerable importance for the detection of the so-called elementary bodies in, for example, vaccinia, variola, herpes, varicella, rabies and psittacosis.[94] Several staining methods were practised to demonstrate the presence of these elementary bodies which are often composed of viral proteins or nucleic acids. The limits of visibility and of resolution would later be further improved by the use of the *dark field* and *fluorescence* microscope. During the 1930s, the electron microscope was developed, whereby a much higher resolution and magnification could be attained by use of electron rays with extremely short wavelengths. Considerable improvements made it possible to obtain photographs of bacteria and viruses magnified 100,000 times with good definition. In Germany, M. Knoll and E. Ruska had built the first

---

94   The agents causing psittacosis are bacteria, but are obligatory intracellular parasites and can be propagated only in living cells.

model of the apparatus in 1930 and had shown it to many interested people (Freundlich, 1963). However, the Siemens & Halske Company owned several patents of which the applications were filed in 1931. Ruska and his friend and co-doctor B. von Borries continued their work on the electron microscope at the Siemens Company, but commercialization of the instrument was slow and cumbersome. Other electron microscope instruments were developed by Marton in Brussels, Martin, Whelpton, Parnum, and Burton in London, and Hillier and Preybus at the University of Toronto, Canada (Van Rooyen and Rhodes, 1948).

The work of the Berlin pioneers aroused interest of Dutch scientists, too. H.B. Dorgelo, professor of technical physics in Delft, and H.B.G. Casimir of Philips Physics Laboratory (NatLab) visited Germany in 1932 in order to learn about the development of the electron microscope (Buiter, 2012, p. 82). In 1935 the investigators W.G. Burgers and J.J.A. Ploos van Amstel of NatLab built a cathode ray tube with a magnetic lens, which in fact represents the first electron microscope in the Netherlands (Van de Schootbrugge, 1991, pp. 36-38). At the Polytechnical School in Delft, A.C. van Dorsten, a co-worker of Dorgelo, was less successful, because the fluorescent material used in the cathode to visualize objects in the electron beam was not appropriate. Van Dorsten moved in 1937 from Delft to the Philips Physics Laboratory. Van de Schootbrugge described a visit of Dorgelo to Siemens in Berlin in July 1939. He was now accompanied by F.G. Waller of the Netherlands Yeast and Spirit Works in Delft and the famous microbiologist A.J. Kluyver, the successor of Beijerinck in Delft. The price of the commercially available Siemens 'Übermikroskop' of more than 70,000 Dutch guilders was too high to purchase an instrument. Furthermore, Dorgelo had the opinion that such an instrument could be 'home' built in Delft. After his visit at Siemens in Berlin in 1939, Waller proposed to found a Dutch cooperation to build an electron microscope. Eventually, his activity resulted in the foundation in 1943 of an electron microscopic institute with the following participants: Netherlands Yeast and Spirits Works, the chocolate factory Van Houten, the Nederlandse Kunstzijdefabriek (Netherlands Artificial Silk Union), and the Heineken Brewery. Later in 1939, a student of Dorgelo named J.B. Le Poole who was unaware of the previous developments proposed to build an electron microscope as the final project for his thesis. To Le Poole's astonishment the latter agreed immediately. In 1941, the Mark I was completed by him, the instrument reaching a magnification of 10,000-fold. Le Poole was appointed technical 'director' of the above-mentioned institute and continued his work with the financial help of the Netherlands Yeast and Spirit Works, among others. A spectacularly improved instrument, the

Figure 19   Presentation of the EM 100 at Philips in 1949

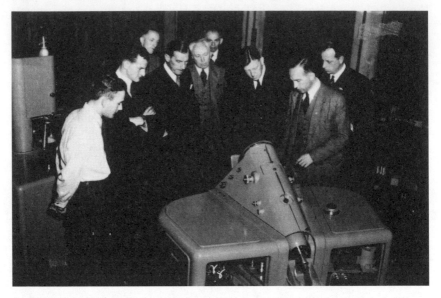

Second from left: J.B. Le Poole; second from right A.C. Van Dorsten
Reproduction courtesy of *Philips Technical Reviews*

Mark II, which had a 100,000-fold magnification, was ready in 1944, but there
were well-founded fears that the German occupiers would take possession
of the instrument. Woutera van Iterson, one of the co-workers of Le Poole,
wrote: 'Then came a day when it seemed advisable to dismantle the electron
microscope to hide the heart of the instrument, i.e. the [magnetic] lenses.
The cooling oil of the high-voltage generator turned out to be a blessing
not intended by Philips: it was distributed for fuel among the workers of
the institute' (Van Delft and Van Helvoort, 2018, p. 158; Van Iterson, 1996).

After World War II, the Philips Company in the person of G. Holst, director of the NatLab, was hesitating to take on the production of an electron
microscope based on the Mark II. H.B.G. Casimir, who succeeded Holst
in 1947 as director of the Natlab together with H. Rinia and E. Verwey,
mentioned in his autobiographical memories that the contact between the
Philips Company and Le Poole at the Polytechnic School was first made
on the initiative of Holst (Casimir, 1983, p. 339). On the other hand, Van de
Schootbrugge described that when Le Poole informed Holst that the Mark
II might offer commercial possibilities, Holst initially refused, as he did not
believe in the economic benefit of scientific instruments. His decision was
revised after talks with Van Dorsten and possibly also after intervention by
Anton Philips himself, who was informed of his reticence by the father of

Woutera van Iterson accompanied by his daughter while they had lunch at Anton Philips home (Van Iterson, 1996). According to Van de Schootbrugge, Van Dorsten, now at Philips, and Le Poole built a more convenient prototype for commercialization; this experimental instrument was well received internationally. Le Poole continued to invent technical improvements for the instrument (Le Poole, 1947/1948). The production of electron microscopes later brought reasonable benefits to the company.

Reception of the electron microscope in the virology field in the Netherlands

Although electron microscopy has been recognized early as a key tool for the detection of virus particles, it did not find wide application for virus identification. The main reasons behind the limited application of electron microscopy as a rapid method for virus detection were: a) the instruments were expensive to buy and maintain; b) experienced operators were needed; c) the method was rather insensitive ($> 10^7$ particles per ml needed); d) viruses with similar morphologies cannot easily be distinguished; and, last but not least, e) biological material could hardly withstand the conditions of operation, namely a vacuum and the electron beam. Therefore, the electron microscope was at first more useful for materials science. This, however, did not last for long when new staining techniques became available, such as negative staining, that showed the surface structure of viral particles.

Van Iterson colourfully reported on the difficulties experienced at the start of the first commercial electron microscope, the EM 100, which was delivered at the University of Amsterdam in January 1951. The instrument was installed in a basement bicycle storage area with a ceiling low enough to bump one's head and without ventilation. Since the institute was without special funds, the microscope films had to be developed by Van Iterson using her own kitchenware (Van Iterson, 1996). In Amsterdam, the NKI received the first electron microscope in the early 1960s and the Amsterdam Laboratory for Hygiene, in the early 1970s. The instrument was mainly used for research. The first paper from investigators of this laboratory describing methods based on electron microscopy was published in 1974 (Walig et al., 1974). The instrument used for electron microscopy was a Philips EM 300 that appeared on the market in 1966 and became a commercial success (in total 1,850 were sold).

In Rotterdam, at the Virology Laboratory of the GGD, an electron microscope was part of the equipment since 1977 when the laboratory moved to the building of the Municipal Health Service at the Schiedamsedijk (R. Woudenberg, personal communication, 2013). In larger institutions, such as the Medical Faculty of the Erasmus University, techniques requiring expensive equipment (such as electron microscopy) were shared with other laboratories, e.g. the Department of Pathology.

To the best of our knowledge, diagnostic electron microscopy has not been used in Groningen as a routinely applied tool in spite of the talk delivered in 1978 by Dick Madeley, a prophet of electron microscopy, to the members of the Department (Madeley, 1992). Madeley referred to this talk at his presentation on the occasion of the valedictory lecture of J.B. Wilterdink in 1992.

The situation in the Netherlands related to the use of electron microscopes in diagnostic virology was different from that in the United Kingdom. By 1976, eighteen of about 50 regional and area laboratories had their own microscopes and thirteen others had ready access to these instruments; they were in particular applied to seeking virus particles in the faeces of patients with non-bacterial gastro-enteritis (Williams, 1985).

Immunofluorescence

While electron microscopy was advocated as the method of choice for rapid virus diagnosis, it remained a selective tool in specific situations, whereas immunofluorescence technique was soon employed for rapidly detecting acute virus infections, particularly in the respiratory tract. A significant technical contribution has been delivered by J.S. Ploem, who introduced the incident light fluorescence microscope (Gardner and McQuillin, 1980, p. 28; Ploem, 1976). An early report on the use of immunofluorescence as a rapid and reliable method for the diagnosis of influenza was published by Hers, Van der Kuip and Masurel in 1968. They described that in seven of eight proven cases of influenza, the diagnosis was established by immunofluorescence: in three cases in three hours by direct staining of sputum; in the other three cases in 36 hours by means of monkey kidney tissue culture or organ culture of throat washings. A fatal case was diagnosed immediately by examination of impression smears of trachea and lung, further confirmed in 24 hours by examining inoculated monkey kidney cells (Hers et al., 1968). In their opinion, it should become the method of choice for the rapid identification of outbreaks, as the one that occurred in 1967-1968.

Over the 1970s, much experience was gained in the investigation of acute respiratory virus infections using immunofluorescence. The technique required carefully testing of the reagents for specificity. When the reagents became commercially available, fluorescence microscopy was brought into use in general hospital laboratories in the Netherlands e.g. for the rapid detection of respiratory syncytial virus in nasal swabs.

Immunological techniques using specific fluorescent antibodies could also be used to detect viral antigens in monolayer cell cultures and immunostaining 48 to 72 hours post inoculation, speeding up virology laboratory diagnosis. Centrifugation of specimens onto cell monolayers was also helpful to reduce the time needed for the detection of the presence of virus replication.

In the Regional Public Health Laboratory in Groningen, which performed virus diagnostics for the University Medical Centre in that city, the techniques of rapid culture of CMV and respiratory viruses using centrifugation and immunofluorescence were developed in the 1980s following the protocols used by P.D. Griffiths in 1984 for CMV (Griffiths et al., 1984; Schirm et al., 1987, 1992). The 'shell vial/monoclonal antibody mixture' approach could also be applied on monolayers cultured in microtiter plates; this method was applied in the diagnostic virology laboratory of the Erasmus Centre in Rotterdam (Rothbarth et al., 1987; Rothbarth et al., 1988).

Through the years 1985 to 1995, these methods were extensively discussed at the meetings of the Dutch Clinical Virology Working Group. A matter of concern was the reliability and specificity of the monoclonal antibodies used in the detection of the viral antigens.

Enzyme-immunoassay or enzyme-linked immunosorbent assay

In the development of the enzyme immunosorbent assay (EIA), also called enzyme-linked immunosorbent assay (ELISA), the Dutchmen A.H.W.M. (Anton) Schuurs and B.K. (Bauke) van Weemen were key players (Barnes, 2016; Tausk, 1978). They applied the use of antigen-, hapten- or antibody-enzyme conjugates in solid phase immunoassays in their research at Organon Research Laboratories in Oss, the Netherlands (Van Weemen and Schuurs, 1971, 1972, 1974). The management had asked to develop a simple dip-read strip giving a colour change technology to replace a successful immuno-chemical pregnancy test based on inhibition of hemagglutination or latex agglutination. It was Anton Schuurs who proposed to explore the potential of enzymes linked to antigens or antibodies for immunochemical reactions with a colorimetric endpoint (Van Weemen, 2005). It has to be noted that the Organon researchers used initially the term 'enzyme-immunoassay'

(EIA) following the term 'radio-immunoassay' (RIA). In the meantime, they had become aware of the ELISA studies by Engvall and Perlmann from Sweden (Engvall and Perlmann, 1971). Together with Eva Engvall and Peter Perlmann at Stockholm University, in Munich in April 1976 they received the Preis Biochemische Analytik offered by the German Society of Clinical Chemistry. The coupling agent used by both groups to conjugate enzymes with proteins was glutaraldehyde; this technique had been reported by S. Avrameas (Avrameas, 1969). For serological assays, the plastic microtiter plates appeared to be useful when testing large numbers of samples. In the EIA technique, specific polyclonal or monoclonal antibodies are labelled with enzymes such as, for instance, peroxidase or alkaline phosphatase. The reaction between (virus) antigen and labelled antibody is carried out on microtiter plates, which are the solid phase. The capacity of the material of the solid phase to bind protein is of crucial importance. The amount of enzyme-labelled antibody bound to the solid phase can be detected after removing unbound material by washing and after adding the specific substrate for the enzyme. The enzyme product detection system measures the development of colour without the need for expensive apparatus (Kemeny and Challacombe, 1988). As Kemeny and Challacombe wrote: 'The solid phase immunometric assay has come a long way since it was first described. The promise of increased sensitivity and ease of performance has largely been realized.'

The ELISA techniques were within a decade widely applied for the detection of antibodies or antigens in the laboratory diagnosis of infectious diseases. The advent of EIA/ELISA has been nicely described in retrospect by Van Weemen (2005). The technology was patented by Organon. The company decided not to monopolize the technology and the licensing conditions were so reasonable that the number of licensees was more than a hundred. In the field of infectious disease diagnosis, the EIA developed at Organon was primarily employed in hepatitis B testing. In the opinion of Van Weemen, the way the Organon management dealt with the invention was a decisive factor in the success of its widespread applicability in laboratory medicine.

Agar gel electrophoresis

Although the eminent molecular biologist P. Borst, who had been trained as a medical doctor, is not considered to be a virologist *pur sang*, in 1963, he and Weissmann published on MS2 phage-induced RNA synthetase, an

Figure 20   A. Schuurs and B. van Weemen on the occasion of the presentation of the Saal van Zwanenberg Prize in Nijmegen, 22 April 1980

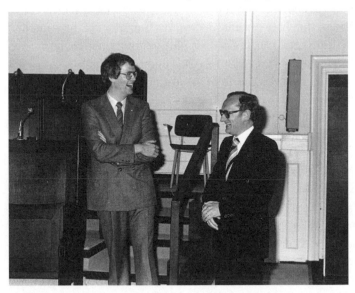

A. Schuurs (right) and B. van Weemen (left) on the occasion of the presentation of the Saal van Zwanenberg prize in Nijmegen on 22 April 1980. The prize was awarded to them for the development of a world-famous enzyme-immuno-assay.
Reproduction courtesy of A. Schuurs and B. van Weemen

RNA-dependent RNA polymerase (Weissmann and Borst, 1963). Their work gave further insight into the replication mechanism of viral RNA.

The technique of the gel electrophoresis that was described by Aaij and Borst in 1972 was another of his contributions to virology; this technique has been used widely to study viral nucleic acid (Aaij and Borst, 1972). Co-workers of Borst, for example, J. ter Schegget and C. Sol, moved in the 1970s from the Borst's Laboratory of Biochemistry to the Laboratory for Hygiene (Laboratorium voor de Gezondheidsleer) at the University of Amsterdam. J. van der Noordaa, head of the laboratory, was convinced that he needed scientists trained in molecular biology to strengthen the research program on SV40 that he initiated.

Introducing DNA into mammalian cells

The Canadian Frank L. Graham had arranged a postdoctoral position at the laboratory of Alex J.A. van der Eb in Leiden, who was interested in human adenoviruses (Graham, 1988). In his application for a fellowship from the National Cancer Institute of Canada, he proposed to work on a problem involving adenovirus and cancer and develop an assay for infectious adenovirus DNA so that he could analyse various fragments of the viral DNA for its ability to infect and transform cells. The method involved formation of DNA-calcium phosphate precipitates that upon addition to cell culture become absorbed by the cells. The DNA uptake occurs during incubation at 37°C in the presence of excess calcium ions (Graham and Van der Eb, 1973). Graham described the serendipity of the many ways in which the discovery of the technique took place:

> Had the DNA solutions not contained just the right amount of phosphate and been at the right pH, no biologically active co-precipitate would have formed. Had the DNA-CaPO$_4$-CaCl$_2$ cocktail not been left in the culture dishes when medium was added back on to the cells, DNA would not have been taken up because the calcium ion concentration would have been too low. Finally, had I seen a precipitate in the first experiment, I may have chucked the mixture down the drain and tried something else. Who would have believed that precipitating DNA out of solution could enhance its biological activity? (Graham, 1988)

Whereas this technique was intended to assay infectivity of adenoviral DNA, it appeared to be also a simple method assessing transformation activity, i.e. genetic alteration of eukaryotic cells caused by introducing foreign DNA into cells, as well as transient expression of pure DNA. As of February 2016, the paper has been cited in 9,314 publications (Publish or Perish, 3 February 2016).

Pepscan and combinatorial chemistry

From the beginning of the 1980s onwards, combinatorial chemistry techniques were developed by the group of R.H. Meloen at the Central Veterinary Institute in Lelystad (now Wageningen Bioveterinary Research), to identify bioactive binding sites. The first steps were achieved by the development of procedures for rapid concurrent synthesis on solid supports of hundreds of peptides, of sufficient purity to react in an enzyme-linked immunosorbent assay (Geysen et al., 1984). The affiliation of the authors of the cited publication hides a later conflict concerning the patents of the techniques between the Commonwealth Serum Laboratories, Melbourne,

Australia, and the Central Veterinary Institute in Lelystad. This conflict was solved with the help of the Dutch government prosecutor (Meloen et al., 1995; Meloen et al., 2001; Meloen, 2001). Three points were important to the success of the technique: automatized production of synthetic peptides, high throughput screening using checkerboard arrays and the combinatorial approach. Epitope mapping is carried out by use of long series of overlapping synthetic peptides of any given protein sequence; each possible epitope is tested separately. The Pepscan method allows fast definition of the bioactive binding sites, for instance, B- and T-cell epitopes. Its superiority to all other available approaches was shown by the first definition of the major neutralizing site of HIV (Goudsmit et al., 1988) and subsequently of B and T-cell epitopes of other agents (for instance: Van Eden et al., 1989; Kast et al., 1989). Furthermore, the method allows the ready development of new diagnostics which was achieved for Epstein-Barr virus (Middeldorp and Meloen, 1988) and prion disease (Schreuder et al., 1996).

The definition of the neutralizing site of parvovirus led to the development of the first synthetic peptide vaccine that was able to fully protect the natural host (dogs and mink) against infection (Langeveld et al., 1994). Since 2000, Pepscan is a privately held company that is still based in Lelystad, the Netherlands.

Nucleic acid purification

Another important Dutch contribution to virology was the description by R. Boom et al. (Amsterdam) of a rapid and simple method for purification of nucleic acids (Boom et al., 1990). The method is based on the lysing and nuclease-inactivating properties of the chaotropic agent guanidinium thiocyanate together with the nucleic acid-binding properties of silica particles or diatoms in the presence of this agent. By using size-fractionated silica particles, nucleic acids (covalently closed circular, relaxed circular and linear double-stranded DNA; single-stranded DNA; and rRNA) could be purified from twelve different specimens in less than one hour and were recovered in the initial reaction vessel. The number of quotations, approximately 4,968 until 2016, of this article indicates how often this technique has been used worldwide (Publish or Perish, February 2016). But of course, this is nothing compared to Lowry's assay (1951) for the quantification of total protein content, which has been cited more than 300,000 times (Garfield, 1990).

Nucleic acid extraction and the isothermal nucleic acid sequence-based amplification

The extraction technique of Boom was combined by researchers at Organon Teknika, Boxtel, with isothermal nucleic acid sequence-based amplification (NASBA) (Kievits et al., 1991). Amplification of target RNA or DNA sequences is accomplished by the simultaneous enzymatic activity of AMV reverse transcriptase, T7 RNA polymerase and RNase H. The NASBA technique is highly suited for the amplification of RNA. The invention of the NASBA technique had not been of Dutch origin, as the concept of this nucleic acid amplification has not been designed by Dutch researchers themselves. The patents were bought by the Dutch company Organon Teknika from Cangene in Canada, while the technique was developed at the Salk Institute Biotechnology/Industrial Associates, La Jolla, CA, USA. The NASBA technique has been a cornerstone of Organon Teknika's NucliSens line of diagnostic virology products for the clinical laboratory (Guatelli et al., 1990; Compton, 1991). Leading figures at Organon Teknika were B. van Gemen, T. Kievits and P. Lens, who worked further on improvement of nucleic acid amplification by NASBA.

Excerpta Medica

A considerable contribution from the Netherlands has been the publishing activities of Excerpta Medica. After the end of World War II, the idea that international science documentation service in the English language would be extremely valuable for the wide distribution of information and coordination of scientific research occurred to scientists at the University of Amsterdam, such as M.W. Woerdeman as well as in Amsterdam-based publishing houses. The initiative led to the establishment of the foundation Excerpta Medica Ltd. in 1946 that would develop its innovative abstracting system. Excerpta Medica was established by five partners: the publishing house J.M. Meulenhoff, The Workers' Press (De Arbeiders Pers), Em. Querido Publishing, Janos Freud and Woerdeman. Woerdeman persuaded the other collaborating partners. According to Andriesse, a Dutch expert on science publishing, one of the founders was also Erich Landsberger, a German Jewish refugee, who joined on the suggestion of Janos Freud, who was born in Hungary and finally settled in 1935 in Amsterdam as a pharmacologist (2008). Already during the war, while hiding in Amsterdam, Landsberger had found some support from Woerdeman and two other professors at the

University of Amsterdam and a few publishers. Nevertheless, a portrait study of the founders of Excerpta Medica painted by the then famous Jean Paul Vroom in the 1960s portrays the following persons: Woerdeman, Fred von Eugen (formerly of Em. Querido and the Workers' Press), Dick Vriesman (an independent cultural entrepreneur), and Coenraad van der Waerden (Workers' Press). Janos Freud had passed away in 1948, and Erich Landsberger had been dismissed in 1953 as director of the foundation, owing to financial problems. The role of Vriesman as founder is not clear (Stichting Bibliotheek van het Boekenvak bij de Amsterdamse Universiteitsbibliotheek – Bijzondere Collecties, 2007: 6.)

The goal of the company was to publish English summaries of all important medical publications from across the world (Andriesse, 2008, p. 148). The collaboration between publishers in the role of entrepreneurs and scientists in the role of editors implied that the former were owners of the company. The network of scientists, including Martinus Woerdeman, Jan Duyff, David de Wied and other medical specialists, was important to the publishers. According to Andriesse, in 1949, alongside Excerpta Medica Ltd (for profit), an Excerpta Medica Foundation (non-profit) was also set up for international recognition as a science documentation service and eligible for project grants. He wrote further: 'In 1965 the foundation took over the capital of Excerpta Medica Ltd, which thenceforth became dormant. In 1971, when the company was sold to Elsevier, the limited liability company had to be brought back to life, for who else was the owner?' Somewhat surprisingly, not the original shareholders, but the six managers of the foundation each received one-sixth of the purchase price (Andriesse, 2008, p. 151). The spreading of the excerpts by Excerpta Medica and the early development of an automatic information system were fruitful also for the development of clinical virology. A.C. Hekker, a medical virologist affiliated at RIVM, was working as an editor at Excerpta Medica during the 1970s and 1980s.

Conclusion: Offstage in the spotlight

This chapter on the Dutch contributions to technical developments in medical virology reflects the 'molecularization' of biology and medicine in the second half of the twentieth century. On the one hand, the contributions of Dutch researchers to the advances of virology have been relatively small through the first half of the twentieth century with the exception of the electron microscope built by Le Poole's group, although the initial aim of the project was not intended for imaging viruses. On the other hand, since the 1950s there was a significant growth in Dutch electron microscopy. Probably the best-known Dutch contribution has come from Philips, with their series EM 75, EM 100, EM 200, EM 300, EM 400, up to the most recent CM series transmission microscopes and XL series scanning microscopes (Kruit et al., 1996).

The successful development of Frenkel's culture method using explanted epithelial tissue from normal bovine tongue mucosa for the preparation of foot-and-mouth disease vaccine was, however, not applied in *clinical* virology. However, the invention of Van Wezel of producing vaccine on a large scale might be seen as a valuable contribution to medical virology. This technique had also the advantage that much smaller numbers of monkeys were required than formerly.

Looking back in summary, the discovery of the EIA/ELISA technique provided worldwide sensitive assays for detection of antibodies and antigens in infectious diseases and immunology. As expressed by R.M. Lequin: 'Given the impact that their [i.e. Schuurs, Van Weemen, Engvall and Perlmann] inventions have had on clinical diagnosis and healthcare in general, as well as on the development of a well-established in vitro diagnostic industry, these inventors deserve to be honored again' (2005).

Agar gel electrophoresis, nucleic acid purification, and introduction of foreign DNA in mammalian cells turned out to be useful tools for biotechnology and virology. The phenotyping of HIV-1 variants offered an important tool to understand the progression of initial HIV infection to the clinical AIDS. While at the beginning of the twentieth century virus infections could mainly be studied by symptoms or when they appeared in epidemics, at the brink of the twenty-first century viruses are diagnosed as specific molecular and immunological targets. In order to transform all the collected data into useful information, molecular biologists, bio-information scientists, epidemiologists, clinicians and clinical virologists together will be the necessary and key players in the development of practical applications in clinical diagnostic laboratories.

7   Dutch virology in the tropics

From colonial to international virology

Besides, every Malayan woman practises medicine and midwifery with facility; so
(I confess that it is the case) I would prefer to submit myself to such hands than to
a half-taught doctor or arrogant surgeon, whose shadow of education was acquired
in schools, being inflated with presumption while having no real experience.
– Johannes Bontius (1931, p. XX and XXI)

The theme of the 1989 symposium 'Dutch Medicine in the Malay Archipelago
1816-1942,' held at the University of Nijmegen to honour of the career of D.
de Moulin, who was retiring as professor of the history of medicine, was
chosen for two main reasons: first to recognize De Moulin's love for the place
of his birth, and, second, to indicate a renewed interest in the Netherlands
in its colonial history (Luyendijk-Elshout et al., 1989). And although Dutch
medical virology was not De Moulin's speciality per se, its history is so
tightly interwoven with that of colonial or tropical medicine that it is not
possible to do either topic justice without giving the other its due attention.
Consequently, we devote this chapter to the history of medical virology in
the Dutch colonies, including in our purview not only the Malay Archipelago
that De Moulin so loved, but also lands in the opposite direction, such as
Suriname and the Dutch Antilles in the Caribbean to the West, where the
early Dutch Republic also had colonies. We give an overview of the medical practices and public health measures in these former Dutch colonies,
focusing primarily on the development of virological laboratories and such
activities as vaccine production and epidemiological studies at these stations
as well as notable contributions of various researchers in this field. With the
decolonization that occurred over the latter half of the twentieth century,
the reach of colonial medicine – also known as tropical medicine due to
the geographic features shared by these far-flung colonies – expanded and
became more international, and, increasingly, more oriented towards Africa,
a facet of the field we also address here.

Therefore, we turn to Dutch virological activities in Africa in the last
part of this chapter. The establishment of the Nairobi Medical Research
Centre in 1964 will be focused on and a special note must also be made
on HIV/AIDS in the context of tropical medicine. Attention will be paid to
the Ethiopian-Netherlands HIV/AIDS Research Project (ENARP) that was

started in 1994. Since the introduction of effective antiretroviral therapy in 1996, an HIV infection transformed very quickly from being a lethal infection to a chronic one in the more affluent and technically advanced countries (in North America or Western Europe, for example). In contrast, in the countries with a low income, especially those in Africa, the global HIV burden in 2001 was still higher than expected at the beginning of the HIV epidemic in Africa. In 2001 Thomas Quinn, a recognized expert on HIV epidemiology looked back to a paper he co-authored in 1986 on AIDS in Africa. Despite all efforts he had to admit: 'We estimated that 1-2 million Africans were HIV-infected in 1986, whereas today 25.3 million Africans are infected and the adult prevalence for the continent is now 8.8%.' He concluded that the recommendations that could be made in 2001 were in fact similar to those we made in 1986. Nevertheless, he was optimistic that with reductions in the price of antiretroviral drugs for Africa – and with the development of the Global Fund for AIDS, Tuberculosis, and Malaria – that antiretroviral drugs might soon be made available to those afflicted with AIDS. In that process J.M.A. (Joep) Lange played an important role.

Dutch colonial history also has deep links to maritime history, as evidenced by the growth of global commercial markets in the two centuries that followed the establishment of the seven United Provinces of the Netherlands during the mid-1580s. Specific connections with the tropics began during the seventeenth century, popularly known as the Dutch Golden Age. During this time, trading companies were given power to negotiate treaties, build fortifications, and enlist soldiers. The Dutch East India Company (VOC) and the West India Company (WIC)[95] set up in 1602 and 1622, respectively, contributed to an exchange of information about medicine and natural history (Cook, 2007,). The VOC was given the right to act as a sovereign power east of the Cape of Good Hope in South Africa and the WIC was given similar powers in the Americas. In 1619 the VOC conquered the city of Jayakarta at the west coast of Java, where it built the Batavia fortification, which became the main Dutch port of call in the region. In 1667 seven ships of the WIC conquered an English settlement along the Suriname River in the north-eastern part of South America and established Suriname (Dutch Guiana) as a Dutch colony.

Although the Dutch colonialism retained a strong business-oriented and technocratic bent, at the turn of the nineteenth century the government in the Netherlands accepted the ethical responsibility for the health of

95 Verenigde Oostindische Compagnie and Westindische Compagnie.

inhabitants of colonies (Raben, 2013). As the medical historian William Bynum rightly observed, whereas most of the so-called 'tropical medicine' prior to World War I was initiated by colonial powers – not just the Netherlands but also Great Britain and France – it is 'historically distorting to write off medical and public health efforts in Imperial dominions as simply exploitative' (2008, p. 139).

Dutch domination ended in rather different ways in its eastern and western colonies. Although Indonesia first proclaimed its independence in August 1945, it was only formally recognized by the Dutch in 1949, until which time the Netherlands maintained its hold over the Malay Archipelago and repeatedly tried to reoccupy Indonesia (Himawan, 1995). The decolonization in the West, in contrast, took a longer and more peaceful course. The largest of the colonies, Suriname, attained independence in 1975. With regard to the Dutch Antilles the process of decolonization had begun even earlier, with the Islands Regulation of the Netherlands Antilles in 1948; under this regulation, the various islands were given broad autonomy within the Kingdom of the Netherlands until 2010. Thereafter, Curaçao and St Maarten became distinct constituent countries alongside Aruba; whereas Bonaire, St Eustatius, and Saba became special municipalities within the Netherlands.

The main sources about medical knowledge and practise in the early years of Dutch colonialism come from accounts of various physicians and scientists who voyaged to these parts. The writings of Jacobus Bontius, for instance, provide a window into the state of medical knowledge and practise in the eastern colonies in the early part of the seventeenth century (see the section following), while the works of the Dutch physician and naturalist Willem Piso and the German cartographer and natural-history illustrator, Georg Marcgraff served as sources for the history of natural history and medicine in the South American tropics in a similar period (Cook, 2007). The proceedings of the Nijmegen symposium provide a fairly comprehensive overview of tropical medicine in nineteenth century. The historical records of the Netherlands Society for Tropical Medicine, which was founded in 1907, are a rich source of material about the twentieth century and beyond. They give the impression that during the time period covered by this book the activities of Dutch tropical medicine were oriented more towards the East rather than the West Indies (Van Bergen, 2007, p. 178). Another major source of information about the Dutch contribution to advancements in tropical medicine and hygiene over the years from 1900 to 1950 is a 1951 review by J.E. Dinger, who succeeded Paul Flu as professor of tropical hygiene in 1947. He mentioned in this report studies on virus diseases: smallpox, dengue, yellow fever, and rabies. With the exception of yellow fever studies in Amsterdam, all studies he referred to were performed in the Dutch East Indies.

Indonesia and the former Dutch East Indies

It was Bontius, while serving simultaneously as physician, apothecary, and overseer of surgeons in the VOC territories, who first began to collect local knowledge about medicine in the East Indies and transformed it into transferable matters of fact (Cook, 2007; Bontius, 1931). He held that many of his local acquaintances in the East Indies were superior in knowledge and skill to any European medical practitioners because of their greater experience, at least in the arena of locally prevalent diseases (Cook, 2007). It was a very unorthodox view, especially for his times, and appeared to have little impact on his compatriots. Even in 1925, E.P. Snijders, newly appointed as professor of tropical medicine, pointed out in his inaugural lecture that medical knowledge had predominantly flowed from West to East with little return traffic until the 1880s, when medical research took shape in the East Indies (see De Knecht-van Eekelen, 1989). Meanwhile, however, Bontius left a lasting legacy in the form of his writings, which earned him his title as one of the fathers of 'tropical medicine' (Jeanselme, 1929): His *Historiae naturalis et medicae Indiae orientalis* (1631), and *De medicina Indorum* (1642), a four-volume collection of his medical observations in the East Indies, which he sent to his brother over the years, and which were collected and published only after his death (Cook, 2007, p. 209). In the series Opuscula Selecta Neerlandicorum de Arte Medica the six books were published in a reprint with the original Latin text together with an English translation (Bontius, 1931). Despite some remarkable 'firsts' – including the first written description of the disease beriberi and a detailed account of a 1628 dysentery outbreak in Java , the six books of Bontius contain virtually no information on diseases that were later recognized to be viral in origin (Bontius, 1931: 180,183, 188, 189; Singh, 2002, p. 682; Van Andel 1931, p. XXX and XXXI).

Tragically and somewhat ironically, Bontius was confronted with diseases in his personal life. He lost his first wife on the voyage to the VOC territories, and his second wife, whom he married three months after the arrival in Batavia, passed away after two and a half years of marriage. In early 1631 his eldest child died of '*kinderpoxkens*' or smallpox (and not measles, as suggested by Cook in his otherwise brilliant book on the history of Dutch medicine and science in the sixteenth and seventeenth century) (Cook, 2007, p. 192; Van Andel, 1931, pp. xiv and xxxiv).

Smallpox

In his detailed article title 'Smallpox, vaccination, and the Pax Neerlandica, Indonesia, 1550-1930', P. Boomgaard, professor of environmental and economic history of Southeast Asia, contended that 'the presence of the smallpox in the archipelago predated the early sixteenth-century arrival of the Europeans' in the islands (Boomgaard, 1989a and b; Boomgaard, 2003, p. 593). Variolation was introduced by the Dutch in Java and by the British in Sumatra during the late 1770s and 1780s. One of the early figures to promote this procedure was Willem van Hogendorp, a member of a rich, aristocratic family, who nearly went bankrupt in 1773 due to a financial crisis and too luxurious a lifestyle. Thereupon, he left for the East in hopes of regaining a fortune. In 1779 he published *Sophronisba: of, de gelukkige moeder door de inëntinge van haare dochters* (Sophronisba; or, The happy mother who had her daughters inoculated) in which he recommended variolation as suitable method for the prevention of smallpox. Although the procedure had been accepted by many people in Batavia, public opinion about it changed due to an unfortunate incident that occurred shortly after Van Hogendorp's first article. He published a second paper in 1780 to defend once again his opinion on the efficacy of the procedure (Van Hogendorp, 1921/1784; Van der Steege, 1921/1779). Meanwhile, he succeeded in regaining his fortune after ten years, and set sail for home in 1783; unfortunately, he never arrived in the Netherlands because he sailed from Ceylon (present-day Sri Lanka) on the vessel *Harmonia*, which was shipwrecked, leaving no survivors.

Following Edward Jenner's 1798 discovery, the cowpox vaccination began to grow rapidly in popularity and was distributed by various colonial powers to their colonies via Baghdad and Basra in the Middle East. Unfortunately, however, the international political situation hampered getting the vaccine specimens to their destinations in time and being still active. For example, although an 1802 shipment of the vaccine successfully reached Bombay and beyond to Ceylon despite transport difficulties, however, it did not make it further to Dutch East Indies due to the political situation. Eventually the French general Charles Decaen shipped a consignment of the vaccine from Isle de France (nowadays Mauritius), which eventually arrived in Batavia in 1804. Unfortunately, by then the vaccine was no longer viable. Then, a ship with a dozen slave children sailed from Java to Isle de France to collect the vaccine that was kept viable using the arm-to-arm method on the children. This approach worked; thereupon the vaccine was distributed first over Java and there upon over the Archipelago (Boomgaard, 2003; Schoute, 1942). The vaccination was rapidly distributed in Java as well, but mainly among the Europeans and their slaves (Boomgaard, 2003).

Figure 21   *Sophronisba: of, de gelukkige moeder door de inëntinge van haare*
dochters (Sophronisba; or, The happy mother who had her daughters
inoculated), 1779

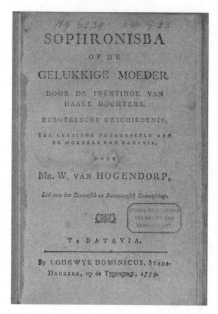

It was not until the British interregnum period, i.e. 1811-1816, that Lieuten-
ant Governor Thomas Stamford Raffles gave the vaccination programme a
sound organizational basis in the region. Boomgaard attributed the success
of the program to the expansion of Pax Neerlandica, that is, the 'law and
order' imposed by the Dutch colonial state in the Indonesian archipelago
(Boomgaard, 2003; Schoute, 1935a and 1935b). Indigenous people – explicitly
Islamic officials or priests – were recruited as smallpox vaccinators due to
the shortage of Dutch physicians (Boomgaard, 2003; Himawan, 1995; Schoute,
1935a and b). The education of the vaccinators was improved by establishing
a medical school in Weltevreden, a suburb of Batavia located in Central Java
in 1851. In Boomgaard's opinion the programme was successful because it
not only attempted to immunize as many very young children as possible,
but it also provided for the surveillance and containment of epidemics
(2003). But it must be noted that the success was somewhat geographically
uneven and less marked in the so-called Outer Islands. For instance, around
1860 the situation was that in comparison to the approximately 350,000
vaccinations carried out annually in Java, vaccinations were administered
to about 20,000 people in Sumatra's West Coast and approximately 10,000 in

the rest of the Outer Islands. Boomgaard attributed this uneven distribution to a parallel unevenness of Pax Neerlandica in the region. Records show that the vaccination of the population against smallpox was quite well organized by 1860. Smallpox had been done away with as a 'big killer' (Boomgaard, 1989a, p. 123; Boomgaard 1989b, p. 127).

In 1879 there was an attempt to set up the production of cowpox vaccine in Batutulis (Bogor or Buitenzorg, part of Batavia), but the experiments using animal lymph from the Netherlands failed for several years (Himawan, 1995). Luckily, in 1884 C.D. Schucking Kool, working in Meester Cornelis (another part of Batavia), succeeded in preparing a vaccine by inoculating human lymph from a smallpox patient in a calf (Kirschner, 1936, p. 258). In 1890 the government decided to establish a Parc Vaccinogène at Weltevreden and production of vaccinia was centralized in the Landskoepokinrichting in 1891. In 1895 this institution merged with the Pasteur Institute (now named Biofarma) in Bandung (West Java), where prophylactic and therapeutic vaccines and sera were produced (Himawan, 1995; Hüsken-Nillissen and De Moulin, 1986; Kirschner, 1936). To maintain the potency of the vaccine, which was dependent on the virulence of the virus strains, the retrovaccination technique developed by Calmette and Guérin was applied since 1905: lymph obtained from the calf was used to inoculate rabbits and subsequently taken back to the calf. The production could be increased by using local *karbouws* (water buffalo) instead of cows. After the 1891 introduction of the so-called animal lymph produced in Parcs Vaccinogènes, the whole population of the Dutch East Indies could be immunized.

In the 1920s L. Otten (1883-1946) at the Pasteur Institute in Bandung developed a method to produce a dried smallpox vaccine that had the advantage that it could be prepared at large batches, and also stored and transported over long distances without losing its potency over significant periods of time (Collier, 1952; Collier, 1954; Otten, 1926 and 1927). This dried vaccine was used in Indonesia since 1921 for vaccinating the local population, and by 1930 smallpox had become a rare infection in the Malay Archipelago. The success was mirrored in the increased reach of the vaccine: for example, the number of doses of vaccine supplied rose from 147,000 in 1931 to 801,700 in 1941 and to more than 26 million by 1949. Before World War II then, the Dutch East Indies had become free of smallpox (Boomgaard, 1996). However, due to World War II the vaccination programme reached a lower percentage of the Indonesian population and there was a weakening of the immunity of the population. As a consequence, a 1947 introduction of smallpox infection resulted in an epidemic that spread over the Indonesian archipelago. The vaccines proved of great service in helping control this epidemic (Collier, 1952).

Figure 22   Institute Pasteur and s'Lands Koepok Inrichting, Bandung

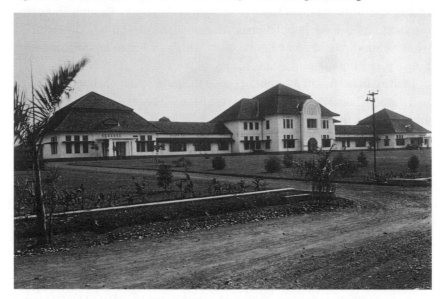

Reproduction courtesy of Collectie Stichting Nationaal Museum van Wereldculturen
Coll.nr. TM-60012974

Yellow fever, dengue and scrub typhus

Although yellow fever did not occur naturally in the East Indies, it was a concern for the colonial powers in the region, largely due to the construction of the Panama Canal, which greatly increased the trade relations between the East and West. Many notable figures, such as Sir Patrick Manson, the father of British tropical medicine, as well as the Dutch researcher J.J. van Loghem, raised concerns about the spread of this dread infection from the Caribbean to the East Indies. In 1914, the same year as the Canal was finally opened, Wickliffe Rose, secretary of the Rockefeller Sanitary Commission, published the report *Yellow fever: Feasibility of its eradication* for which he sought opinions from both figures. Manson in 1903 had insistently expressed his concerns about conveying yellow fever to the Far East, which had remained free of the disease until that time, and in 1914 Van Loghem had declared that 'so long as yellow fever exists in America the danger remains for Asia' (quoted in Rose, 1914).

As a result of Rose's report, the government of the Netherlands addressed a communication to the government of the United States, suggesting that a Dutch initiative to appoint an international commission to institute a system of preventive measures against the spread of yellow fever to the Pacific and South Sea Islands due to the opening of the Panama Canal. The statement of the report was based on the evidence provided by Van Loghem in 1908/1909 that the *Aedes aegypti* mosquito, the principal vector in transmitting yellow fever, was present in the East Indies. Flu later established that an infected mosquito from the Americas that accidentally introduced aboard a ship to the East Indies could survive long enough to spread the infection at the destination (Dinger et al., 1929a). Therefore, Dinger and his colleagues carried out an investigation in Amsterdam in 1929 to gauge whether the mosquitoes from the East Indies were biologically capable of serving as a vector and whether or not East Indian monkeys, e.g. *Macacus cynomolgus*, were susceptible to the yellow fever virus. The result of the experiments proved that the East Indian *Aedes aegypti* mosquitoes could be a vector for yellow fever virus, and that the *Macacus cynomolgus* monkeys were susceptible for the virus, which made the earlier concerns of Manson and Van Loghem all the more valid. Meanwhile, quite by accident researchers also found that humans could be infected via this chain of transmission (Dinger et al., 1929a, 1929b, and 1929c). As one of Dinger's co-authors later revealed, it was Dinger himself who contracted a yellow fever infection, although luckily, he recovered (Swellengrebel, 1955). Although the reasons still remain unknown, this transmission did not seem to have occurred in nature. Asia to this day remains free of epidemic yellow fever, while in 2016 for the first time in history confirmed yellow fever virus was imported in China from Angola, where the patient had acquired the infection (Song et al., 2018; Wilder-Smith and Leong, 2017; Wilder-Smith et al., 2019).

Around the same time as Van Hogendorp had advocated variolation, David Beylon, the municipal barber-surgeon in Batavia, published a report in the *Proceedings of the Batavian Society of Arts and Sciences* in which he described an epidemic of 'knuckle fever'[96] (1921/1780). Although it appeared to be a well-known disease in the area, Beylon reported that the disease never had been known to reach epidemic proportions among the people in Batavia before then. A footnote to the paper mentions a much longer rainy season, suggesting that weather conditions might have influenced the outbreak. Although relatively obscure, Beylon's report must be regarded as having given the first account of the disease, what we now know as dengue fever. Ten years after this publication, the American physician Benjamin Rush published a monograph entitled 'Account on the bilious, remitting fever' (1789), where he described the epidemic of knuckle fever that struck Philadelphia in 1780 (Packard, 2016). More than a century later A. van der Scheer, a Dutch military doctor in the East Indies, described various fever

96   *knokkelkoorts* (dengue).

patterns; he distinguished the 'five-day fever' (*vijfdaagse koorts*) as a pattern typical of dengue (Bonne, 1936). In what is perhaps a dubious honour, this fever type is now named 'Van der Scheerse koorts' after him. In 1918 Australian microbiologists Cleland and Bradley demonstrated that the mosquito *Stegomyia fasciata* (now *Aedes aegypti*) transmitted both dengue as well yellow fever.

Another infectious disease that received considerable attention from European medical doctors working in the East Indies was later revealed to be a rickettsial infection. At a meeting of the Society of Tropical Medicine in 1913 in The Hague, W. Schüffner presented a paper on an infectious disease he called 'pseudo-typhus', which he had encountered while working in Deli in the northern part of Sumatra. He found that the disease resembled the Japanese 'kedani fever' that was assumed to be transmitted by the kedani mite. Later, it was shown that this disease was scrub typhus; a mite-borne infectious disease caused by an intracellular microorganism *Orientia tsutsugamushi* that was previously called *Rickettsia tsutsugamushi* (Schüffner, 1913).

Poliomyelitis

According to K.T. Lie of the Pasteur Institute of Bandung, poliomyelitis has presented a relatively minor public health problem in Indonesia, especially compared to other parts of the world where it has wreaked considerable havoc. Despite the paucity of complete and reliable statistical data, he assumed poliomyelitis to be endemic in the region with low morbidity (Lie, 1960). We, too, found very little source material about poliomyelitis in the Dutch East Indies and are therefore not able to draw too many further conclusions. It is possible that disease was not even endemic in all the islands and that, depending on the density of the population or the intensity of contacts with other populations, many remained free of the diseases altogether. Anyway, outbreaks were reported in the 1950s from several regions in Java and Sumatra (Lie, 1960; Van Erp, 1958). Following these episodes, Lie conducted a cross-sectional study in Bandung (West Java) among preschool children, schoolchildren and adults. All sera were tested on neutralizing antibodies against poliovirus type 1, 2, and 3, using prototypes provided by J.D. Verlinde of Leiden. Fifty per cent of the sera obtained from one-year-old children contained antibodies against type 3, whereas those at age three years had antibodies against type 2 and 3 viruses. This indicated that they had also acquired poliovirus type 2 in the meantime. By age six, some 74 per cent of the children had acquired antibodies against all three types. It has to be taken into account that on the average only 1 per cent of the infected children will show clinical symptoms of poliomyelitis. It was assumed that paralytic poliomyelitis was a rare occurrence among the very young children and that the antibodies-positive children would be protected against infection and did not need protection by immunization. After the age of six the percentage of persons with antibody to each of the three types remained high. Based on these finding, Lie recommended in 1960 the following: Poliomyelitis is a major endemic disease in Indonesia but at present the amount of clinical damage is relatively small. There are many more important diseases which need to be placed higher in the priority list for money and resources (Lie, 1960). Paradoxically, as it happens in the case of polio, the improved conditions of hygiene and living environments might actually increase the number of susceptible children and adults. In that case, the decision on vaccinations may need to be re-evaluated based on serologic surveys among representative groups of three-year-old children and six-year-old children. Luckily, in 1988, Indonesia adopted the goal of eradicating poliomyelitis by the year 2000.

Rabies

A series of communications in the NTvG between Dutch veterinarians W.C. Schimmel and C.A. Penning show rather different opinions on the status of rabies in the Dutch East Indies at the end of the nineteenth century. Whereas Schimmel believed that the human incidence was low despite the widespread occurrence of rabies among dogs in the kampongs of Java and Sumatra, Penning was convinced that the death rate due to rabies among indigenous people in these kampongs was actually significant, and these figures were not entered into the statistics because Dutch doctors had not been consulted (Schimmel, 1889). This exchange throws some doubt on modern-day statements, such as that of the veterinary epidemiologist M.P. Ward that the Dutch East Indies had been infected only since the 1890s (Ward, 2014). After 1890, however, there are regular reports of rabies from Java and the east coast of Sumatra. In 1895 the Pasteur Institute administered some of the first treatments against rabies in the islands. Different techniques were used in succession for preparing the vaccines: from 1895 to 1905, they relied on Pasteur's original method of using dried canine spinal cord, but in 1906 they switched to the dilution method developed by the Hungarian scientist E. Högyes using monkey brains to propagate the virus (Kirschner, 1936; Van Loghem, 1935). Then in the 1930s Maria J. Otten-van Stockum developed a method whereby a 10 per cent suspension of monkey brain infected with 'virus fixe' was inactivated by incubating with 1.5 per cent formaldehyde for five days at 37°C. Advantageously this last preparation could be stored at 5°C without loss of activity and was hence more durable and portable. From 1933 this vaccine became the standard treatment of patients who were bitten by rabid dogs (Van Stockum, 1935; Van Loghem, 1935; Van Stockum, 1941).

The last Dutch head of the Department for rabies and the Smallpox Department of the Pasteur Institute in Bandung was W.A. Collier, a parasitologist and tropical medicine expert of considerable renown. Of German descent, Collier first studied medicine and then joined the Ehrlich Institute in Frankfurt am Main and the Koch Institute in Berlin. He also spent time in South America in the mid-1920s, working as a parasitologist in Venezuela, Buenos Aires and Brazil. Due to the changing political climate in Germany, he left his homeland for good in 1935 and moved to the Netherlands, where he continued as volunteer his research on chemotherapy and cancer at the Institute for Preventive Medicine in Leiden (Bijl, 1954). In 1937 he embarked for the East Indies and joined the Pasteur Institute in 1941. Despite his German nationality he and his family were interned by the Japanese occupation forces from 1942 until 1945, because he refused to declare himself in favour of Adolf Hitler. After the war he was granted Dutch citizenship in 1947, the unfortunate and unpleasant consequence of which was that he had to be coerced to leave Indonesia in 1950. But he continued to pursue tropical medicine as he was then appointed head of the Public Health Laboratory for Bacteriology, Paramaribo, Suriname. His research activities had a wide scope, besides virology – rabies, smallpox, yellow fever – and his research fields comprised parasitology, cancer, chemotherapy. He was also interested in Western psychology and Indian philosophy and psychology (Adhin, 1960; Ruys, 1960; Wolff, 1961).

Suriname and the Netherlands Antilles, former West Indies

The Dutch colonies in the West comprised both islands and parts of the mainland of the South American continent. Suriname, on the north-eastern coast of South America, came under Dutch rule in the late seventeenth century. The majority of its population lives in the coastal regions and the savannah zone. South of the savannah is the third region, roughly 80 per cent of the country, where dense tropical forests intersected by a variety of streams, is home to only a small minority of the population. The Netherlands Antilles are composed of two groups of islands in the Caribbean;

the distance from Paramaribo, capital of Suriname, to each of the groups is approximately 1,600 km north-westwards and north-eastwards from Suriname, respectively. The Leeward Antilles[97] Curaçao, Aruba, and Bonaire belong to the Curaçao group in the southern part of the Caribbean near the north-west coast of Venezuela. The three smaller islands St Maarten, St Eustatius, and Saba are located within the Leeward Islands[98] of the Lesser Antilles in the north-eastern part of the Caribbean at a distance of 900 km from the Curaçao group (Goslinga, 1979).

The early history of Suriname was first described in 1789 by David de Isaac Cohen Nassy, S.H. Brandon, M.P. de Leon, S.J.V. de la Parra and J. de la Parra in their *Essai historique sur la colonie de Surinam*. The work appeared first anonymously but with a dedication to the directors of the colony of Suriname (Bijlsma, 1982). More recently, historian C.C. Goslinga published an account of the history of both Suriname and the Netherlands Antilles (1979). Soon after the Spanish invasion of the Caribbean, the original inhabitants were killed or removed from the islands, and a century later, at the time of the occupation of the Dutch, most of the remaining Indians scattered to the mainland (Goslinga, 1979, p. 6). After a first unsuccessful attempt the Dutch had gained control of Suriname in 1667 from the English, exchanging it for the North American island, New Amsterdam (later New York). The history of the region is deeply intertwined with that of the slave trade; Black Africans were brought in as enslaved labourers from Congo, Angola, and West Africa (Goslinga, 1979). While fairly widespread, slavery played in Suriname a more important role in the economy than in the Curaçao islands and the Dutch Leeward Islands. It also had its consequences for the transmission of viral diseases as smallpox and yellow fever from Africa to the Americas.

Smallpox

Smallpox is believed to have been introduced into the Americas by the European invaders after the 1492 discovery of the continents by Christopher Columbus. Smallpox was imported into the Caribbean Islands and South America by the Spanish and Portuguese, either directly from Europe or from Africa (Fenner, 1988b). As far as one can tell, the first smallpox epidemic hit Paramaribo in 1743, and subsequent outbreaks occurred in 1763/64, 1785, 1800, and 1806. Perhaps the worst epidemic to affect the region was that of 1819-1820, which claimed the lives of at least 10,000 slaves (Van Andel,

97 Benedenwindse eilanden (Leeward Islands).
98 Bovenwindse eilanden (Windward Islands).

1947, p. 151; Benjamins and Snelleman, 1914-1917, pp. 281-283). According to Oudschans Dentz, vaccinations were first administered in 1801 by Dr Walther Cadell at the Amsterdam plantation in the Perica, but despite its success, the example was not followed by owners of other plantations (Oudschans Dentz, 1943).

It should be noted that the British occupied Suriname between 1799 and 1816. After the French revolution and during the Napoleonic era the constitution of the Republic of the Seven United Provinces also underwent significant changes. In 1795 the United Provinces was replaced by the Batavian Republic, which was subsequently changed to the Kingdom of Holland, which was incorporated within France in 1810. It was under this governmental structure that in 1805 Dr Wölfing, Paramaribo's municipal physician, first vaccinated some children against smallpox (Hallewas, 1981, p. 35). Then in 1812 an English merchant named Carstairs brought the cowpox vaccine from England and let his children be inoculated by a local physician. The English governor, Pinson Bonham, strongly advocated vaccination, and he provided the Collegium Medicum with vaccine (Oudschans Dentz, 1943). From then onwards vaccination was practiced more extensively. According this author, the first subsequent epidemic in 1819 was small. His report sounds somewhat contrary to the communication by Benjamins and Snelleman, who reported that in 1819 and 1820 more than 10,000 slaves succumbed to smallpox during this epidemic (1814-1817). But no subsequent serious epidemic was observed. Two Parcs Vaccinogènes were established in the region for the continuous production of cowpox vaccine, in Curaçao and Venezuela in 1882, and in Suriname in 1884 (Lampe, 1927 and 1936).

Yellow fever

One of the earliest European accounts of yellow fever in the Americas comes to us from A. Schlaprizi, who reported a 1741 outbreak of what he called the 'chocolate disease'[99] that occurred aboard a Dutch man-of-war in the harbour of Curaçao, near Venezuela (Prakken, 1975). Suriname did play a somewhat indirect part in the early history of the understanding of yellow fever, specifically through the person of one of its citizens, a Portuguese Jewish physician named David (de Isaac Cohen) Nassy, although he was not recognized as a physician by the Collegium Medicum, which had been established in 1781 (Cohen, 1991; Simons, 1947). Nassy cared for yellow fever patients during the 1793 epidemic in Philadelphia that was also described

99 *chocolaadziekte.*

by Benjamin Rush (Packard, 2016). Nassy argued in favour of a mild therapy instead of a therapy with healing, bleeding and purging (Nassy, 1793). He was credited for his care of the Philadelphian citizens by George Washington, and he was invited to be member of the prestigious American Philosophical Society (1843).

In mainland Suriname a barber-surgeon named Edward B. Bancroft was the first to describe a case of yellow fever in 1782, but as far as we know, there were no reports of major outbreaks for some decades (De Haas et al., 1971). The first report of a full epidemic of yellow fever in Suriname itself dates to 1793; thereafter, in the nineteenth century a dozen epidemics were reported (De Haas et al., 1971; Flu, 1910; Hallewas, 1981; Van Leent, 1881). The microbiologist Paul Flu, who was from Suriname, provided an exact, firsthand description of an epidemic that struck in 1908-1909 (Flu, 1910; see also Flu, 1937; Van der Kuyp, 1958). Since 1911, Flu found several Hindustanis and Europeans in the area afflicted with a disease whose symptoms were similar, but which could not be confirmed as yellow fever (Flu, 1937; Van der Kuyp, 1958). In 1937 Suriname was declared free of yellow fever, after which no clear cases of the disease have been reported officially. Nevertheless, still in 1993 Chippaux et al. reported cases of yellow fever in French Guiana that were imported from Suriname.

More information on the epidemiology and vaccinations of yellow fever in the western colonies of the Netherlands can be found in the doctoral thesis of M.F. Polak (1944/1945). Based on serological data from patients in the area, Polak concluded that yellow fever did not prevail after the epidemics of 1902 and 1908/1909 in and around Paramaribo, where *Aedes aegypti* mosquitoes – the natural vectors of urban yellow fever – were prevalent. Studies among the aboriginal Indian peoples in the jungle area, and those living in the Maroon[100] villages, revealed that about 25 to 30 per cent of the Indians had antibodies against yellow fever virus, but that the distribution among the Maroons was heavily weighted towards the male populations: 21 per cent of the samples collected from the Maroon males was reactive in contrast to 4 per cent found among Maroon females. This phenomenon was seen as characteristic of jungle yellow fever which was contracted out of doors, and Polak concluded that male Maroon Indians spent more time outdoors in the tropical forests than did the female members of the communities. This is the so-called jungle or sylvatic fever.[101] He concluded:

---

100 Polak used the old term 'Bushnegro'.
101 Sylvatic yellow fever: human infection occurs from the enzootic forest cycle between primates or other animals.

'We cannot but accept at the moment that the yellow fever virus keeps in Surinamese jungle independent of the *Aëdes aegypti* and man, though human infections do occur.' At that time the vector of the sylvatic yellow fever was not yet known. His opinion on the matter of administering vaccinations against yellow fever was to practice restraint, in part because he was unable to predict which of the two recommended methods of vaccination would be preferable in the long run: the French method, with the neurotropic virus, or the American method, with the virus attenuated in tissue culture. At that time vaccine preparation had just commenced at the Institute for Tropical Hygiene at Amsterdam using a virus strain received from Brazil, where they had not yet resolved or traced certain difficulties that had arisen in the preparation methods (Polak, 1944/1945).

Serological surveys after World War II revealed that jungle yellow fever remained prevalent in the interior of Suriname (Snijders et al., 1947; Van der Kuyp, 1958; Wolff et al., 1958). In 1971 De Haas et al. reported a 1968 case of yellow fever in a patient who had worked at the government Forestry Department in the hinterland of Suriname for nearly three years (De Haas et al., 1971). Although there were no or very few monkeys at the pine (pinus) plantation where the patient worked, the serological findings hinted at jungle fever rather than urban yellow fever. That the latter was even a consideration was due to the fact that the patient was found to be part of a group of labourers who, every fortnight or so, spent a long weekend in Paramaribo town. Consequently, the investigators hesitantly proposed the idea that the virus was maintained through a basic cycle that did not necessarily involve monkeys, the population of which was too sparse to sustainably maintain the monkey-*Haemagogus* [mosquito]-monkey cycle of propagation. The laboratory diagnosis yellow fever was made by A.H. Jonkers of the Trinidad Regional Virus Laboratory in the British West Indies, who had received material obtained at autopsy – primarily liver tissue – of the patient collected. He reported to De Haas that the specimen received was positive for yellow fever virus.

Certain surveys were conducted in the population that lived around the construction of a barrage near the town Afobaka in the Brokopondo province between 1961 and 1964, in order to create a storage lake for generating hydroelectricity (Van Tongeren, 1965). The authors paid no attention in their conclusion to the question of whether or not the prevalence of antibodies against not only yellow fever but also dengue 2 and Ilhéus viruses had any association with the storage lake. Neutralizing antibody tests showed that such viral infections as yellow fever, dengue 2 and Ilhéus had high antibody ratios more or less across the population, whereas Bussuquara and St Louis encephalitis virus were consistently present in lower ratios.

Dengue

Dengue is known to have been widespread in the Caribbean and Suriname for many years. As mentioned earlier, the first description of a dengue-like epidemic (in 1780) in the Americas was published by Benjamin Rush in 1789 (Packard, 2016). Serological and epidemiological investigations on this disease were carried out both in Suriname as well on the Dutch Antilles during the second half of the twentieth century. A serologic survey on St Eustatius in 1979 led to the hypothesis that dengue virus type 1 was present around 1900 and overtaken by dengue virus 2 of late (Van der Sar et al., 1979). This is remarkable as only dengue type 2 was reported before 1963 (Allicock et al., 2012). Another serologic survey indicated that dengue 2 was endemic on Curaçao, but not on Aruba (Weiland et al., 1978).

Other arboviruses

In 1962 the Public Health Service of Suriname requested the Medical Faculty of the University in Leiden for support to set up a virology laboratory in addition to the bacteriology laboratory already in place. Verlinde, the head of the medical microbiology department, invited Dirk Metselaar to implement the plans for establishing a self-sufficient unit with laboratories for cells culture as well as animal facilities for mice and guinea pigs. Metselaar had accomplished creditable work on malaria in Western New Guinea (Irian Jaya). He had just started a traineeship in virology and was interested in insect-borne diseases; he arrived in Paramaribo at the Central Public Health Laboratory in 1962. Towards the end of that very year, he had to deal with an outbreak of polio in Suriname, but meanwhile he did not neglect his personal goals of studying the arboviruses (P.J. van der Maas, personal communication, 2013).

Within months of his arrival Metselaar had succeeded in establishing tissue culture laboratories for virus cultivation and setting up the equipment for isolating viruses in suckling mice. The laboratory began to routinely handle diagnostics of Dutch military men posted to Suriname, who often fell ill with fevers upon returning from training patrols in forested areas. Until the establishment of this virus facility, there had been just a single report of the isolation of an arbovirus from Suriname (Metselaar, 1966). But with the newly equipped laboratory in place, there was a dramatic increase in the number of publications reporting the isolation of many other arboviruses: Mayaro virus, Oriboca virus, Caraparu virus, and two Mucambo strains were isolated by inoculating suckling mice (Jonkers et al., 1967; Metselaar et al., 1964a; Metselaar, 1966). Another three strains eventually found to be identical to each other and to strains in Trinidad were also isolated around the same time. They represented a new Arbovirus Group C agent that was described as Restan virus in a separate paper (Jonkers et al., 1967). Still another newly reported virus was found to be a member of the group of arboviruses on the basis of serological tests. Because it was not clear whether it deserved its own place or had to be classified as a strain of Semliki Forest virus, it was temporarily named Paramaribo virus, but later was confirmed as the Semliki Forest virus, the first such isolation from a human (Metselaar et al., 1964a). Two decades later, in 1987, during an outbreak of mild febrile illness in Bangui, Central African Republic, the Semliki Forest virus was isolated from mosquitoes for the first time and found in the sera of 22 patients as well (Mathiot et al., 1990). Unfortunately, to the best of our knowledge no further reports on the identification of Paramaribo virus can be found.

Since human arbovirus infections were observed and could be confirmed by laboratory assays in Suriname, it seemed expedient to start an investigation program which would also include studies of their insect vectors. Since the beginning of this program in 1964, dozens of virus strains have been isolated from man as well from mosquitoes or sentinel mice. The Kwatta virus was isolated from *Culex* mosquitoes, but none of the 78 sera collected from residents living in the neighbourhood neutralized this virus (De Haas et al., 1966). De Haas's group also reported the isolation of eight viruses belonging to the Guama group in 1971 (De Haas and De Kruyf, 1971). Six strains originated from sentinel mice and two from *Culex portesi* mosquitoes.

Poliomyelitis

There are no written accounts of clinical poliomyelitis in Suriname before the twentieth century, as neither the annual reports of the Military Hospital, Paramaribo, nor Lampe's study on the health situation in Suriname mentioned the disease (Wilterdink et al., 1964). A few suspected cases were reported sporadically between 1929 and 1947, and one imported case each in 1947, 1951, and 1952, respectively. The above-mentioned Collier reported on an outbreak of seventeen cases of an 'infantile paralysis' in 1954, three of the cases proved to be caused by the Coxsackie A-10 rather than the poliomyelitis virus (Collier et al., 1954). In 1960 Hofman and Wilterdink conducted a large scale sero-epidemiologic study on 4,155 sera samples collected from patients in the Netherlands (2,073), Curaçao (1,669), Suriname (46), St Eustatius (20), and Netherlands New Guinea (347), attempting to gauge the exposure to the poliomyelitis virus in these regions before the large-scale introduction of poliomyelitis vaccines. The results showed that all three types of poliovirus circulated in the Netherlands, Curaçao, St Eustatius, Suriname and Netherlands New Guinea and those infections took place at an earlier age in Curaçao than in the Netherlands. The sample size from Suriname, St Eustatius, and New Guinea the number of sera proved too small for a clear evaluation.

Another serological and epidemiological survey of poliomyelitis in Suriname was executed in 1961 by the famous virologist and epidemiologist Joseph Melnick (Melnick et al., 1962). The American team found a solid immunity to all three types of poliovirus by the age of 20 years; 82 per cent of the children aged five to nine had antibody to types 1 and 2, and 59 per cent to type 3. Forty per cent in the same age group were triple positive, and the number rose to 72 per cent in the 10- to 14-year-old age group.

In 1962, a polio virus type 1 outbreak spread from the neighbouring British Guiana to Suriname resulting in 40 traceable cases of paralytic disease. Not a single case was reported from the Nickerie district at the border between Suriname and British Guiana, where the vaccination campaign with the trivalent oral Sabin-type poliovirus was started early in the course of the epidemic. Most cases occurred in the Suriname district around Paramaribo, about 230 km from Nickerie (Wilterdink et al., 1964; Metselaar et al., 1964b). As mentioned earlier, Metselaar was stationed in Paramaribo for about a year during this outbreak. Having set up the virological lab by then he was able to examine sera as well as stool samples from children in the age group of 0-4 years of age, whose immune status was unknown. An increasing number of poliovirus type 1 positive stool specimens towards the end of 1962 announced the approaching outbreak. The proportion of children possessing the antibody against type 1 increased from 12 per cent up to 74 per cent after the outbreak. From 1964 until 1969 the distribution of polioviruses in the region was monitored by regular virological examination of stool specimens from children of the 1- to 5-year-old age group (De Haas, 1971). All three types were found to circulate continuously, and a correlation was found between an increased level of poliovirus circulation and the appearance of clinical poliomyelitis. The application of trivalent oral vaccine at times had only a partial effect on the level of circulation because the acceptance rate for the vaccine was too low. For the application of the first dose only 55, 48, and 25 per cent of the children were presented in 1963, 1965, and 1967, respectively. The proportion of children receiving a second or a third dose was still lower.

Rabies

It was only in the beginning of the twentieth century that it came to be
known that insectivorous, frugivorous and hematophagous bats act as
wildlife reservoirs for the rabies virus (Johnson et al., 2010). In Suriname,
Desmodus rotundus, common vampire bats, functioned as the main reservoirs and transmitters of the virus, which were maintained in epidemiologic
sylvatic cycles for a very long time. In contrast to the mainland, however,
these vampire bats are absent from most of the Caribbean islands with
the exception of Trinidad, Tobago, and Margarita Island (Lee et al., 2012).
Although capable of feeding off any mammal, these bats tend most readily
to feed on the blood of cattle. Consequently, vampire bat-transmitted rabies
is primarily a problem in livestock, but seldom transmitted to humans.

With regard to rabies, a contribution of another member of the above-
mentioned Nassy family to the history of Dutch virology in the tropics might
be mentioned. In 1918 Jacques George Nassy defended in Amsterdam his
doctoral thesis entitled *Preservation of 'virus fixe' with regard to the fight
against rabies in the tropics*. He investigated immunization against rabies using
an inactivated vaccine which could be shipped to remote places in the tropics
instead of transporting the patient over a long distance to a central hospital
where the living attenuated virus fixe was available (Van Driel, 1921). We could
not retrieve information whether this vaccine has been used in Suriname.

The first laboratory-confirmed outbreak of vampire bat-transmitted rabies
of cattle in Suriname was reported by W.A. Collier and V.A.H. Tiggelman-van
Krugten (1955). The source of the initial infection seems to have been a
large swamp, approximately 100 square km in area, about 5 km south of
the capital Paramaribo, where rabies was epizootic. Public health officials
quickly responded to the outbreak with a mass – not just cattle, but also
donkeys and horses – vaccination programme, the results of which were
tracked until 1960. New cases of rabies ceased within four months of the
administration of the first vaccines, and none were reported thereafter until
the end of the observation period (Bush, 1961). A second outbreak occurred
in 1967 (Verlinde, 1969b; Verlinde et al., 1970). These authors compared two
strains isolated from Surinamese cattle with Strain Amsterdam III isolated
from a case of human rabies acquired from a street dog, and the Pasteur
strain of fixed rabies virus. The main results were that the Surinamese
strain occupied an intermediate position between the Pasteur strain and
the strain of the European street virus. Therefore, it was quite reasonable
to expect that vaccination or treatment using the *virus fixe* rabies virus be
effective against rabies with the Suriname viruses.

Seven years after the epizootic outbreak of rabies, an epidemic of ascending flaccid paralysis among children – killing seven – was reported in a Maroon village alongside the Suriname River (Verlinde et al., 1975). The clinical picture of the disease was not recognized as rabies, at least at first, although it was known that the neuropathological picture of vampire bat rabies presented most mostly with paralysis but without hydrophobia. Indeed, despite the high numbers of vampire bats in the area, most indications ran contrary to what one expected of a bat-transmitted infection. At first, a virological examination of stool specimens of the affected children revealed coxsackie A4 virus. But upon further examination, suspensions of brain and spinal cord from three autopsied children were found to be pathogenic both for suckling mice and weaning mice, producing histological lesions of encephalomyelitis, but no muscular lesions. The surprising outcome was therefore, that the investigators had isolated the lyssa virus from the central nervous system of three autopsied children (Verlinde et al., 1975). Upon closer questioning, it was found that the mothers of the first two children infected had been bitten by a rat. Furthermore, about one month before the epidemic a number of 'pingoes' – the white-lip peccary, hog-like animal also known to harbour the rabies virus – had been slaughtered and almost all children had assisted in the ceremony. But since none of the adult males had contracted rabies nobody made the connection at first. Although the laboratory diagnosis of the case of death was rabies, the probable source of which might be the white-lip peccary; this could not be proved by lack of specimens of these animals.

Africa: Kenya, Uganda and Ethiopia and West Africa

The geographical focus of Dutch virologists to Africa was related with the position of tropical medicine and hygiene in the former Dutch colonies. According to the medical historian L. van Bergen, Dutch specialists in tropical medicine began to move their primary working area from both the East and the West Indies to Africa sometime around the 1960s (2007, p. 120). Events such as the 1949 transfer of Indonesia's sovereignty and of Western New Guinea to United Nations Temporary Executive Authority (UNTEA) in 1962 marked a significant change for tropical hygienists working in the Dutch colonies in the East and West Indies. They greatly diminished these scientists' prospects for research on diseases peculiar to these regions (Kranendonk, 1967, pp. 151-157). Fortunately, however, at the same time, development cooperation began to attract political attention, due to which a direction of technical assistance

(DTA) was created within the Ministry of Foreign Affairs. The director of the Department for Tropical Hygiene of the Royal Tropical Institute, Prof. Dr Otto Kranendonk, was invited by the DTA to reconnoitre in Africa, where, it was imagined, the medical scientific expertise of the Dutch scientists from the Indies could be combined with the needs of the African countries. Thus, an important impetus for this initiative was the continuation of tropical hygiene-related research for the Dutch specialists from the East Indies who would have otherwise either lose their expertise or find themselves without occupation. A Medical Research Centre as a department of the Royal Tropical Institute, Amsterdam, was established in Kenya in which a virology laboratory should be set up. Since the 1970s the ideas of the aim of tropical medicine changed from curative and preventive medicine to more social-economic issues, from tropical medicine to international healthcare. The advent of the AIDS pandemic towards the later part of the century unfortunately caused a shift towards much more attention for Africa as exemplified by the international conferences on AIDS in Africa that started in 1985 in Brussels.

Kenya

The Medical Research Centre was located between the Jomo Kenyatta Hospital and the Division of Vector-Borne Diseases of the Ministry of Health. Dirk Metselaar, already well regarded for his work on insect-borne diseases and poliomyelitis in Paramaribo, was appointed as the head of the Laboratory for Virology of the Nairobi Medical Research Centre in 1964 before the centre was opened officially. President Mzee Jomo Kenyatta performed the inauguration in 1966 by unveiling a plaque.

In Nairobi just like in the Paramaribo, Metselaar performed very valuable work, beginning with the setting up of facilities for the laboratory diagnosis of various virus diseases. In his first year he spent some time at the East African Virus Research Institute (EAVRI) in Entebbe, Uganda, to familiarize himself with colleagues and build a network (P.J. van der Maas, personal communication, 2013). Research by himself in Kenya concerned the epidemiology of a variety of arboviruses that were isolated from both mosquitoes and patient specimens (Rodhain et al., 1975). He was also responsible for isolating an arbovirus called Akabane virus, since found to be related to the rather better-known Schmallenberg virus (Metselaar et al. 1976). These latter studies were conducted in collaboration with reference laboratories outside Kenya, notably the East African Virus Research Institute at Entebbe, Uganda. Another topic of interest was the spread of poliomyelitis as observed in Kenya and in Western Europe (Metselaar 1976;

Figure 23   Nairobi Medical Research Centre

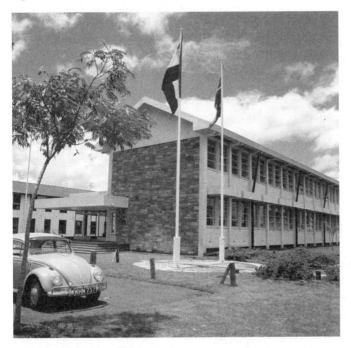

Reproduction courtesy of Collectie Nationaal Museum van Wereldculturen
Coll.nr. TM nr. 20038579

Metselaar et al. 1977a; Metselaar et al., 1977b; Metselaar, 1978). With regard
to these studies the epidemiologist A.S. (Lex) Muller, head of the Department of Epidemiology of the Medical Research Centre in Nairobi, was an
important figure. He was the driving force behind the so-called Machakos
Studies Project within which Metselaar carried out his poliomyelitis studies
(Muller et al., 1977).

To explain the rapid development of polio from being a relatively rare
disease to one of considerable public health importance concurrent with
increase in incidence of paralysis, Metselaar (1976) proposed the hypothesis
of selection of virulent viruses at the expense of less virulent ones. He
also initiated the organization of a vaccination campaign in the Kiambu
District (nowadays Kiambu County) at the northern border of Nairobi
County, whereby vaccination centres were located at such distances that
no mother would have had to walk more than 3 km to bring their children
in (Metselaar, 1977). The vaccines were administered by well-instructed, if
non-medical personnel. The outcome was that the overall immunization
coverage against polio was more than 90 per cent in this region.

Metselaar also described a new member of the rhabdovirus group, the Mount Elton bat virus. In addition, during the 1969-1971 pandemic of haemorrhagic conjunctivitis, his group isolated an enterovirus that was later found to be identical to the prototype enterovirus 70, known to the etiologic agent of pandemic acute haemorrhagic conjunctivitis (Metselaar et al., 1976). Although the first published report of successful isolation of the prototype came from Japan, the virus was, in fact, earlier isolated in Nairobi. Unfortunately, the typing results of this strain were not published until later and hence the group missed getting their due priority (P.J. van der Maas, personal communication, 2014). He was also involved in handling and investigating smallpox material, especially around the time when eradication appeared imminent. In 1977 the laboratory received a specimen from a surveillance team at the Mandera triangle (at the joint border of Kenya, Ethiopia, and Somalia. Rather than immediately notifying the WHO and sending the specimen the headquarters in Geneva, for further investigation, Metselaar first cultured the material in fertile eggs and isolated a poxvirus, information that he sent to Geneva together with the specimen (Henderson and Ježek, 1988, p. 1051; Foster et al., 1978; P.J. van der Maas, personal communication, 2014; Metselaar, 1977, p. S16). Many years later, he would mention the incident, saying that the WHO officials blamed him for the possible delay. He retired in 1978 from active laboratory work, but would subsequently publish a well-received book – in cooperation with his former colleague in Entebbe, Uganda, D.I.H. Simpson – entitled *Practical virology for medical students and practitioners in tropical countries* (1982).

Although the MRC in Nairobi was principally staffed by Dutch scientists until 1977, it served as the de facto National Public Health Virus Laboratory in Kenya. Researchers there initiated fruitful collaborations with the Medical Faculty of the University of Nairobi, and also built up a network with various other national and regional research facilities, such as the East African Virus Research Institute in Entebbe, Uganda, as well as with international institutes and organizations (Metselaar, 1977). Following the collapse of the East African Community in 1977, the Kenyan government decided to bring all foreign institutes under Kenyan authority, and it was agreed that the Royal Tropical Institute should transfer the Nairobi MRC in 1982 to the Republic of Kenya. In 1979 the institute was incorporated as the Kenyan Medical Research Institute (KEMRI). Meanwhile, however, the upper-level political and bureaucratic changes did not result in the ousting of the foreign staff from Kenyan research projects. For example, in a study on the epidemiology of haemorrhagic fever viruses by Peter Muhumuza Tukei, the American Bruce K. Johnson headed a part of the

Figure 24   D. Metselaar (1914-2006) in northern Kenya

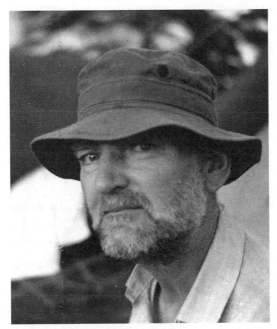

Reproduction courtesy of P.J. van der Maas

project in collaboration with the Dutch young medical doctor Pieter Petit who played the role of a fieldworker, taking detailed histories and clinical finding in patients suspected of haemorrhagic fevers (Tukei, 1988). Later, Tukei was nominated to head the Virus Research Centre of the Kenyan Medical Research Institute, in which capacity he continued to conduct collaborative studies. For example, in 1992 he performed a study on the efficacy of orally administered OPV and the injectable, inactivated IPV in stimulating humoral and intestinal immunity in children who lived in a rural community in Kenya in collaboration with the Royal Tropical Institute in Amsterdam and RIVM in Bilthoven (Kok et al., 1992). This study was funded by the WHO and carried out within the framework of the Joint Project Machakos, which concluded in 1988, the same project within which Metselaar had performed his studies in the 1970s.

Uganda

The institute now known as the Uganda Virus Research Institute (UVRI) in Entebbe has a long history. It was first established in 1936 by the International

Division of the Rockefeller Foundation (USA) as the Yellow Fever Institute. The main focus then was on yellow fever epidemiology, with particular emphasis laid on investigating the extent of spread of the virus from West Africa eastwards. Over the years, UVRI was the home of the discovery and isolation of a number of other, previously unknown, arboviruses, some of which proved to be of considerable medical importance. In 1950, the Institute was renamed as the East African Virus Research Institute (EAVRI) and was then designated as a World Health Organization (WHO) Regional Centre for Arboviruses Reference and Research. After the collapse of the East African community there was a period of deterioration, but the Institute pulled through after the return of political stability and due to help from international funding agencies such as the NIH and the WHO.

Worth mentioning in connections with later activities at the UVRI are the contributions of D.W. (Daan) Mulder. Trained in medicine in Groningen, Mulder went first to Tanzania in 1978 where he started first as a general clinical officer and later as the coordinator for tuberculosis and leprosy research. In 1988 he joined the Medical Research Council in the UK and in this capacity helped to initiate a collaborative effort between the MRC and UVRI to combat AIDS, which he directed until 1994 (Mulder, 1996). Mulder's work on AIDS was critically important to understanding the epidemiology of this devastating disease in Africa, where in contrast to the Western world – the high-risk groups first identified were intravenous drug users and male homosexuals – there was high incidence of heterosexual transmission. Tragically Mulder died an early death in the October of 1998. A supplement of the journal *Tropical Medicine and International Health* dedicated to his memory was published in 2000, where his friends and colleagues mourned and celebrated the career of 'someone who made critically important contributions to our knowledge of the epidemic of AIDS which is devastating populations in large areas of Africa' (Smith and Muller, 2000).

Ethiopia

In 1992 Amsterdam hosted the eighth International AIDS Conference, themed 'A World United against AIDS'. During the conference, Jan Pronk, the Netherlands's Minister of Developing Cooperation, became especially attentive to the necessity of setting up HIV research in developing countries (Sanders et al., 2001). Dutch AIDS researchers of the Amsterdam Cohort Studies were invited to make a proposal for setting up an HIV reference centre in Africa. The result was the establishment of Ethiopian-Netherlands HIV/AIDS Research Project (ENARP) in 1994. The goals of the project were to investigate

HIV and AIDS in Ethiopia, train Ethiopian researchers in epidemiology, immunology and virology, and to establish an HIV reference laboratory for Ethiopia and surrounding countries, with the aim of gradually transferring ownership (Sanders et al., 2003). This aim was markedly different from that of the above-mentioned Nairobi Medical Research Institute. Despite commendable goals, differences in both the vision and priorities gradually became evident amongst the various participants and stakeholders of the ENARP. For instance, different parties could not agree on whether to emphasize the development of high-tech laboratories or divert the resources towards a regional and national surveillance system. Thus, despite some tangible gains, there was a stalemate in the cooperation between ENARP and such other stakeholders as the Federal Ministry of Health, which could not be resolved. Eventually, the financial support sustaining this bilateral project came to an end in 2003. Fortunately, however, HIV/AIDS activities themselves did not come to a similar end as they were integrated within Ethiopian Health and Nutrition Research Institute (EHNRI) (Sanders et al., 2003).

West Africa

One Dutch medical researcher who deserves special recognition in the context of medical virology in West Africa is M.F. Schim van der Loeff, specifically for his epidemiological work on HIV-2. This virus type was first described in 1986 and appeared to be more closely related to simian immunodeficiency virus (SIV) than to HIV-1 (Clavel et al., 1986). Compared to HIV-1 infection, HIV-2 is less transmissible and the progression to AIDS is slower, but at the time Schim van der Loeff began his studies at the MRC laboratories in Gambia in 1995, very little information was available about HIV-2. At the time it was also not possible to conduct the type of trials and cohort studies in Africa, which were needed to identify appropriate treatment regimens. Despite these considerable hurdles Schim van der Loeff used the available material from three cohort studies that had already been built in Gambia and was able to conclude that the stable prevalence of HIV-2 was either low enough or declining so as to not pose a global threat (Schim van der Loeff, 2003).

Accessibility of essential medicines

In the introduction of this chapter we referred to the wish of Thomas Quinn that antiretroviral drugs might soon be made available to those afflicted with AIDS in Africa. A Dutch contribution to improve the accessibility to cheaper drugs by people in low-income countries was made by J.M.A. Lange (1954-2014). His name was already mentioned in Chapter 5 as one of the investigators within the Amsterdam Cohort Studies. He was also involved in quite a number of international studies on antiretroviral drugs. Judging by a comment in the journal AIDS he took already in 1993 interest in the HIV epidemic in Africa. He argued in favour of prophylaxis against cerebral toxoplasmosis and *Pneumocystis carinii* pneumonia in asymptomatic African HIV-infected individuals. He announced that the Steering Committee on Clinical Research and Drug Development of the Global Programme on AIDS had given priority to studies on the combined chemoprophylaxis with isoniazid and cotrimoxazole in African HIV-infected patients. After the introduction of the successful combined antiretroviral therapy, he aimed to make this therapy also accessible for HIV-infected individuals in low-income countries. This resulted in the establishment of the PharmAccess foundation in 2000, which aims to remove barriers to AIDS treatment in Africa. The thesis of Stefaan van der Borght (2011) shows examples of projects with the private sector – Heineken Brewery – in which the PharmAccess International foundation collaborated with the Accelerating Access Initiative (AAI), an initiative of six pharmaceutical companies and five United Nations agencies offering the possibility of obtaining brand antiretroviral drugs (ARVs) at 10 per cent of the commercial price. PharmAccess helped to establish an HIV policy and treatment guidelines and a workplace programme. Tragically, his life ended in harness so he was unable to finish the job. Joep perished on 17 July 2014, together with his beloved partner, Jacqueline van Tongeren, while flying from Amsterdam to the International AIDS Conference in Melbourne aboard Malaysia Airlines Flight 17 (Hankins et al., 2014).

8 From cancer mice in the roaring 1920s to oncogenes and signalling molecules in the booming 1990s

> Once upon a time there was a family of viruses, much like other viruses. Some
> of them liked mutton, others poultry. Some of them multiplied wantonly in
> the cells they inhabited and smashed up their homes; others, more restrained,
> practiced a magic which caused their homes to proliferate.
> *C.H. Andrewes (1935, cited in Sankaran and Van Helvoort, 2016)*[102]

Today, it is appreciated that at least 20 per cent of the global burden of human cancer has an infectious aetiology of which two-thirds is viral (Parkin, 2006; Zur Hausen, 2006). 'The percentage of infection-attributable cancer is higher in developing countries (26.3 per cent) than in developed countries (7.7 per cent), reflecting the high prevalence of infection with hepatitis B and C viruses, human papillomaviruses (HPV), *Helicobacter pylori*, and human immunodeficiency viruses' (Parkin, 2006). In women, high-risk HPV infections are the main contributors to gynaecological cancers, whereas in men, the bacterium *H. pylori* and hepatitis B and hepatitis C viruses are the main causes of gastric cancer and hepatocellular cancer, respectively.

A few landmarks characterize the history of tumour virology (Javier and Butel, 2008; Rubin, 2011). About a decade after the discovery by Beijerinck and Ivanowski that infectious diseases may be caused by ultramicroscopic microorganisms, F. Peyton Rous at the Rockefeller Institute proposed a viral agent behind the transmissibility of fowl sarcoma. He did not, however, exclude agents of other kinds (Rous, 1911). He wrote:

> The first tendency will be to regard the self-perpetuating agent active in this sarcoma of the fowl as a *minute parasitic organism*. Analogy with several infectious diseases of man and the lower animals caused by ultramicroscopic organisms gives support to this view of the findings, and at present work is being directed to its experimental verification. But an agent of another sort is not out of the question. It is conceivable that a *chemical stimulant*, elaborated by the neoplastic cells, might cause

102 Also used by Creager, 2014.

the tumour in another host and bring about in consequence a further
production of the same stimulant. For the moment we have not adopted
either hypothesis.

The importance of his discovery was not evident until the 1960s. According
to his colleague Thomas M. Rivers, this was a watershed in cancer as well
as in virus research. In 1967, Rivers declared, 'Virologists, particularly those
down at the National Institutes of Health, are hell bent on proving that a
virus is the cause of cancer in man' (Benison and Rivers, 1967, p. 87). In the
opinion of Waterson and Wilkinson, however, there was far from general
approbation of Rous's results and conclusion (Waterson and Wilkinson,
1978). Due to lack of support, Rous ended his research on fowl sarcoma a few
years after publishing his report. During World War I, he moved to solving
issues related to the preservation of blood. Yet, he returned to virus research
in 1933 when his Rockefeller Institute colleague R.E. Shope discovered the
virus that induced natural papilloma in the wild North American rabbit.
Rous initially confirmed the benign character of the warts in the natural
host, but later proved the potential malignancy of the warts in cottontail
rabbits (Rous et al., 1936; Benison and Rivers, 1967).

In the Netherlands, the Netherlands Cancer Institute-Antoni van Leeuwenhoek Hospital[103] in Amsterdam was and still is a prominent laboratory
where cancer research was carried out during the twentieth century. Genetic
studies on mouse mammary carcinoma started in 1931. Later on, in the
second half of the twentieth century, the availability of mouse strains with
high incidences of mammary tumours provided the opportunity to study
the genetic basis of cancer development. In 1968, Bentvelzen, working at
the NKI-AVL, formulated the hypothesis that the so-called GR mouse strain
contained genetic information from a cancer-causing RNA tumour virus,
the mouse mammary tumour virus (MMTV), in its own cellular DNA. The
discovery of viral RNA-dependent DNA polymerase by Temin and Mizutani
of the University of Wisconsin and by Baltimore of MIT in 1970 opened a
new perspective for the identification of RNA tumour viruses in cancers. It
demonstrated the molecular mechanism bridging viral RNA-coded information and host cell DNA-based hereditary material and, subsequently, the
cellular origin of so-called retroviral oncogenes.

In his publication on infectious causes of human cancers, and later
during his 2008 Nobel Laureate lecture, Zur Hausen defined this period
as the difficult 1970s (Zur Hausen, 2006, 2008). Many reports suggesting

103 Nederlands Kanker Instituut (NKI); Antoni van Leeuwenhoek-Huis (AVL).

an association between tumour viruses and human cancers could not be confirmed by other groups. Furthermore, another mechanism driving cellular transformation was proposed at that time. Knudson demonstrated the existence of tumour suppressor genes, which may result in cancer when they lose – not gain – function (Knudson, 1971).

However, it became clear that the viral induction of malignant tumours was associated with a long period of persistency of an oncogenic virus, independently of its generic make-up, be it a DNA or an RNA virus. Viruses that were identified possessing oncogenic potential were the herpesviruses (Epstein-Barr virus, human herpesvirus type 8), human papillomaviruses (HPV), hepadnaviruses (hepatitis B virus), flaviviruses (hepatitis C virus), retroviruses (HTLV-1), and polyomaviruses (BK virus and SV40 virus as model, JC virus).

In this chapter, we will focus on the developments of the field of tumour virology in the Netherlands.

Amsterdam

Netherlands Cancer Institute

Two years after the discovery of Rous in 1911, the Netherlands Cancer Institute (NKI) and the Antoni van Leeuwenhoek Ziekenhuis (AVL) were founded in Amsterdam from a private initiative of Professor J. Rotgans, a surgeon at the University of Amsterdam, and of publisher J.H. de Bussy. The latter approached business acquaintances with the proposal to found a specialist cancer institute. The aim was to establish a centralized institute in which both a hospital and a research laboratory were erected, similarly to the institute founded in 1906 by Vincent Czerny in Heidelberg, Germany (Bakker et al., 2015; Jongkees, 1963). A building that had formerly housed a bank was thus renovated and adapted for the treatment of patients and for scientific research. In 1922, thirteen Dutch and ten international experts attended a meeting at the NKI-AVL to discuss the then current topics, such as tar-induced neoplasms. During the meeting, the Van Leeuwenhoek Association[104] was launched to promote international cooperation with all present participants as members (NKI-AVL Annual Reports (A), 1922). This society may be considered as one of the predecessors of the International

---

104 Van Leeuwenhoek Vereeniging.

Figure 25   R. Korteweg (1884-1961)

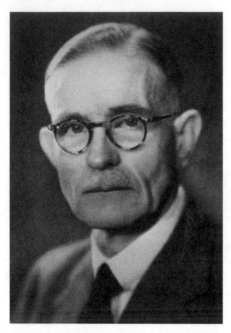

Reproduction courtesy NKI-AVL

Association to Combat Cancer, or the Union Internationale contre le Cancer (UICC), that was founded in 1933 (Van Lier, 2004). By the end of the 1920s, the NKI-AVL moved to facilities that had previously hosted the Military Hospital and central depot for military uniforms in the Sarphatistraat in Amsterdam. This new site provided enough space to host the hospital, the living-in staff and the laboratory departments of Biochemistry-Serology (head, Dr N. Waterman), Biology (head, R. Korteweg, MD) and Tissue Culture (head, Ms Dr W.M. de Bruyn). The pathologist Korteweg was appointed head of the pathology laboratory in 1927; he fell under the spell of genetic research to study the origin of cancer. Mice models were used to unravel the question of heredity of cancer (Lesterhuis and Houwaart, 2000). The experimental setup required large numbers of mice, as standardized test animals, which were bred in collaboration with Clarence C. Little at the Jackson Memorial Laboratory (Bar Harbor, Maine, USA).

Little started in 1909 brother-sister inbreeding of mice with a high incidence of mammary cancer leading 20 to 30 generations later to a genetically homogenous population. In 1930, Little visited the NKI-AVL and promised Korteweg to send diverse mouse strains. Thanks to the conciliatory attitude of the management of the Holland-Amerika Line, the animals promised by Little could be shipped, and they arrived in Amsterdam in March 1931 (NKI-AVL Annual Reports (A), 1931). The shipment contained two mouse strains: a strain inbred from 1909 on (dilute brown) in which about half of the virgin females above the age of eight months die of mammary cancer, and another strain (C.57 Black) that had been brother-sister inbred since 1920 and in which no mammary tumours are observed (Korteweg, 1933). Korteweg concluded in 1934 that the heredity of mammary tumours in the dilute brown mice could not be explained by a dominant Mendelian gene for developing mammary tumours that was received from the mother, or exclusively by a recessive factor. He hypothesized a higher disposition for cancer due to circulating agents during embryogenesis or by an extrachromosomal agent in the protoplasm of the female gamete. He considered, however, the possibility of transmission of the mammary tumour causing agent by breast milk less probable because of the short fostering period (Korteweg, 1934a, 1934b). However, Little, with whom Korteweg corresponded on his research results, had claimed earlier in November 1933 on behalf of the staff of the Roscoe B. Jackson Memorial Laboratory the existence of a non-chromosomal influence in the incidence of mammary tumours in mice (1933). Nevertheless, Little recognized the research of Korteweg in a later publication (Murray and Little, 1935).

This heralded a new and long-lasting era of tumour virus research in the Netherlands. J.J. Bittner, a co-worker of Little, reported surprisingly in 1936 that an extrachromosomal factor present in the milk of cancer-prone mice transmitted the disease to new-borne mice of a strain with low cancer incidence when fostered by high-risk mice (Bittner, 1936; Bittner and Little, 1937; Bittner, 1939). Korteweg then confirmed the results of Bittner, as he carried out similar experiments (Korteweg, 1936a, 1936b, 1937a, 1937b). The strains of mice used by both investigators were almost identical, according to the information given by Little (Bittner, 1936; Korteweg, 1933, 1934a and b, 1936a and b, 1937a and b). Still in 1946, Korteweg hesitated whether this factor called 'mammary tumour inciter' (MTI) was a virus or an agent of a different nature (Korteweg, 1946). However, this factor was later proven a true virus, christened as the 'mouse mammary tumour virus' (MMTV).

The preservation of the mice strains during the winter of starvation in World War II was a source of great concern to Korteweg. Thanks to his dedication, the mice survived and the animal facility of Korteweg largely contributed to the further development of the field of tumour virology in the Netherlands. Shortly before his retirement he visited Little in Bar Harbor during a study tour in the US in 1947. Some weeks after his visit the laboratory was completely destroyed by wildfire that swept through

New England (Korteweg, 1948). In 1949 on the occasion of his farewell from the NKI-AVL he was honoured by the University of Groningen, where he received an honorary medical degree. His promoter was Prof. Dr J.J.T. Vos, who had succeeded Landsteiner as pathologist in The Hague in 1922 (Vos, 1949; Arends et al., 1961).

O.F.E. Mühlbock, who had joined the institute as an assistant to Korteweg in 1946, became his successor as head of the laboratory. Mühlbock was a gynaecologist (MD, 1933) and also trained as a chemist (PhD, 1927) in Berlin; he left Germany in 1934 for political reasons and worked at the pharmacology laboratory of Professor E. Laqueur in Amsterdam until 1940 (Boot, 1980). In 1948, he was appointed head of the NKI-AVL biology department, where he started investigating the hormonal induction of tumours in various organs. Later, he concentrated on the genetic, viral and environmental factors of carcinogenesis of mouse mammary tumours; his work successfully built on the mouse strains of the animal facility set up by Korteweg. As L.M. Boot wrote in the obituary of Mühlbock: 'He developed the European GRS strain, which proved to be of special interest because it carries a MMTV variant which can be transmitted not only through the milk but also genetically, by both sperm and ova. This provided one of the first models for the study of a viral genome incorporated into mammalian DNA' (Boot, 1980; Mühlbock, 1965). Mühlbock sought cooperation with other investigators and foreign institutes which were engaged in research on the genesis of mammary tumours. He notably had fruitful contacts with the National Cancer Institute in Bethesda, Maryland, and the Cancer Research Genetics Laboratory in Berkeley, California, both in the USA (Boot, 1980). He also pursued collaborations in the laboratory and clinical study of cancer.

New instruments that had been developed since the 1930s were introduced to the NKI-AVL only by the second half of the 1950s. An ultracentrifuge was ordered in 1957 and delivered in 1958. It took even more time for E.L. Benedetti, appointed in 1959, to set up a modified Philips 100 kV electron microscope, which was operational by mid-1960. The instrument was installed in a small, dilapidated building provided by the neighbouring military authorities. Luckily, in the meantime, Benedetti and his staff were welcome at the Department of Electron Microscopy of the University of Amsterdam that was headed by Miss Woutera van Iterson (NKI-AVL Annual Reports (A), 1960). The use of the electron microscope and the ultracentrifuge were instrumental for NKI-AVL's cancer research.

In 1962, a virology working unit dedicated to the study of tumour viruses was established at the NKI-AVL, which became, from 1966 onwards, a section of the Biochemistry Department. At the same time, under the guidance of Mühlbock, an interdisciplinary working unit on the mouse mammary tumour virus (MMTV) was initiated, combining the cooperation of NKI-AVL biology, immunology, biochemistry, and electron microscopy departments. By the mid-1960s, after nearly half a century of existence, the NKI-AVL and its laboratory staff had made a series of internationally respected discoveries. MMTV was shown to be an RNA virus in which genetic material was converted into a DNA copy in mice and inserted into the animal's DNA. Based on genetic studies combined with imaging studies using immunofluorescence and electron microscopical techniques, and after discussions with F. Jacob and J. Monod at the Institut Pasteur in Paris, P.A. Bentvelzen and J.H. Daams proposed the concept of provirus to describe these processes (Bentvelzen and Daams, 1969). They wrote: 'According to this hypothesis, in one of the chromosomes of the GR and the C3Hf mouse strains, a DNA copy of the whole viral genome is present which, under circumstances, can be transcribed, so that it gives rise to a giant messenger RNA molecule, the viral RNA.' With this hypothesis of genetic transmission of MMTV, they could explain the vertical transmission of the mammary tumours in these mouse strains.

Before defending his thesis in 1968, Bentvelzen worked briefly at the Laboratory of Biology of the National Cancer Institute, Bethesda, MD, USA. He thereafter moved to the Radiobiological Institute (TNO), in Rijswijk, the Netherlands, where he continued his studies on the origin of cancer. An illustration of the importance of his work lies in the following quote of Heston and Parks, who wrote in 1977: 'It was of special interest to us when Bentvelzen in 1968 and 1972 suggested from his data that the GR virus was genetically transmitted as a structural gene, the provirus, controlled by a regulator gene. From tumour non-tumour segregation ratios Bentvelzen concluded that single gene segregation accounted for mammary tumori-genesis' (Heston and Parks, 1977).

Such findings brought Amsterdam at the forefront of international cancer research. The spectacular progress on deciphering oncogenetic mechanisms had been made possible by multidisciplinary research efforts. In fact, these were fuelled by a prevailing trend in the life sciences in the 1960s and 1970s, in response to the development of new branches of science and techniques, such as biochemistry, biophysics, electron microscopy, molecular biology, and immunology.

Topics for discussion at the international symposium 'RNA Viruses and Host Genome in Oncogenesis' organized by the NKI-AVL on the occasion of the retirement of Mühlbock in Amsterdam in 1971 included the genetics of avian and murine leukaemia viruses, the mouse mammary tumour virus, and biochemical aspects of their pathogenesis. The meeting resulted in an overview of the state of cancer research in the Netherlands. Although cancer research was restricted to animal studies, it was considered of great importance for understanding the role of viruses in human cancers. The editors of the proceedings summarized the work of Mühlbock as follows: 'He and his collaborators paid much attention to the analysis and investigation of the various factors concerned, viz. viruses, hormones, genes and environmental conditions. A very important aspect of their work is the emphasis on the interrelation between these factors in the cancerous process' (Emmelot and Bentvelzen, 1972, p. vii). An overview of the state of knowledge on the genetic aspects of the origin of tumour cell was given at a symposium in 1978 (Cleton and Simons, 1980).

Admittedly, even a small-scale institute does not always guarantee peaceful cohabitation among clinicians and researchers. In the past, Korteweg, head of the laboratory, was not always on good speaking terms with his colleagues N. Waterman of the Biochemistry-Serology Department and W.F. Wassink, head of the clinic, due to their marked and different individualities (De Bruyn, 1961). The presence of the hospital and laboratory settings at one location at Sarphatistraat, however, resulted in a typical small-scale institute where overall, everybody knew each other personally, with a high level of cross-fertilization between departments. This was to change when the clinic – the AVL part – moved to a brand-new complex in the Slotervaart district on the periphery of town in 1973, five years before the laboratory – the NKI part.

By the time the laboratory moved to the Slotervaart district, its reputation had deteriorated considerably. The wave of 'democratizing', with innumerable meetings, endless deliberations, and lack of leadership may have been among the causes of the decline. As described by Van Lier: 'About 1980 an institute of international reputation in an old and dilapidated building was changed into an institute with fading esteem in a brand-new state-of-the-art accommodation' (Van Lier, 2004). The situation improved when the medical doctor, yet not a clinician, and famous biochemist P. Borst was appointed research director of NKI-AVL in 1982. Borst had received his medical degree from the University of Amsterdam, and thereafter engaged into biochemical research. He became a well-known scientist who also acquired experience with administrative and managerial tasks at the University of Amsterdam.

Borst managed to breathe new life into the NKI-AVL experimental agenda, based on the old mouse laboratory, for instance, by concentrating research efforts on genetically modified mouse models. He recruited young and talented researchers, such as the biochemist H.L. Ploegh, the molecular geneticist A. Berns with his expertise on genetic modification of mice, the immunologist C.J.M. Melief, and, later, R.A.H. Plasterk. As a result, the laboratory fully regained its former status as a state-of-the-art cancer laboratory.

Nonetheless, it must be noted that high-quality research was also carried out during the 'dark' period. For example, starting in 1975, R. Nusse prepared his thesis *Mouse mammary tumour virus proteins: mechanism of synthesis and antigenic expression in experimental animals*, which he defended in 1980. Further work in cooperation with H.E. Varmus at the University of California showed evidence in 1982 that an MMTV provirus which was integrated at the cellular *int* locus strongly favoured tumorigenesis. After a post-doctoral position at the laboratory of H. Varmus in 1980, Nusse returned to the NKI. It took another six-year quest for the function of the *int-1* oncogene to witness an interesting and gratifying denouement in 1987. The gene appeared to be a homologue of the wingless gene in fruit flies. In 2012, Nusse and Varmus described in retrospect how *int-1* was recognized as belonging to the *Wnt* gene family and the importance of the Wnt pathway in human cancers. Nusse and Varmus noted with satisfaction the growth of the Wnt field from the finding of a single cancer gene in a mouse model to a rich system branching out to fields as diverse as embryogenesis, growth of organs, regeneration of injured organs, and maintenance of stem cells. Nusse was awarded the 2017 Breakthrough Prize in Life Sciences for his contributions to the understanding of the Wnt signalling molecule.

Nusse left the NKI in 1990 when he joined the Department of Development Biology at Stanford University. As mentioned in an NKI-AVL annual report, he took with him most of his research team, which encompassed half of the Molecular Biology Division (NKI-AVL Annual Reports (D), 1990). When Nusse left the institute, R.H.A. Plasterk was appointed as head of the Molecular Biology section until 2000, when he was offered to move to the Hubrecht Laboratories in Utrecht.

In 1985, A.J.M. Berns, a molecular biologist from Radboud University in Nijmegen, who discovered the *pim-1* oncogene, and C.J.M. Melief, an immunologist at the neighbouring Central Laboratory of the Blood Transfusion Service, joined the NKI-AVL. The research of both Melief and Berns on inbred mouse strains and their transfer to the institute led to an optimal use of NKI-AVL mouse facilities (NKI-AVL Annual Reports (D), 1985). In 1990, Melief was appointed in Leiden as professor in internal medicine, in particular, in

Figure 26   A working map of the mouse *int-1* locus as drawn by Roel Nusse used from 1982 to 1984

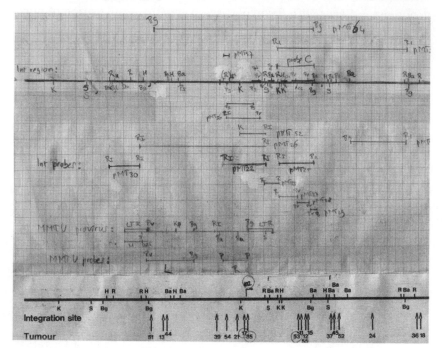

With the position of various cloned genomic restriction fragments. Red lines indicate the presence of int1 exons, mapped in 1984. Note the location of Probe C, a genomic fragment hybridizing with int1 mRNA in mouse mammary tumours. At the bottom, the position of MMTV proviruses mapped in different tumours, with the position of the provirus in tumour #18, the starting point of the cloning of the locus, indicated at the right hand end.

Reproduction courtesy of EMBO and Wiley-VCH Verlag GmbH & Co.

immune-haematology, where he worked on tumour immunology, cancer immunotherapy, and cancer vaccination.

As described by Berns, the NKI-AVL metamorphosed under the leadership of Piet Borst from 1983 until 1999, when he stepped down as director of research, from an organization that had lost contact with the fast-developing area of molecular and cellular biology back into a high-profile research institute. In the laboratory, the mouse tumour models and mouse (reverse) genetics still played a key role in cancer research (NKI-AVL Annual Reports (E), 1999). Even nowadays, mouse mammary tumour virus and murine leukaemia virus are the most relevant models to study DNA integration elements in many areas of molecular biology, e.g. gene therapy, oncogene discovery, gene regulation, and functional genetics (De Jong et al., 2014).

Major developments of the last two decades are reflected in the changes of the research program of the laboratories and the number of permanent staff members. In 1980, the laboratories were: Biochemistry I and II, Biology I/Radiology and Biology II, Electron Microscopy, Experimental Animals, Experimental Cytology, Immunology, Physics, Radionuclides and Virology. In 2000, molecular-biological techniques were introduced and cell biology was an important research topic. According to the scientific report for 2000, the laboratory covered all major areas of cancer research, with special emphasis on mouse tumour models, mouse (reverse) genetics, cell biology, immunology and translational research requiring close collaboration between clinical and fundamental scientists (NKI-AVL Annual Reports (E), 2000). In 2000, the basic research laboratories, now called divisions, were: I Cell Biology, II Division of Molecular Carcinogenesis, III Division of Cellular Biochemistry, IV Division of Immunology, V Division of Molecular Biology, VI Division of Tumor Biology, and VII Division of Molecular Genetics. Remarkably, the number of permanent staff members dropped from 74 in 1980 to 40 in 2000.

Looking back, NKI-AVL research programs in the 1970s and 1980s followed more or less the pattern foreseen by Renato Dulbecco in a talk entitled 'Oncogenic viruses: The last twelve years', presented at a Cold Spring Harbor symposium in 1974 (Dulbecco, 1974). Forecasting the next twelve years of cancer research, he predicted that after the discovery of the reverse transcription by Baltimore, Temin and Mizutami in 1970, the mechanisms of the so-called oncogenes would be elucidated. In essence, Dulbecco's predictions for the following twelve years were the sequencing of oncogenic viruses and the determination of the structure of viral proteins. In his opinion, predicting the role of cellular proteins was to prove more difficult. Progress there would probably depend on technological breakthroughs in the methodologies for studying the genome of eukaryotic cells.

At the turn of the twentieth century, A. Berns, director of NKI-AVL research, wrote that the last fifty years yielded fabulous insights into the works of nature and declared: 'We now know in some detail how cancer arises, and have identified many of the genetic lesions instrumental in causing cancer. However, there are still many unknowns. The understanding of the genetic traits determining the level of susceptibility or resistance of individuals to the development of malignancies remained limited. A more detailed insight was required for effective intervention strategies'. He stated also: 'While expressing this optimism for the future, we have to realize that current successful cancer treatments depend almost entirely on surgery, radiotherapy, and chemotherapy' (NKI-AVL Annual Reports (E), 1999).

Coming back to one of the first research subjects of Korteweg, namely breast cancer, the scientific report for 2000 reveals continuing joint efforts of the NKI-AVL in this field. At that time, eight of the thirteen research divisions were carrying out studies on breast cancer: fundamental research divisions as Molecular Carcinogenesis, Tumor Biology, Experimental Therapy (Molecular Pathology), together with clinical divisions, such as Radiotherapy, Medical Oncology, Surgical Oncology, Psychosocial Research and Epidemiology, and Diagnostic Oncology. The search for a tumour virus as the cause of breast cancer progressively evolved towards the generation of key insights into the contribution of BRCA germline mutational status to breast cancer patients' prognosis.

Laboratory for Hygiene, later the Department of Medical Microbiology and the Department of Virology, University of Amsterdam

Besides the research on tumour virology at the NKI-AVL, the association between persistent virus infections and carcinogenesis was also studied at laboratories of the University of Amsterdam. At the end of the 1960s, J. van der Noordaa initiated research at the Laboratory for Hygiene using the SV40 model to investigate virus-induced transformation and oncogenesis. His first steps in the field of DNA tumour viruses were taken in 1965-1966 at the laboratory of J.F. Enders, where he worked as a post-doctoral researcher on herpes viruses and SV40. He befriended other researchers at the laboratory of the 'Chief' and remained in contact with them all his life (Van der Noordaa, personal archive). Having realized that the expertise of research on SV40-mediated oncogenesis offered opportunities for fruitful research on papillomaviruses, the group of J. ter Schegget turned to the etiologic role of human papillomavirus in anogenital cancers from 1984 onwards. In the final decade of the twentieth century, the relationships between cutaneous papillomavirus infections and squamous cell carcinoma and basal cell carcinoma were an important research focus, in cooperation with J.N. Bouwes Bavinck and B.J. Vermeer of the Department of Dermatology of Leiden University. Based on studies on the function of SV40 small-t in transformation of human cells, another line of investigation was initiated, namely on the role of a putative 'small-t antigen' (a subunit of protein phosphatase 2A) in the transformation of human cells. This factor was highly expressed in human cells with a deletion in chromosome 11 (del11 cells) but not in diploid cells. Cooperation in the 1990s with the group of C. Melief, then in Leiden, opened a door to study the immunology of HPV infections and to investigate the possibility to treat genital cancer patients by vaccination with cytotoxic T lymphocyte epitope-containing peptides.

Department of Pathology, Free University of Amsterdam

J.M.M. Walboomers joined the Department of Pathology of the Medical Faculty of the Free University of Amsterdam (head, C.J.L.M. Meijer) in 1987, where he founded the laboratory for molecular pathology. In 1997, he was appointed professor of pathology to address the molecular aspects of viral oncogenesis. His main objective was the detection of oncogenic viruses, in particular human papillomaviruses. In the early days, much work was performed by his PhD students A.J. van den Brule and P.J.F. Snijders. Rather soon, Walboomers was convinced of the advantages of screening cervical cancer by detection of oncogenic human papillomavirus by molecular techniques. His sustained efforts to switch from cytology to HPV detection for cervical cancer screening were interrupted by his sudden passing away in 2000. Yet, his line of work continued through the involvement of Meijer and his co-workers.

J.M. Middeldorp joined the Department of Pathology of the Free University of Amsterdam in 1996; his teaching commitment was the molecular immunopathogenesis of Epstein-Barr virus-associated malignancies. At the beginning of his career, at the Department of Clinical Immunology at the University Hospital Groningen, he carried out research on CMV- and EBV-related diseases after transplantation. Thereafter, he moved to Organon International, Oss (1987-1994), for the development of diagnostic tests. After his appointment at the Free University of Amsterdam, he focused particularly on EBV-associated nasopharyngeal carcinoma that shows a peculiar high incidence in East Asia among Cantonese males and among the Inuit population in the Northwest Territories of Canada.

Leiden

Laboratory of Physiological Chemistry, Leiden University

After studying biology in Leiden and microbiology in Delft, A.J. van der Eb was posted by colonel Beunders at the Laboratory of Virology of the Leiden Academic Hospital to perform his military service. His work there, on smallpox virus and vaccination of the military, was of overriding importance for his future career, through his contact with Professor J.A. Cohen at the

Medical Biology Laboratory in Rijswijk, where he could carry out his PhD studies on the structure and biological properties of adenovirus DNA. It was then recently known that some adenoviruses could cause cancer. In 1968, he obtained a post-doctoral position at the California Institute of Technology but came back to Leiden in 1970 following the invitation by his former promotor to set up a new research group on the molecular biology of oncogenic viruses.

At the Laboratory for Physiological Chemistry at Leiden University, cancer research focused mainly on adenoviruses. The publication in 1973 by F.L. Graham and Van der Eb on the calcium phosphate precipitation method for transfection of cells with adenovirus may be considered as pioneering research in tumour virology. With the help of C. Mulder, a Dutchman who worked at Cold Spring Harbor Laboratory in New York, they obtained restriction enzymes and demonstrated the biological activity of isolated DNA fragments in mammalian cells. Besides viral oncogenesis, other mechanisms of cancer induction were studied, such as those associated with tumour suppressor genes and radiation. As adenoviruses can be used to introduce other gene fragments in mammalian cells, a group to study gene therapy was also formed (Meijer van Putten, 1998). Although it falls beyond the scope of this chapter on tumour virology, the work on gene therapy by Van der Eb's co-workers D. Valerio, R.C. Hoeben, and H. van Ormondt is to be mentioned (Hoeben et al., 1992). An interesting change would be later the shift from oncogenic to oncolytic viruses (Belcaid et al., 2014). In 1993 Valerio founded a commercial company, IntroGene, which merged in 2000 with UbiSys from Utrecht to form a new company, Crucell. After the retirement of Van der Eb in 1999, Hoeben was appointed professor in 2000 to teach virus and stem cell biology.

Laboratory of Immuno-haematology, Leiden University

The arrival of Melief from the NKI-AVL to Leiden Medical Faculty in 1990 initiated a new line of immunological research on therapy against cervical cancers caused by human papillomavirus. His interest in the immunology of human papillomaviruses causing cervical cancer started in cooperation with the group of J. ter Schegget at the Department for Virology of the AMC in Amsterdam. Experiments exploring the possibility of antiviral vaccination with short MHC class I binding peptides were performed by M. (Mariet) Feltkamp and B. de Jongh at the AMC together with M. Kast and others of Melief's group in Leiden. The results showed that a cytotoxic lymphocyte (CTL) line raised against the subdominant CTL epitope offered as a synthetic peptide E7 49-57, eradicated established HPV16-induced tumours in mice. Therefore, the possibility of anti-viral and anti-cancer vaccination was demonstrated (in mice). This promised to be a long line of research (Melief et al., 2014).

Utrecht

Laboratory of Physiological Chemistry, Utrecht University

When tumour virology started involving the fields of cell biology and molecular biology, research on the interactions with nucleic acids gained much importance. Van Kammen recently wrote an objective and compressive review of the history of nucleic acid research in the Netherlands (Van Kammen, 2004). The career of H.S. Jansz is an example of the importance of pioneering work on nucleic acids for the field of tumour virology. Jansz, who was trained as a chemist at the Free University of Amsterdam, was appointed professor in physiological chemistry in 1967 in Utrecht, where he introduced molecular biology and DNA research (Van der Vliet, 2005). Jansz became interested in DNA research in the USA following contact with A. Kornberg, discoverer of the DNA polymerase. Back in the Netherlands, Jansz worked at the Medical-Biological Laboratory (Medisch-Biologisch Laboratorium) of TNO-RVO (head, J.A. Cohen) on the effect of ionizing radiation on DNA using as model bacteriophage ØX174. This small circular bacteriophage continued to retain his attention in Leiden at the Laboratory of Physiological Chemistry, where he came in contact with the adenovirus work of A.J. van der Eb. During his inaugural address in 1968, he predicted optimistically that the synthesis of viruses would occur within two years (Jansz, 1968; Van der Vliet, 2005). However, this did not occur until 2002, one year before he passed away. In that year, Cello, Paul and Wimmer reported on the generation of infectious poliovirus in the absence of a natural template (Cello et al., 2002). In Utrecht, Jansz initiated a line of research on the 'structure and replication of DNA'. The studies on bacteriophage ØX174 DNA as well as adenovirus DNA were key to understand the mechanisms of virus-induced cancer. The names of J.S. Sussenbach and P.C. van der Vliet among others have to be mentioned. Their work on the details of adenovirus replication in eukaryotic cells resulted in proposing a model that describes the dynamics of initiation and elongation as well as the assembly and disassembly of the preinitiation complex (De Jong and Van der Vliet, 1999).

Van der Vliet was the last known chairman of the Working Group on Persistent Virus Infections and Oncogenesis from 1987 until 1992 (see below).

Nijmegen

Laboratory for Biochemistry, Department of Biochemistry, Radboud University

A depiction of the beginning of tumour virus research in Nijmegen has been given by H.P. Bloemers in a memorial on the occasion of the 75th anniversary of the Roman Catholic Radboud University, now Radboud University (Bloemers, 1998). In 1965, H. Bloemendal and S. Bonting were appointed professors of biochemistry, both at the Medical Faculty and the Faculty of Mathematics and Science. It is remarkable that they both were not of Catholic origin; Bonting was an ordained priest in the Anglican Church and the Old Catholic Church, and Bloemendal was cantor (chazzan) in the Jewish Community of Amsterdam (Nederlands-Israëlitische Hoofdsynagoge). Bloemendal attended a course on chemistry in Amsterdam and was attached to the NKI-AVL after his doctorate on lens proteins. After his appointment in Nijmegen, he continued research on the regulation of the synthesis of messenger RNA that resulted later in one of the first isolations of eukaryotic messenger RNA. Besides investigating crystalline proteins, Bloemendal initiated studies on Rauscher-leukaemia virus (Van Kammen, 2004). The pioneering molecular biological work at the NKI on the oncogenesis of MMTV by Nusse and Michalides stimulated the development of research of the same kind in Nijmegen, where the group of A.J.M. Berns at the Laboratory of Biochemistry of Bloemendal discovered the *pim-1* oncogene. Berns was also involved in the production of 'transgenic' mice by introducing purified genes into mouse egg cells, a technique that had great potentials for the study of oncogenesis. In 1972, H.P. Bloemers joined the Laboratory of Biochemistry of Radboud University, where he contributed to the understanding of the molecular biology of cancer processes. Initially, his work focused on animal RNA tumour viruses and their oncogenes. Together with W.J.M. van de Ven, and in cooperation with the Frederick Cancer Research and Development Center, part of the National Institutes of Health, USA, he investigated the presence and function of animal cellular genes related to the viral oncogenes. He was appointed professor of biochemistry at the Faculty of Science in 1980 and at the Faculty of Medicine in 1987.

Rijswijk

Radiobiological Institute and Primate Centre

The Radiobiological Institute TNO (RBI) was founded in 1956 as part of the Dutch Health Organisation (TNO-NGO) in part due to the civil applications of nuclear energy and expected increase in possible side effects. Although the institute earned an international reputation in several fields, such as bone marrow transplants and haemopoietic stem cells, it did not survive the structural overhaul of the 1980s. After merging with the Primate Centre and the Medical Biological Laboratory, it closed down in 1993.

D.W. van Bekkum, who was director from 1960 until 1990, and the pathologist M.J. de Vries were interested in the potential induction of tumour viruses by ionizing radiation. After his groundbreaking work at the NKI, P. Bentvelzen joined the institute in Rijswijk in 1968. There he continued to study MMTV and the interaction between host and viral genomes (1980 and 1982). He also attempted to isolate a possible human leukaemia virus in the 1970s. Before publishing his findings in a scientific journal, the results were divulged in a daily paper. This led to a comment in the NTvG by J. van der Noordaa, who warned about drawing too early a conclusion and that contamination could not be excluded (Van der Noordaa, 1975). In a reply, Bentvelzen pointed out that further work had to be done, in cooperation with R.C. Gallo (Bentvelzen, 1975). According to the TNO expert Van de Schootbrugge, it was still not clear in 1993 whether contamination had occurred or whether a human leukaemia virus had been isolated, indeed (Van de Schootbrugge, 2016).

It was at the Primate Centre TNO that H. Schellekens carried out a series of studies on interferon, hepatitis B, and acquired immunodeficiencies. The number of the chimpanzees used in these experiments was as limited as possible.

Rotterdam

Erasmus MC

Erasmus MC came into existence following the merging of the Academic Hospital, the Daniel den Hoed Clinic and the Medical Faculty in Rotterdam. Although cancer research was and is a main topic of research in several departments of Erasmus MC, studies designated as tumour virus research in a strict sense started to be published only by the last decade of the twentieth century. The clinical departments involved in these studies covered a wide range of disciplines, including haematology, gynaecology, hepatology, neurosurgery, medical oncology, urology, clinical bacteriology and pathology. Research on Epstein-Barr virus and the association with EBV-lymphoproliferative disease (EBV-LPD) was carried out by J.W. Gratama at the Daniel den Hoed Clinic. Gratama completed his doctoral and post-doctoral studies at the Department of Immunohematology and Blood Bank in Leiden in the 1980s, at the Department of Tumour Biology, Karolinska Institute, Stockholm, Sweden, from 1988 to 1991 and at the Department of Immunology of the Daniel den Hoed Cancer Centre in Rotterdam from 1992 onwards; a department that became associated with the Academic Hospital in 1993. His studies focused mainly on the role of Epstein-Barr virus in lymphoproliferative diseases after allogeneic stem cell transplantation.

Groningen

Laboratory of Molecular Virology, State University of Groningen

Before his appointment in 1999 at the Laboratory of Molecular Virology, J.C. Wilschut was affiliated to the Laboratory of Physiological Chemistry of the University of Groningen. He investigated model systems of fusion processes between endosomal cellular membranes and reconstituted viral envelope membranes (virosomes) after internalization through receptor-mediated endocytosis. The virosomes can be used for intracellular delivery of antigens for the induction of immune responses as well as drugs for treatment of tumours. The majority of the studies on such applications were executed after the turn of the century together with his co-workers C.A.H.H. Daemen and A. Huckriede, who were both appointed professor in 2008 and 2011, respectively. The clinical part of their studies was carried out in collaboration with clinicians as A.G. van der Zee of the Department of Gynaecology.

Delft/Rijswijk

Delft Diagnostic Laboratory

J. Lindeman, pathologist at the regional diagnostic centre of the joined general hospitals in Delft,[105] initiated the formation of a Laboratory of Mo-

---

105   Stichting Samenwerkende Delftse Ziekenhuizen (SSDZ).

lecular Biology in the beginning of the 1980s. From 1985 onwards, molecular diagnostic assays were performed in collaboration with the Departments of Microbiology, Clinical Chemistry and Pathology. W.G.V. Quint became head of the Molecular Biology laboratory in 1986. Quint trained at Radboud University in Nijmegen, where he defended his doctoral thesis 'Endogenous murine leukaemia viruses: germline transmission and involvement in generation of recombinant viruses' in 1984. Both Lindeman and Quint were keen to perform scientific research besides daily diagnostics for the clinic. Their research program was intended to develop novel molecular assays and encompassed studies on human papillomavirus. Since 1989, there also was an active collaboration between the laboratory and Innogenetics N.V (Ghent, Belgium) in the field of diagnostics for infectious diseases. This resulted in the founding of Delft Diagnostic Laboratory (DDL), which participated in phase II and III clinical trials, in particular related to HPV screening and development of HPV vaccines; and hepatitis C virus.

Working Group on Persistent Virus Infections and Oncogenesis

At the end of the 1960s, a need for more cooperation between laboratories performing research in the field of tumour virology started to emerge. In 1968, Prof. Mühlbock at the NKI was granted permission by the Queen Wilhelmina Fund (KWF) or Dutch Cancer Society, to set up a KWF working group on 'oncogenic viruses'. Van der Noordaa of the Laboratory for Hygiene in Amsterdam was proposed to act as secretary and organizer (Mühlbock, 1968). Members of the working group came from Amsterdam, Bilthoven, Leiden, Nijmegen, Rijswijk, Rotterdam, Soesterberg and Utrecht and origi-nated from various disciplines: cancer researchers, virologists, pathologists, biochemists, veterinarians, and radiobiologists. The KWF, founded in 1949 and closely related to the NKI-AVL, is a charitable foundation raising funds; the basic activities are financing cancer research and providing patient information and patient support.

In the 1970s, the working group on oncogenic viruses was brought under the umbrella of FUNGO[106] (Fundamental Medical Research), a division of the government-subsidized Netherlands Organisation for Pure Scientific Research (ZWO).[107] It was then renamed the Working Group on Persistent Virus Infections and Oncogenesis. The major aims of ZWO working groups

---

106 Stichting voor Fundamenteel Geneeskundig Onderzoek (FUNGO).
107 Nederlandse Organisatie voor Zuiver Wetenschappelijk Onderzoek (ZWO).

were the coordination of research projects, research cooperation, and exchange of ideas and results. However, the evaluation of the submitted projects and the decision to grant a project seemed to be a rather closed system according to Borst (Borst in Van Helvoort, 2004; Van Helvoort et al., 2004). The topics of the proposals submitted in 1984 illustrate well the main objects of studies subsidized by ZWO/FUNGO: detection of oncogenes in well-defined tumour cell lines with Rauscher mouse leukaemia virus induced malignancies (Rotterdam), introduction of the *pim* oncogene in the germ line of fertilized mouse eggs and study of the influence on the tissue-specific expression (Nijmegen); cell transformation by herpes virus type 2 DNA fragments (cervical cancer) (Amsterdam, pathology); isolation, characterization and possible diagnostic application of oncogenes from hereditary colon carcinoma (Amsterdam, pathology); molecular, biological and genetic aspects of virus-induced mouse mammary tumours (Amsterdam, NKI); mechanisms of cell transformation by oncogenic DNA viruses (adenovirus, SV40 and BK virus), and a concerted project by laboratories in Amsterdam, Leiden and Utrecht (Archief Nederlandse Kankerbestrijding/ Koningin Wilhelmina Fonds, Noord-Hollands Archief, Haarlem: 426, 701).

With the transition of ZWO into the Dutch Research Council (or the Netherlands Organisation for Scientific Research)[108] (NWO) in 1988, and changes in financing research programs via Medigon,[109] a subsidiary foundation of the NWO, the working group petered out in the course of the 1990s. Another factor might have been the foundation of the Research Schools in 1991 which were accredited by the Royal Netherlands Academy of Arts and Sciences[110] (KNAW) and not the NWO. In any case, the causes of the dissolution of the working group remain unclear, as the records of NWO/Medigon filed at the institutions and at the National Archive do not contain any information on the working group in question (A.E. Kersten and D. van Waarde, personal communication, 2014 and 2015, respectively).

Conclusion

There are at least four lessons to be learnt from this chapter. The first is that the concept of virus changed enormously during the twentieth century. At the beginnings of the century, a virus was defined as an infectious agent

---

108 Nederlandse Organisatie voor Wetenschappelijk Onderzoek (NWO).
109 Stichting voor Medisch Wetenschappelijk Onderzoek Medigon.
110 Koninklijke Nederlandse Akademie van Wetenschappen (KNAW).

which multiplied and caused pathological changes in cells and tissues. It escaped the methods of isolation and culture that were applied so successfully and usefully with bacteria. Supposed virus aetiology of cancer was deemed improbable because the consensus opinion was that cancer was not transmissible. In the 1950s and 1960s, many experimental models pointed out that a virus can have an infectious phase as well as an 'hidden' phase in which case genetic predisposition (*Anlage*) may be incorporated into the genetic material of the host cell and may sometimes lead to excessive growth, i.e. cancer. Such a mechanism can also explain the phenomenon of persistent viruses, i.e. the spontaneous rise of virus particles *de novo*. This, apparently, was at odds with one of Pasteur's theses that a microorganism always arises from an earlier microorganism.

These major changes in the definition and understanding of viruses introduce us to the second lesson, i.e. the growing importance of the experimental laboratory sciences for cancer studies, as opposed to a classical approach via pathology. Of course, the struggle against cancer in the patient was fought in the clinics but since the 1930s, it was felt that in order to defeat cancer in humans one had to begin with studying these phenomena in animals. Although there is a qualitative gap between cancer in man on the one hand and cancer in animals on the other, it was only logical to explore experimental findings in 'laboratory animals' (such as mice or guinea pigs) and 'translate' this to the therapeutic repertory for cancer in man (i.e. the Holy Grail of cancer vaccines). This holds especially true for the spectacular results on the molecular mechanisms of cancer genesis.

The third lesson is that the enormous growth of tumour virus work since the 1960s offered many hundreds of Dutch scientists a chance to be educated in the new field of molecular genetics. The centres in this emerging field at Amsterdam, Leiden, Utrecht, Nijmegen, Groningen, Rotterdam and Rijswijk became all well known internationally.

This leads us to the fourth lesson, namely that via the international recognition of laboratory leaders in the Netherlands, new generations of Dutch scientists were offered post-doctoral positions at outstanding laboratories abroad.

Contemplating about the past, there is no other conclusion than that tumour viruses are magnificent looking glasses to study the finite riddles of cancer. Research at the Dutch NKI-AVL on the genetics of mouse mammary carcinoma that started in the 1930s resulted about fifty years later in the important discovery that MMTV provirus integrated at the cellular *int* locus, strongly favouring tumorigenesis in mice. Even though the existence of a human mammary tumour virus was not established, mutations in the BRCA1 or BRCA2-genes were demonstrated to be associated with mammary cancer. Work on the epidemiology of cervical cancer and HPV led to the recognition that some forms of human cancer are of infectious origins, indeed, resulting in screening programs on cervical cancer using HPV detection assays, and to the introduction of HPV vaccines as a mean to combat gynaecological cancer. This closes the circle of cancer virus studies that had started in the beginning of the twentieth century. Dutch virologists were witnesses as well as *actors* in these astonishing stories.

The developments of cancer research at the NKI-AVL between the 1950s and mid-1970s differed from the 'molecularization' in cancer research in the post-war United States as described by Jean-Paul Gaudillière (1998). In common was the role of new instruments and techniques (such as ultracentrifugation, electron microscopy, and electrophoresis) to study animal tumour viruses. The differences, however, encompassed first the philanthropic and political processes which took place in the United States in the post-war 'biomedical complex', and second the scientific management that in the Netherlands was not modelled on industrial research practices After the heydays of cancer viruses was over in the second half of the 1970s, the emerging 'DNA revolution' superseded the focus on classical tumour viruses, leading to increased attention on oncogenes and tumour suppressor genes. But it should be remembered that viruses gave conception to these new 'operators'.

9 Virus vaccines and immunization programmes

> I have a dream that one day through scientific endeavour, experimentation and inspiration we will produce those new and better vaccines to combat the rampant infectious diseases that cause such mortality and morbidity throughout the world.
> *– Geoffrey F. Smith (2018)*

Introduction

The purpose of this chapter is to present an overview of virus vaccines within the Dutch national immunization programme (Rijksvaccinatieprogramma, RVP), its organization and the level of public acceptance. In 1957, the Ministry of Social Affairs and Public Health initiated the RVP with the vaccination of children with a combination vaccine against diphtheria, pertussis, and tetanus (DPT, Dutch DKT) and with the vaccination against poliomyelitis (Lindner and Blume, 2006). Before 1953, the diphtheria vaccine was already made available free of costs by the National Institute of Public Health[111] (Hoogendoorn, 1948). In 1954, a combination vaccine against diphtheria and DTP was offered, also produced by RIV (Health Inspectorate, 1953). However, a national programme for the vaccination of all children was lacking.

The immediate reason for further regulation of a vaccination programme were the polio epidemics in the early 1950s. The total numbers of cases of paralytic poliomyelitis reported to the health authorities were 1,338 and 1,829 in the epidemic years 1952 and 1956, respectively (Kalwij, 1959). Answering questions of B.S. Polak, a general practitioner and member of the Senate, the Minister of Social Affairs and Public Health H.G. Suurhoff proposed a framework for the structural organization of the RVP (Suurhoff, 1957). From 1957 onwards, provincial organizations, the so-called Provincial Immunisation Communities,[112] would provide leadership and coordinate the implementation of the RVP, together with municipal health services, local authorities, paediatricians, and general practitioners. The Health Inspectorate was made responsible as supervisor of the programme. From its inception to this day, the RVP has been voluntary and all recommended immunizations

---

111 Rijksinstituut voor de Volksgezondheid (RIV, from 1984 onwards RIVM).
112 Provinciale Entgemeenschappen.

are provided free of charge. In the Netherlands, the Minister of Social Affairs and Public Health has the authority to decide on the composition of the RVP, based on advice of the Health Council (Gezondheidsraad), an independent advisory body of the government. An overview of the history of the RVP can be found in Burgmeijer, Hoppenbrouwers and Bolscher (eds), *Handboek vaccinaties* (2006), of which, regrettably, an English edition is not available.

In 1955, the Salk inactivated poliomyelitis vaccine was licensed for use in the United States; the Health Council immediately established a 'Polio Committee' to advise on the relevance of this newly available vaccine for the Netherlands. The committee met for the first time in May 1955 (Lindner and Blume, 2006; Rigter, 1992). After initial hesitation and a preference of the committee for the live attenuated oral vaccine in December 1956, the Minister of Social Affairs and Public Health announced the importation of the inactivated polio vaccine, to be distributed by RIV. In 1957, the government decided that the country should produce the vaccine itself. It is beyond the scope of this book to analyse the considerations behind the decision of some European countries (Denmark, Sweden, the Netherlands) to have the polio vaccine produced by a state institution and that of other countries (United Kingdom, Germany, France) to have it produced by private companies (Böttiger et al., 1972; Böttiger, 1993; Lindner and Blume, 2006). Anyway, as a result of having RIV be responsible for the production and distribution of the polio vaccine, and requesting the Health Inspectorate to develop a plan for national polio vaccination, the organization, implementation and surveillance of the RVP became centralized and strengthened. Establishment of regional vaccination authorities, under the supervision of the health inspectorates, guaranteed standard procedures for the implementation and surveillance of polio vaccination (Lindner and Blume, 2006). Lindner and Blume remarked appropriately that this programme was very effective from the beginning. By 1960, 87 per cent of children born between 1945 and 1957 had been vaccinated with the inactivated polio vaccine (IVP). The number of reported cases of polio fell dramatically, from 203 in 1957 to around ten after 1965 (Lindner and Blume, 2006).

RIV played a pivotal role in the development of vaccines, together with its tasks in epidemiology, public health microbiology and reference services. In 1919, the Dutch State had taken over the Bacterio-Therapeutic Institute from Professor C.H.H. Spronck, with its vaccine-production facilities. A complication was the presence of the Laboratory for Serum and Vaccine controls within RIV. This situation could cause conflict of interests as this laboratory was charged with both the quality control and the market release of sera and vaccines in the Netherlands. Therefore, in 1939, the head of the laboratory was formally made independent from the director of RIV to exclude possible conflicts of interest. The establishment of the legal responsibility and associated laws for the approval and registration of new medication was nevertheless slow. The Medicines Evaluation Board[113] was established only by 1963, and was legally charged with this responsibility.

The structure of RIV was nearly unaltered from 1961 to 1984, except for some adjustments in 1967. However, the production and control of virus vaccines over this period were separated. We will not delve into the details – they can be found in Van Zon's history of RIV (1990). From 1967 on there was a diagnostic laboratory for virus diseases and rickettsioses, and a laboratory for serum and vaccine control. Furthermore, the laboratories in Sector IV, Immunology, focused on the production of vaccines: bacterial vaccines, smallpox vaccines (production and control of the production process were separate), measles, and poliomyelitis (Van Zon, 1990, pp. 211-221). With the merger of RIV and two other government institutes (Rijksinstituut voor Drinkwatervoorziening and Instituut voor Afvalstoffenonderzoek[114]) forming the new National Institute for Public Health and the Environment (RIVM) in 1984, the functions of the former RIV were classed under Sector I, Microbiology and Immunology. For infectious diseases there were separate laboratories for development, production, and control of vaccines. To separate the production of vaccines and the control of vaccines, the Foundation for the Advancement of Public Health and the Environment[115] (SVM) was established in 1988 (RIVM, 1988, p. 99; Van Zon, 1990, p. 378).[116] This foundation was formally responsible for the so-called end production of vaccines (formulation, filling, freeze-drying, labelling, packaging, and sale). Although SVM was a non-profit legal body it was intimately connected with RIVM: the governing body of the foundation consisted of the members of the directorate of RIVM. Later, all activities on the filling and formulation of vaccines were transferred to SVM; simultaneous transfer of personnel from RIVM to SVM contributed to the reduction of RIVM personnel, as required by the government. In 1998, all remaining vaccine-production activities at RIVM were transferred to SVM, which became officially a contract manufacturer of RIVM. In the following years, the continuation of vaccine development and production as part of the public domain was questioned. In early 2002, the Dutch cabinet

113 College ter beoordeling van Geneesmiddelen (CBG).
114 National Institute for Drinking Water Supply and Institute for Waste Research.
115 Stichting tot Bevordering van de Volksgezondheid en Milieuhygiëne (SVM).
116 According to the RIVM-organogram, the laboratories for control of bacterial and virus vaccines fell under the authority of the head of the Sector Vaccine Production in 1991 (Van Zon, 1990, p. 406).

approved the responsibility of the state to ensure a stable vaccine supply. At this point, we sneak over the self-chosen time limit of the year 2000 for this book, because it should end in the closing of vaccine production within the public sector. In 2003, a new agency named the Netherlands Vaccine Institute (NVI), a merger between SVM and relevant parts of RIVM, was established for this task. However, in 2009, vaccine production at NVI was discontinued because of NVI's limited resources and facilities. In 2011, the public tasks of vaccine development and production went back to RIVM. In 2012, ownership of RIVM vaccine-production facilities was sold to the Serum Institute of India, but the facility remained in Bilthoven under the name Bilthoven Biologicals BV. The public and research activities continued under the hospice of Intravacc, a commercial organization with public tasks, which operates under the Dutch Ministry for Public Health and the Environment. It was the intention of the then minister to privatize Intravacc after 2016 (Schippers, 2016). At the present time (1 January 2018), Intravacc operates under the Dutch Ministry of Public Health, Welfare and Sport. For a detailed report on the developments of the public sector vaccine production in the Netherlands we refer to the thesis of J.T. Hendriks (2017) and an essay by S. Blume, who was the supervisor of Hendriks's thesis.

After this brief overview, the following will focus on key vaccines used in the Netherlands.

Smallpox vaccine

The long history of vaccination started empirically. As described in Chapter 1, variolation by cutaneous application was applied in the Netherlands for the first time in 1748 by T. Tronchin. It remained, however, infrequently implemented, with e.g. only 64 inoculations performed in Rotterdam in 1764 (Gispen, 1953). In contrast to the situation in the United Kingdom, variolation mainly occurred in the upper classes. The variolation material had to be obtained from a patient with smallpox. Under dry conditions, poxviruses are stable and can be stored for a long time (Nakano, 1979, p. 267). After the introduction of vaccination in 1801, the practice of variolation was discontinued. Initially, the vaccine material was taken from a vesicle of a cow suffering from cowpox and the fluid was applied by scarification on the arm of a human individual. Thereafter, the vaccine material was transferred from arm to arm, through multiple generations, thus removing reliance on the cow material.

Continuous production of cowpox vaccine on the skin of calves, developed in 1848 by G. Negri in Naples, was introduced in the Netherlands relatively late, in 1868 (Buonaguro et al., 2015; Veldhuyzen, 1957, p. 42). Eventually, thirteen Parcs Vaccinogènes where the so-called animal lymph was produced on a large scale were officially recognized by the Dutch authorities. In 1934, the number of the parcs was reduced to three, located in Amsterdam, Rotterdam and Groningen, respectively. After the death of the director of the parc in Amsterdam, centralization was discussed in order to improve the quality of the vaccine. The decision was made to set up a centralized production facility at RIV in Utrecht, but it took two decades until, in 1954, the production was initiated at the Smallpox Vaccine Laboratory of RIV in Bilthoven (Van Zon, 1990, pp. 211, 251, 283).

With regards to the overseas territories of the Dutch kingdom, the whole of the Dutch Indies were provided since 1928 by one central production facility, the Landskoepokinrichting on Java, for the production of vacuo-dried vaccine. The technique was developed in 1926 in the East Indies by L. Otten whereby the lymph was dried in thin layers in vacuo (Collier LH, 1954; Collier WA, 1952; Otten, 1926, 1927). The dried material was then removed from the desiccator and ground to a fine powder, which could be transferred to glass tubes, vacuumed and sealed.

Based on comparative studies among young adults and infants in 1962, the decision was taken to use the third calf skin passage of the Elstree strain, obtained from the Lister Institute of Preventive Medicine, Elstree, Hertfordshire, UK, as a 'seed lot'. The Elstree strain was selected because it caused less adverse effect than other strains (Polak and Brans, 1962; Polak et al., 1963; Polak et al., 1964; Rigter, 1992). Seed lots of the strain were then globally distributed to other countries, after the recognition of RIV as a WHO International Reference Centre for Smallpox Vaccine in 1967 (Arita, 1988, p. 547).

After the global eradication of smallpox in 1979, the smallpox virus strains present at RIV were shipped to the Centers for Disease Control, Atlanta, GA, USA. The head of the Smallpox Laboratory, A.C. Hekker, personally transported, under police escort, the containers to Schiphol Airport.

The decision to abandon smallpox vaccination had been taken earlier, in 1974, following the advice of the Dutch Health Council. Yet, the votes of the council advisory committee had been equally divided for and against this advice. Thus, contrary to the usual practice and against the express wish of the chairman, the secretary, J. Huisman, exercised his right to vote to settle the discontinuation of smallpox vaccination (Huisman, 2002a).

However, the vaccinia virus stocks have been preserved up to today. Thus, using the old production protocols, new virus stocks were produced after the terrorist attack on the Twin Towers in New York in 2001, to protect against potential attacks by bioterrorists. Protocols and virus stocks are in place to vaccinate the whole of the Dutch population within a week.

Rabies vaccine

As early as in 1886, free rabies vaccination in Paris, including travel expenses and accommodation, was offered to selected Dutch citizens; permission was required from a district veterinarian in consultation with the district medical doctor of the Medical Inspectorate. The Pasteur Institute in Paris administered the vaccine, prepared according to the method developed by Louis Pasteur and co-workers. From 1907 onwards, rabies vaccination could be administered closer to home, in Belgium, at the 'Institut antirabique' of Bordet in Brussels. After the occupation of Belgium by the Germans in 1914, the Dutch-Belgian border was closed and a clinic in Utrecht was opened for rabies vaccination using a vaccine purchased from the Robert Koch Institute in Berlin. In the 1950s, a rabies vaccine developed by the Hungarian E. Högyes was used. The immunization schedule consisted of subsequent injections with preparations of increasing concentration of suspended virus diluted in a bactericidal solution (Verlinde, 1957, p. 610; Van Loghem et al., 1956, p. 254). Högyes developed this method in Budapest, Hungary, where he replaced dried spinal cords with a diluted 'virus fixe'. The dilution did not alter the quality of the virus but only its quantity. A vaccine prepared according to this technique was produced by Philips-Roxane under the name Högyes-Philips vaccine, under the quality control of RIV (Van Loghem et al., 1956, p. 254). In 1962, a new rabies vaccine was developed at RIV in Bilthoven by Gispen and Saathof. It was prepared in suckling rat brains and had advantages of potency, stability and apparent freedom from encephalotigens. But a clear disadvantage was the large number of animals needed for its production. Also, aseptically harvesting the rabies antigen from the brains was difficult (Gispen et al., 1965). Another inactivated rabies vaccine, derived from brain tissue from 4- to 5-day-old suckling rabbits, was also used in 1962, during a rabies epidemic (Gispen, 1975). Later, the development of rabies vaccine from virus grown in embryonated eggs or cell cultures opened the door to large-scale production of rabies vaccine with such a high potency that administration of three instead of fourteen doses was sufficient (Kaplan, 1971; Van Wezel et al., 1978; Van Steenis et al., 1984). By about 1980, a 'dog kidney cell vaccine' (DKCV) produced at RIV was made available.

In the Dutch East Indies, M.J. Otten-van Stockum developed in the mid-1930s a vaccine that consisted of a suspension of 'virus fixe'-infected monkey brain cells incubated with formalin. An advantage was that this vaccine could be stored at 5°C without noticeable loss of effect (Verlinde, 1957, p. 610). The efficacy of this and other vaccines was critically analysed by her (Dinger, 1951; Gispen, 1951; Otten, 1947; Otten-van Stockum, 1941; Van Loghem et al., 1956, pp. 254-255; Van Stockum, 1935).

Poliomyelitis vaccine

In April 1955, the results of a large-scale trial in the USA with the Salk vaccine were presented, demonstrating a vaccine efficacy of 90 per cent against poliovirus type 1 and 2, and 60-70 per cent against poliovirus type 3. Within two hours after the announcement, the Salk vaccine, consisting of inactivated virus and therefore called inactivated polio vaccine or IPV, was licensed for use, with five million American children vaccinated that year (Lindner and Blume, 2006).

In May 1955, the vaccination programme had been briefly suspended in the USA because of the so-called Cutter incident. Shortly after the release of the vaccine, children in California and Idaho who received the vaccine prepared by Cutter Laboratories (founded by E.A. Cutter in 1897) developed paralysis in the arm that received the inoculation (Nathanson and Langmuir, 1963; Offit, 2005). Two production pools of the Cutter vaccine appeared to be inappropriately inactivated and contained a high dose of live poliovirus. These lots had been used for about 120,000 inoculations, with the great majority of the vaccinees receiving only one inoculation shot. About 40,000 children developed an asymptomatic or abortive polio virus infection, and 60 cases of poliomyelitis occurred in vaccinees while 89 cases were reported in family contacts. As a consequence, inoculation with the inactivated Salk vaccine was temporally suspended, and the live attenuated polio vaccine, developed by A. Sabin and H. Koprowski, and that had to be administered orally (oral polio vaccine or OPV), was used during the suspension. Thereupon, the Dutch Health Council established a 'Polio committee' to advise on the relevance of the newly available polio vaccines for the Netherlands. In the reports produced in June 1955 and May 1956, the committee expressed doubts as to the adequacy and safety of the Salk vaccine (Lindner and Blume, 2006; Rigter, 1992). It was thus advised that adequate immunity could be provided only by a vaccine containing live, attenuated virus.

The Netherlands had faced a major poliomyelitis epidemic in 1952, with a total of 1,712 notified paralytic and non-paralytic cases, and saw again in 1956 an epidemic with a total of 2,206 notified cases of which 1,829 were paralytic (Kalwij, 1959). Then in December 1956, the government was thus advised by the Health Council to organize a mass vaccination programme and allowed the importation of polio vaccine. At this time, preference was given to the inactivated polio vaccine prepared according the technique designed by J. Salk. At first, the polio vaccine was imported from the USA (1957-1959). Yet, the Salk vaccine could not be delivered continuously by the manufacturer in the USA. Furthermore, the standards that IPV preparations were required to meet in the USA were felt to be inadequate. The Cutter incident of spring 1955 naturally made the Dutch wary of importing the vaccine from the USA. In 1957, the medical journal *Medisch Contact* announced that in accordance with the American export permits, the Salk vaccine could no longer be imported. Later DAGRA N.V., importer of the Pitman-Moore Company, put an advertisement in which it was announced that the vaccine should only be used within approved vaccination schemes, meanwhile Pharmachemie extolled the virtues of the R.I.T.[117] Poliomyelitis vaccine (Medisch Contact, 1958). From 1958 to 1961, inactivated vaccine produced by the Belgian company R.I.T. in Rixensart (later GlaxoSmithKline), which had to meet higher standards for safety, was used. This successfully avoided any major public health crises.

In 1957, the Dutch government decided that the country should produce polio vaccine itself (Lindner and Blume, 2006). RIV had already experience with the production of a combined bacterial vaccine against diphtheria, pertussis, and tetanus, although production at an industrial scale posed problems that had to be improved. With the production of inactivated polio vaccine containing Mahoney b type 1, M.E.F.1 type 2, and Saukett type 3 strains of poliovirus, a combined diphtheria, pertussis, tetanus and polio vaccine was developed (Brandwijk et al., 1961; Lindner and Blume, 2006). H.H. Cohen (head of vaccine production and later director of RIV) was the driving force behind the concept of the quadruple vaccine; he predicted that the coverage of the vaccination would increase by decreasing the number of injections from seven or eight to four. In a relatively short time, the plain polio vaccine was developed. By the end of 1958, sufficient combined vaccine had been produced for a trial to be held in the city of Leeuwarden. After further safety trials completed by 1961, the combined vaccine was ready to be introduced at a national scale. In 1961, sufficient

---

117   Recherche et Industrie Therapeutique (Research and Therapeutic Industry).

formalin-inactivated polio vaccine was produced by RIV, and used in the RVP. In 1962, the combined vaccine replaced the separate diphtheria, pertussis, and tetanus and inactivated polio vaccines in the RVP. From 1965 onwards, the combined vaccine was produced at sufficient quantities for annual cohorts of babies (Hofman, 1967, 1972).

One of the advocates of the live attenuated vaccine was J.D. Verlinde, who was an acquaintance of Sabin (Sabin, 1957). It is quite possible that they met each other during the Second International Poliomyelitis Conference in Copenhagen in 1951, which they both attended. In 1958, Verlinde and co-workers received Sabin live attenuated vaccine and performed small field studies in the Netherlands (Verlinde, 1958; Verlinde et al., 1958). In an address delivered at a symposium organized by the Princess Beatrix-Polio Fund in Utrecht (and also at other occasions), he described the considerations that had led to the development of inactivated and live attenuated vaccines (Verlinde, 1961, 1962). In his public talk, with Princess Beatrix present in the audience, he acknowledged the reduction of 80-90 per cent of cases of paralytic poliomyelitis thanks to immunization with the Salk vaccine. At the same time, he pointed at the fact that the inactivated vaccine induces only antibodies, whereas the live attenuated vaccine also leads to an increased resistance of the intestinal wall, limiting or even abrogating wild virus replication upon subsequent infection. He admitted 'that insufficient information had been obtained (according to some authors) whether a slight increased neurovirulence of the virus used for vaccination after human passage might constitute a danger to subjects who are thought to be increasingly sensitive to poliomyelitis for some reason, if the virus is disseminated among a population with relatively high number of non-immune subjects'. Therefore, he made a plea to administer a live vaccine only to subjects who had acquired a basic immunity by means of the inactivated Salk vaccine.

R. Gispen and H.H. Cohen of RIV were decisive for the Dutch choice of the inactivated polio vaccine (Gispen, 1957; Cohen, 1987). Later, J. Huisman acknowledged that economic factors had been taken into consideration in the decision to advise the use of an inactivated vaccine (Huisman, 2002b). Gispen based his arguments partly on economic, but also on practical grounds. The Salk vaccination could be integrated into the existing scheme for the immunization of infants; and a quadruple vaccine against diphtheria, pertussis, tetanus and poliomyelitis (DTP-IPV) could be developed at RIV. To address the lower response of infants in the first six months of life, a scheme of three primary injections and boosters given at the ages of three, four, five, and eleven months, respectively, was implemented (Gispen, 1961). The effect of eight vaccination years (1958-1965) has been described by Hofman: the overall reduction of the morbidity rate was 96 per cent in the 1- to 4-year-old children, who are considered the most vulnerable age group, and paralytic poliomyelitis was reduced by about 97 per cent (Hofman, 1967).

By 1964 the overall acceptance rate was almost 90 per cent of those eligible, but there were population pockets with lower rates because of religion based non-compliance. In the late decades of the twentieth century, the coverage rates for immunization remained high, of at least 90 per cent (RIVM, 2014). Despite the high coverage of the DTP-IPV vaccination, two outbreaks of poliomyelitis occurred in 1978 and 1992-1993 (Rümke et al., 1995). In an area stretching from the south-west to the north-east of the Netherlands, several communities refused vaccination on religious grounds. These communities in the so-called Bible belt were infected with poliovirus introduced by visitors from abroad. They contracted the disease while the general population remained protected by vaccination or herd immunity. Control measures during the epidemics were taken by offering OPV (live attenuated virus) to contacts and people who lived in a wide area around the village where the index patient lived, and had never been vaccinated.

Rubella, mumps, measles combination vaccine

The combination measles-mumps-rubella (MMR) vaccine was introduced through incremental steps in the Netherlands. This process has been described in a, cogent and informative article by Blume and Tump (2010).

A selective immunization programme to prevent congenital rubella started in 1974 in the Netherlands, initially restricted to schoolgirls of the age of eleven years. A similar strategy was implemented in the United Kingdom, but despite school-age and pre-pregnancy vaccination, the incidence of rubella in pregnancy remained unacceptably high during outbreaks. Mathematical models predicted that rubella could be eradicated within 40 years or so if 80 per cent to 85 per cent of children were to be vaccinated at the age of two years, in addition to vaccination of girls between the ages of ten and fifteen years (Anderson and May, 1992). Based on these findings, the Dutch vaccination strategy was modified. In 1984, the Dutch Health Council advocated vaccination of girls and boys at the age of fourteen months and re-vaccination at the age of nine years (Van der Veen, 1984). This advice was approved by the government and implemented in 1987.

In the nineteenth century, the death rate attributed to measles was about 72-84 per 100,000 inhabitants, higher than the death rate due to smallpox and scarlet fever (Ballot, 1871). In the second half of the twentieth century, the mean death rate remained high at 1.6 per 10,000 cases (Van der Zwan et al., 1994). For the advisory committee of the Health Council, it was clear that the measles vaccine should be offered to all children in their first year of life and that a live vaccine should be used. In 1976, immunization against measles was included in the RVP. It was based on a live attenuated measles vaccine containing the so-called Moraten (More attenuated Enders) strain purchased from Merck, since RIV could only produce inactivated vaccines (Blume and Tump, 2010). RIV changed its research-and-development strategy, and by 1981, the Merck vaccine was replaced by a RIV vaccine using the same strain obtained in license from Merck.

The advice of the Health Council to include immunization against mumps in the RVP took more time. After years of deliberations by the consultative body on immunization of the Health Council, recommendation was finally given to switch to a combined trivalent vaccine, including measles, mumps and rubella viruses, in 1982. Mumps in children was considered relatively innocuous, and the duration of protection was unknown. Ultimately in 1987, the trivalent combination mumps-measles-rubella (MMR) vaccine replaced the bivalent combination measles-rubella vaccine; to achieve reduction in circulating rubella virus, this trivalent vaccine was offered to both girls and boys at the age of fourteen months and nine years. RIVM produced the trivalent vaccine under license of Merck; according to Ruitenberg, then head of RIVM's vaccine-production department, they had to forget about their own measles and rubella vaccines (Blume and Tump, 2010; Ruitenberg, 1984).

Special Department Immunobiology

In 1984 this department was established with the aim to study fundamental questions related with development of new vaccines under the leadership of A.D.M.E. Osterhaus. As described above measles, mumps and rubella vaccinations (MMR) were introduced in the national vaccination scheme and further development of these vaccines was one of the aims of this department. Furthermore, research on an HIV vaccine was considered a public health sector task. In spite of optimistic hope and expectations of many experts it was reported in 1990 that this field was not yet in a phase to report successes and that one had to wait to at least the year 2000 (Van Zon, 1990, p. 379). Other topics of research at this department were herpes virus and morbillivirus infections in seals, human hantaviruses in the Netherlands, and use of immunostimulating complexes (ISCOMS) as a vaccine adjuvant. In 1992 the greater part of this group moved to Erasmus MC, where Osterhaus was appointed at the chair of virology.

Influenza vaccine

Influenza immunization in specific risk groups

Since the 1950s, influenza vaccine trials have not been particularly encouraging. On the one hand, some influenza vaccine trials found evidence of benefit; while on the other, a long series of studies, indicated that annual vaccination had no long-term advantage. After the major influenza pandemic of 1957 (H2N2), and the severe epidemics of 1969-1970 (H3N2) and 1976 (H1N1), and maybe also in the context of persisting memories of the 1918-1919 devastating (H1N1) pandemic, studies were carried out to estimate excess mortality attributable to influenza in the early 1980s. Based on a cost-effectiveness analysis by Riddiough et al. in Chicago, Beyer and Masurel argued for annual vaccination of elderly persons of 65 years of age or older, besides vaccination of the risk groups, such as individuals with chronic heart or lung disease, metabolic disorders, of which diabetes was the most prevalent, renal disease, or immunodeficiency diseases (Beyer and Masurel, 1983; Riddiough et al., 1983). Masurel was an internationally acknowledged expert on influenza from his thesis work in which he suggested and proved that from 1918 to 1957, an 'era of swine influenza A virus' may have prevailed in man, in which periodically antigenic strains successively emerged from each other (Masurel, 1962).

To increase the low coverage rate for influenza immunization in the defined at-risk groups, a television campaign was deployed in 1992, based on collaborations between the Dutch Ministry of Health, the National Association of General Practitioners (Landelijke Huisartsen Vereniging, LHV), the Royal Dutch Pharmacists Association (Koninklijke Nederlandse Maatschappij ter bevordering der Pharmacie, KNMP), and the Netherlands Influenza Foundation (Sprenger and Masurel, 1992). To create a national coordinated approach, the National Programme for Influenza Prevention (Nationaal Programma Grieppreventie, NPG) was founded in 1997. It established that RIVM was responsible for purchasing influenza vaccines and for their delivery to general practitioners (GPs), who would invite eligible individuals for immunization. The process was to be computerised, with submission of an immunization form by the GP, so that, for instance, local coverage could easily be calculated. This national programme is a commendable initiative; however, the efficacy of influenza vaccines continues to be a major issue that remains to be solved (Darvishian et al., 2017; Osterholm et al., 2012).

Commercial production of influenza vaccines

As mentioned in Chapter 4, influenza vaccines were produced surprisingly early in the Netherlands. Soon after World War II, the Philips van Houten Company was involved in the production of virus vaccines (Klein and Hertzberger, 1951). The optimistic prediction of Klein and Hertzberger, 'the production of virus vaccines, a peculiar form of mass production taking place partly in some large egg hatcheries and promising to be of great importance not only for the Netherlands but also far beyond its frontiers' was to be fulfilled.

The start of manufacturing was a classic example of an (informal?) network between industry and academia. Leading figures were E.H. Reerink, director of the company Philips Van Houten and J. Mulder, professor of internal medicine at Leiden University (W. Rakhorst, personal communication, 2018). Mulder, together with L. Bijlmer, had investigated influenza epidemics in Groningen. When he was nominated professor of internal medicine in Leiden in 1946, Mulder continued to pursue influenza research. During that year, he spent two and a half months in the USA to study viral diseases and influenza, in particular. We do not know when Reerink and Mulder met each other for the first time; in any case, this encounter was fruitful. Mulder initiated the compilation of advices by the Health Council on public health measures for the prevention of influenza epidemics, while Reerink requested the permission to manufacture an influenza vaccine. In 1949, the first vaccine that was cultivated in embryonated chicken eggs was available for the public; the Netherlands became the first country after the USA to produce mass quantities of influenza vaccines. In spite of attempts to grow the vaccine virus on cell cultures, the culture of sufficiently large amounts of influenza virus for vaccines continued to largely occur in embryonated chicken eggs up to the beginning of the twenty-first century; cell culture-derived vaccines are nowadays offering promising alternatives. Through the years, the manufacturing process changed and improved considerably, especially the steps after inactivation of the virus, including ultrafiltration, splitting in subunits (hemagglutinin and neuraminidase), sterile filtration, and addition of preservatives.

Hepatitis B vaccine

In 1989, a screening programme among pregnant women was implemented in the Netherlands to prevent maternal-foetal transmission of hepatitis B.

Figure 27   Inoculation of fertilized eggs for the cultivation of influenza virus

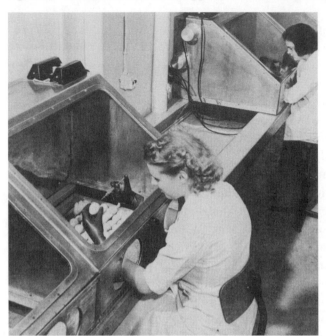

Reproduction courtesy of *Philips Technical Reviews*

The screening was added to the existing routine testing for ABO, rhesus blood groups, and syphilis in the first trimester of pregnancy. Babies born to women positive for hepatitis B surface antigen receive, immediately after delivery, hepatitis B immunoglobulins administered by the person who was in care of the delivery. The active hepatitis B immunization is implemented in combination with the national childhood vaccination programme. This appeared to be a feasible and satisfactory approach (Grosheide et al., 1991, 1995).

The decision process on general vaccination for the prevention of hepatitis B endured many deliberations. An interim advice was published by the Health Council in 1982. People who qualified for immunization were categorized into infected patients and otherwise healthy individuals at risk of infection (Van der Heide, 1982). In 1996, the Minister of Health was advised by the Health Council to initiate procedures to prepare for the addition of general hepatitis B vaccination to the RVP. In 2000, the Minister of Health decided temporarily not to include hepatitis B vaccination in the RVP, based on a suitability study. However, as a result of discussions in the Parliament, the minister asked the Health Council to reconsider the advice of 1996. Based on the low prevalence of hepatitis B in the Netherlands and thus low levels of pre-existing immunity, the Health Council advocated in 2001 to extend the hepatitis B immunization recommendation to include all children with at least one parent originating from a hepatitis B intermediate- or high-endemic country (Health Council, 2001).

Production of hepatitis B vaccine in the Netherlands

At the Central Laboratory of the Netherlands Red Cross Blood Transfusion Service in Amsterdam a vaccine containing plasma-derived, heat-inactivated hepatitis B surface antigen (HBsAg) was developed in the 1970s (Coutinho et al., 1983; Lelie et al., 1984; Reerink-Brongers et al., 1983). The antigen was derived from the plasma of asymptomatic, chronic carriers. The vaccine became available for clinical trials after the required safety and immunogenicity studies, in 1980-1982. The trials were conducted among different populations: low risk volunteers, patients treated with chronic haemodialysis, and among male homosexuals or more general men having sex with men (MSM) living in the Netherlands, a country with low prevalence of hepatitis B. The latter group is at high risk of acquiring hepatitis B infections. Although the efficacy of the vaccine was comparable with other plasma-derived, formalin-inactivated vaccines, the choice to isolate hepatitis-B-surface antigen from plasma was born under an unlucky star. About the same time, in 1982, the HIV epidemic broke out and a considerable number of plasma donors not only belonged to the group of asymptomatic chronic HbsAg carriers, but were also at high risk of HIV-positivity. Recombinant technologies soon superseded human plasma as source of the HBsAg. As a consequence, the plasma-derived vaccine did not reach the market. Another product developed by CLB, nowadays Sanquin, was the plasma-derived hepatitis B immunoglobulin which is still available to be administered when required, e.g. upon needle-stick incidents or immediately after delivery of babies born to mothers positive for the hepatitis B antigen.

Occupationally acquired infections in vaccine-production laboratories

In spite of effective codes of practices, precaution principles and personal protection, viral infections acquired during laboratory research or production of virus vaccines occasionally occurred during the twentieth century in the Netherlands. Although published reports are scarce and scattered, some examples illustrate their importance.

In Chapter 3, experiments were described that were carried out in the Laboratory for Hygiene in Amsterdam with yellow fever virus which was obtained via Petit in Paris and originated from laboratories of the Commission on Yellow Fever, International Health Division of the Rockefeller Foundation, Lagos, Nigeria, West Africa. *Aedes aegypti* mosquitoes were shipped by S.L. Brug from the East Indies. *Macaca cynomolgus* monkeys from the Dutch Indies were already present in the laboratory. The aim of the experiment was to investigate why yellow fever was not present in Asia. The researchers did not want to perform the experiments in Dutch East India because of the risk of spreading yellow fever virus among a susceptible population. Yellow fever was acquired by one of the researchers. This is an example of a laboratory-acquired infection that resulted from work with yellow fever virus, and corroborated their precaution against possible introduction of yellow fever virus in Asia. It must be noted that a yellow fever vaccine was not available at the time the experiments were carried out.

In 1952, A. Pondman reported on the development at RIV of a vaccine against epidemic typhus caused by *Rickettsia prowazeki*. Between 1940 and 1945, he and his co-workers produced a vaccine in the typhus laboratory of RIV that was used for a rather large section of the Dutch population (Pondman, 1952). However, he failed to mention either the number of people having received the vaccine or the fact that he and a technician acquired and recovered from an infection while working with the parasite in 1942 (Van Zon, 1990, p. 1964; Westendorp Boerma, 1960). The story did not end there. When Pondman moved from Utrecht to Groningen in 1946, his successor continued working on epidemic typhus, apparently without sufficient protection; in 1948 he also acquired typhus from the lab and died.

A third case of laboratory-acquired infection occurred in the late twentieth century; a report on the incident was veiled in a publication on the genetic analysis of a wild-type poliovirus in the Netherlands (Mulders et al., 1997). In 1992, in the middle of the type 3 poliomyelitis epidemic, a poliovirus type 1 was isolated from a faecal specimen of 19-month-old boy with transient synovitis of the hip (coxitis fugax) and a respiratory disorder. 'The father of the child worked at a polio vaccine-production facility; he had been accidentally exposed to a high amount of Mahoney prototype vaccine virus'. The isolation of a poliovirus in the Netherlands had to be reported to the Health Inspectorate. The latter may have decided to give no publicity to this particular case to avoid unrest among the general public.

Figure 28 A cell culture forming a monolayer four days after inoculation

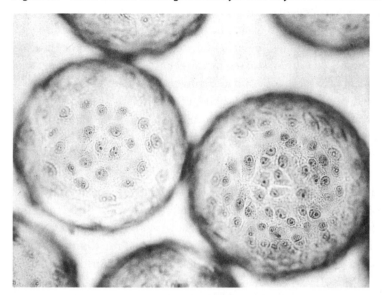

The layer covers the surface of a so-called microcarrier. The use of these small plastic balls in a 'Bilthoven unit' leads to a drastic enlargement of the surface area available for cell culture. This is a prerequisite for scaling up during vaccine preparation.
Reproduction courtesy of RIVM and Natuur en Techniek

Cooperation in the development of vaccine-production methods

Besides investigators as R. Gispen, H.H. Cohen and B. van der Zeijst many other people contributed to the development of viral vaccines in the Netherlands, but too many to be all mentioned. Considerable innovations came from the cooperation between different disciplines, such as chemistry, clinical medicine, public health, and veterinary medicine, represented by A.L. van Wezel (chemist), C.A. Hannik (paediatrician), B. Hofman (medical microbiologist), M.F. Polak (epidemiologist), and G. van Steenis (veterinarian). The latter was head of the Virus Vaccine Control Unit, where he pioneered in the field of development and implementation virus vaccines controls. Van Wezel invented several cell-culture systems to manufacture viral vaccines. Van Wezel's microcarrier cell culture method was used for vaccine production of inactivated polio vaccine, inactivated rabies vaccine and live attenuated measles virus vaccine, in large-volume bioreactors (Cohen and Hofman, 2002).

After training as paediatrician, Charlotte Hannik joined the Office of the Chief Medical Officer (Geneeskundige Hoofd Inspectie), where she organized the 1957 polio-vaccination campaign. The result was a high participation percentage: over 90 per cent of the children at risk received the polio vaccine at least three times. After 1962, she moved to RIV, where she investigated adverse reactions to vaccines, in particular, to the pertussis vaccine (Rümke and Cohen, 1996). B. Hofman started his career as a junior bacteriologist at the Department of Bacteriology and Experimental Pathology of the Institute for Preventive Medicine in Leiden (head, J.D. Verlinde), where he carried out studies on poliovirus. At the beginning of the 1960s he moved to RIV and addressed the epidemiology of poliomyelitis; he became head of the poliomyelitis vaccine laboratory. M.F. Polak obtained his medical degree in Amsterdam in 1940; during World War II he prepared his thesis, resulting in a PhD awarded in August 1945. His dissertation had already been printed in 1944, it had to have been secretly approved by the committee by then, because the University of Amsterdam was, however not formally, closed in 1944. During the 1950s, he was the right-hand man to Prof. Charlotte Ruys in Amsterdam and specialized in the epidemiology of infectious diseases. In 1960, he joined RIV, where he served as an epidemiologist and focused on viral infections. Remarkably, after he left RIV, he passed the notary's examination at Radboud University in 1983.

G. van Steenis was a veterinary pathologist involved in developing vaccine production and manufacturing technologies at RIV. He contributed to the microcarrier production system of Van Wezel by developing a perfusion technique of monkey kidneys using trypsinization (Van Wezel et al., 1979). The benefit of this method is the reduction of the number of animals needed, as well as improvement of the yields and quality of kidney cells. At the same time, he was responsible for the quality control of virological vaccines; and he served as a counsellor to the World Health Organization.

Ultimate sale of public health sector vaccine production

As mentioned above, R. Gispen and H.H. Cohen were leading decision makers at RIV for initiating vaccine production and establishing the RVP. As described by S. Blume, RIVM was a significant participant in vaccine development and production in the 1960s and 1970s (Blume, 2017). However, over the last two decades of the twentieth century the production of vaccines in the public sector had to give way to multinational companies. This period was characterized by changes in production processes patented by the industry and the growing belief in free-market principles in the Dutch government. Vaccine production was no longer seen as the core business of RIVM. At the end of the twentieth century, B.A.M. van der Zeijst played an important role in setting the future of vaccine production in the Netherlands. Trained as a virologist, he worked at the Laboratory for Virology of the Veterinary Faculty of the University of Utrecht, where he became involved in vaccine research; he was appointed professor of bacteriology in 1985. Around 1997, he was invited by RIVM to become director of its Vaccine Division. His task was to align current vaccine research with public health priorities. On the occasion of his formal farewell from the Netherlands Vaccine Institute, he wrote: 'The first task was the easiest. I killed a number of research projects. This was much to the chagrin of researchers, but I confronted them with the certainty that their research, however elegant it was, would not sufficiently reduce burden of disease' (Van der Zeijst, 2011). A priority list was then made based on the potential of vaccination to reduce the burden of infectious diseases (Van der Zeijst et al., 2000). He also was involved in the separation of responsibilities between RIVM and SVM. This ultimately resulted in the foundation of the Netherlands Vaccine Institute (NVI) in 2003 (Minister van Volksgezondheid, Welzijn en Sport, 2003). For the description of the developments after 2000 we refer to the thesis of J.T. Hendriks (2017) in which he clarifies the process of gradual decline and privatization in the 1990s and the takeover by Serum Institute of India Ltd (SIIL) in 2012. This company plays a key role in the supply of affordable vaccines for developing countries made available through the global UN procurement system. Hendriks reaches a remarkable conclusion in this regard as he states that the 2012 takeover has by some insiders been described as 'the ultimate success of technology transfer' (Hendriks, 2017).

Success of the RVP

Of course, the success of an immunization programme depends not only on the quality of the offered vaccines, but also of the processes for the delivery and implementation of the programme. Vaccination is thus as well a scientific as a political and communicative issue. In the Netherlands there has always been a group of citizens that rejects immunization on religious grounds, as we have already seen in the first chapter on the nineteenth century. At the introduction of the RVP, and still nowadays, these groups live mainly in small, closed communities in the so-called Bible belt, and infectious diseases can be transmitted easily within these communities because of a lack of herd immunity. Since the 1950s, several epidemics of polio and measles have been observed within these communities without spread to the general population.

Since the 1980s, another group of opponents to immunization emerged consisting of anthroposophists and adherents of 'natural' and 'alternative healing' (Rümke and Visser, 2004). The Dutch Association Critically Giving a Jab (Nederlandse Vereniging Kritisch Prikken) established in 1994 aims to support parents in making their own personal decisions regarding the vaccination of their children. The association nonetheless claims not to be affiliated with any alternative view of medicine (Blume, 2006). The low vaccine uptake, in particular of the MMR vaccine, within these groups is less noticeable because they live among the general society and are protected by herd immunity generated by high immunization levels of the surrounding population.

Besides coverage rates, another important factor for the success of the RVP is the efficacy of the vaccines. In an evaluation of the vaccination programme, De Melker et al. concluded that all together the programme induces good protection and that herd immunity is sufficient among the general population, but not among orthodox reformed individuals (De Melker et al., 2003; Van den Hof et al., 2002). However, the authors warned for changes that may occur in the long term, such as the waning of immunity.

The growing resistance against vaccination, especially among the educated public, is worrisome and widespread (Betsch et al., 2017). Probably this has more to do with a deep aversion against pharmaceutical industry (Big Pharma) and fear of alleged adverse effects than with doubt about vaccine efficacy. It would be tragic if it turns out that a severe viral epidemic is necessary for the public concerns about the safety of vaccination to be rebuffed. Society does have the means at hand to prevent mortality and morbidity caused by major viral infections thanks to the vaccines and public health measures mentioned in this chapter.

10 Conclusions

Fortunate are those who are starting now.
– *M.W. Beijerinck (1926)*[118]

Blessed is he who carries within him a god, an ideal of beauty and who obeys it: ideal
of art, ideal of science, ideal of the homeland, ideal of the virtues of the Gospel.[119]
– *Louis Pasteur (1882)*

In his opening address at the Twelfth Congress on Physics and Medicine[120] that took place in April 1909, C.Λ. Pekelharing, professor of pathology at the University of Utrecht, spoke on the importance of the advancement of medicine since the time it was incorporated into the natural sciences by the work of Pasteur, Lister, Koch and their followers (1909). More than a century later, we might well echo his words with the mere expediency of transmuting the actors. His claim underlines that the progress of medicine and science is not the result of accomplishments by individuals but of an extension, and integration, of the work of communities of scholars over a wide range of applied sciences. The medical profession will continue to be changed by science; and science itself will keep evolving. Here, we emphasize that medical virology is greatly indebted to physics, chemistry, biology, biochemistry, immunology, technical science, and information technology.

Since at least the mid-nineteenth century, the germ theory has operated on the assumption that infectious diseases were transmitted by contagion and were caused by 'seeds' or 'animalculae' described by Van Leeuwenhoek in the preceding century. A concurrent explanation for the spread of epidemics of such diseases was the miasmatic theory. Miasmata were conceived as poisons spread through the atmosphere and that were causes of disease, besides the traditional environmental factors, such as damp and cold. Unfortunately, we did not meet in our rambles through the history of Dutch virology any travellers with the stature of John Tyndall, the famous Irish/English scientist who studied the floating matter of the air in relation to putrefaction and infection during his exercises in the Alps (Tyndall, 1882).

118 Quoted in Van Iterson, Den Dooren de Jong, Kluyver, 1940: p. 189.
119 Heureux celui qui porte en soi un dieu, un idéal de beauté et qui lui obéit : idéal de l'art, idéal de la science, idéal de la patrie, idéal des vertus de l'Évangile.
120 Het 12ᵉ Nederlandsch Natuur- en Geneeskundig Congres.

Advocating the germ theory, Tyndall wrote that putrefaction and epidemic disease both arose from something contained in the air. This 'something' was a *particle*; he draws the distinction between molecules and particles as follows: the atom or the molecule, if free, is always part of a gas, the particle is never so. A particle is a bit of liquid or solid matter, formed by the aggregation of atoms or molecules (Tyndall, 1882, p. 27). By the end of the century, however, there was sufficient evidence linking specific infectious diseases to specific microbes. But although bacteriology was established as a science, the causative agents of a number of infectious diseases could not be demonstrated, due in many cases, as we now know, to inadequate laboratory techniques and instruments. Some of these diseases – smallpox, rabies, measles, influenza, and poliomyelitis – could be recognized by their clinical symptoms and epidemiology, well before the identification of their causative agents. Such matters as infectivity and routes of transmission of smallpox, rabies, and measles, for example, were already well defined by the nineteenth century or earlier. Consequently, preventive measures could be taken and were promulgated by the local or provincial authorities when epidemics of these diseases struck.

Indeed, preventive practices against smallpox (such as variolation) had been introduced in Western Europe as early as 1721. By the middle of the eighteenth century, following the examples of neighbouring Great Britain and Switzerland, similar measures were adopted in the Netherlands as well, mainly by well-to-do families. The practice of vaccination, inoculating fluid originating from a cowpox vesicle, developed by the English physician Edward Jenner in 1798, enjoyed a much faster and wider response. Regardless, due to various factors (such as laxity and anti-vaccination movements primarily based on religious principles), smallpox – that 'most terrible of all harpies' (Rutten, 1997) – remained endemic in the Netherlands until the early twentieth century.

Rabies, another horrific disease, occurred much less frequently in the Netherlands. Before the availability of vaccination, preventive measures at the level of the rabid animal, such as detainment and observation followed by the killing of the rabid animal, were taken and for the bitten person, extensive treatment with immediate cauterization of the wound was recommended. Soon after the discovery of therapeutic vaccination by Pasteur in 1886, public initiative engaged the government to authorize free access of Dutch inhabitants to treatment at the Institut Pasteur in Paris, at the governments expense. While health and prevention of disease clearly fall under the responsibilities of the government, such private actions were not exceptional phenomena in the nineteenth century.

Then, in the closing years of the nineteenth century, the dawn of virology was announced by the Dutchman M.W. Beijerinck. In 1898, Beijerinck demonstrated that the agent causing tobacco mosaic disease was a *contagium vivum fluidum*. The disease-causing agent was living (*vivum*) because it replicated in living cells and it was fluid (*fluidum*) because it penetrated to a certain depth into agar. Infection experiments performed with these deeper layers of the agar plate caused the disease just as had those using the porcelain filter. He concluded that the contagium must be fit for diffusion and consequently considered as fluid. It appeared that Ivanowski already showed in 1892 that the agent passed through a filter. Beijerinck reportedly admitted that he was not aware of Ivanowski's work. There is no doubt that Ivanowski made the first observations as Thomas Rivers later describes, but the difference between their contributions to this crucial discovery lays in the interpretation of their experiments. Ivanowski concluded that the agent must have been a small bacterium. In contrast, Beijerinck expanded his experiments to prove that the agent was neither an aerobic or anaerobic bacterium nor a bacterial spore. He further drew an analogy to organisms causing other infectious diseases, which lose their virulence through culture outside of the organism and increase it by repeated passages through susceptible animals. Beijerinck realized that it was a new kind of infectious agent. Therefore, we consider his conclusion being a breakthrough comparable with that of the work of Van Leeuwenhoek.

However, Dutch medical doctors appeared like spectators witnessing this remarkable sunrise while standing on the summit of a cloudy mountain. Based on the scarcity of communications in the *Netherlands Journal of Medicine*, we have to conclude that little attention was paid at the time to this major discovery in the Netherlands. In contrast, Beijerinck's interpretations were scrutinized by contemporaries from all over the world, from Russia to the United States. In other words, a Dutch finding about a filterable disease agent had international repercussions, yet little national recognition.

It is nevertheless not fully surprising that wide support from Dutch medical circles could not be observed, because the available technology did not offer techniques to settle further questions in human medicine on diagnostics, aetiology, or development of vaccines. Twenty years later, the phenomenon of bacteriophagy by viruses infecting bacteria as described by Twort (1915) and D'Herelle (1917) enjoyed a better reception. The discussions on the nature of the bacteriophages were in fact similar to the conflicting interpretations of the nature of viruses. The hope raised by phage therapy – the clinical use of phage antagonism to bacteria – as propagated by D'Herelle aroused the scientific and public interest in an innovative antimicrobial treatment using bacteriophages against diseases, such as cholera and plague. Nonetheless, both Beijerinck and D'Herelle received the prestigious Leeuwenhoek Medal in 1905 and 1925, respectively, which was granted by the Royal Netherlands Academy of Science every ten years to the scientist judged to have made the most significant contribution to microbiology during the preceding decade.

From 1930 onwards, advancements in technology reversed the nature of the criteria defining viruses, until then characterized by negative properties: invisibility by ordinary microscopic methods, failure to be retained by filters impervious to well-known bacteria, and the inability to propagate themselves in the absence of susceptible cells. From then on, viruses became visible by electron microscopy as well as X-ray crystallography; ultracentrifuges and electrophoresis enabled the purification of ultrafiltrable virus particles; and viruses could be propagated in fertile chicken embryos and on some cultured cell lines. Symposia organized around the end of the 1930s give evidence of the great interest of the Dutch scientific community in nascent virology. Two years after the end of World War II, the symposium organized by the Dutch biochemistry society was once more exemplary for the interdisciplinary approach advocated in virus research. Four of the speakers were biochemists, two were veterinarians (one of them was working in a medical setting), and the last one was a plant virologist.

This period also witnessed the transition in the use of the term 'virus' from a generic label in the nineteenth century and before as causative agent of any infectious disease, to a separate category of infectious disease agents with specific distinguishing properties of their own. Because these agents were invisible, they could not be characterized until development of the aforementioned special instruments and methods to visualize and analyse them. Thus, we see the first tentative steps of an entry of new biological entities into the worlds of biophysics and biochemistry; initiating an interdisciplinary approach that would become so successful after World War II that it would eventually lead to the molecular biology 'revolution' of the second half of the twentieth century.

Returning to specific viral diseases for which public health measures were heartedly discussed over the nineteenth century, a further look was taken at their general epidemiology during the first half of the twentieth century. Answering a questionnaire on the events associated with the 1889-1890 influenza epidemic, only one respondent declared that he had examined sputum for the presence of bacteria. At the time of the Spanish influenza pandemic of 1918-1920, Dutch scientists were but focused on finding a bacterial agent causing influenza. Some of them suspected a virus as causative agent, but to the best of our knowledge, no further investigations were performed in that direction. In contrast, in the United Kingdom, the Medical Research Council announced in 1922 a policy to encourage research on viruses (Thomson, 1987). In 1933, at the then recently founded Institute for Preventive Hygiene in Leiden, G. Elkeles was invited to perform extensive experiments using human influenza strains. Elkeles obtained the viruses from Smith, Andrewes and Laidlaw from the National Institute for Medical Research, London – earlier that year they had isolated the influenza virus for the first time in ferrets. In his search for other susceptible laboratory animals, Elkeles discovered that human influenza strains can also be transmitted to the piglet, but he warned that they resist with great strength, ferocity and deafening screams and he advocated mild anaesthesia during instillation of virus-containing material. Soon after these experiments, Elkeles left for Argentina in fear of the political developments in Germany. The institute maintained this research line and at the end of the 1930s funded influenza research that was conducted at the University of Groningen by the internist Mulder and the biologist Bijlmer.

It is outside the scope of this book to analyse why non-Dutch scientists such as Elkeles (1934) as well as Landsteiner (1919-1924), and D'Herelle (1922-1924) moved to the Netherlands but did not remain to stay in the Netherlands. The very fact that they came to the Netherlands to spend a part of their careers indicates the international connections Dutch scientists had in those days. Concerning Elkeles, and possibly also Landsteiner, we could think of their sojourns in the Netherlands as being comparable to those of German Jewish writers who came to the Netherlands in the 1930s and published with Querido Verlag N.V. in Amsterdam, where they had the opportunity to issue their works in the German language. This is the so-called *Exilliteratur* (Exile literature) by writers who were not able to work as writers in Nazi Germany and later in Austria.

Regarding the prevention or treatment of rabies and smallpox, there were no new or important developments in the Netherlands to report over the first half of the twentieth century. But modifications of the original methods for the production of rabies vaccine were introduced among others in the Dutch East Indies. With regards to smallpox, prevention research on post-vaccination encephalitis was initiated by J.P. Bijl at the Laboratory for Preventive Medicine in Leiden, who was suggesting from the beginning of the 1930s to centralize the production of cowpox vaccine. The number of Parcs Vaccinogènes was already diminished from thirteen to three locations, but remained rather inefficient. The decision to centralize the production at RIV was made in 1938 and finally executed in 1955. It might be questioned whether this was only a sign of the slow-moving wheels of bureaucracy, or something else.

Concerning measles, the practice of seroprophylaxis for the prevention of this disease was introduced rather soon in the Netherlands. In the absence of a vaccine, this method was applied for the prevention of measles among contacts; it was employed for the first time in 1922. Convalescent measles serum has the property of preventing infection, if injected in the incubation period (within 5-6 days of exposure to infection), while it results in attenuation of the disease, if injected between 6-9 days after exposure. The National Institute of Public Health (RIV) had an elaborate scheme for collection, storage, and supply of the sera. General practitioners bled donors selected among their own patients. RIV prepared the serum and issued the serum to practitioners and hospitals. This was a good example of cooperation between local practitioners and a public health corporation. Rubella convalescent gammaglobuline for the prevention of congenital rubella syndrome was first used in the Netherlands in 1947 (Kamerbeek et al., 1947; Kamerbeek, 1953; Van Gilse and Hildernisse, 1947).

Remarkably, medical virus research in the Netherlands was performed at the institutes for tropical hygiene in Amsterdam and Leiden, on yellow fever and bacteriophagy, respectively, over the first half of the twentieth century, and at the laboratory of the Netherlands Institute for Preventive Medicine in Leiden, on influenza after 1930. Although the State Veterinary Research Institute was not focused on medical virology, the work and ideas of H.S. Frenkel and L.W. Janssen also influenced and contributed indirectly to medical virology since the end of the 1930s. The research of Janssen is an example of the biochemical approach to viruses, made possible through technical advances in electrophoresis, ultracentrifugation, crystallography, and electron microscopy in the 1930s. At the same time, Janssen himself is an example of a scientist who chose the right route to climb the mountain but encountered obstacles halfway through, preventing him from ever reaching the summit.

The advances over the latter half of the twentieth century can be divided according to progress in biological techniques, such as cell culture, on the one hand, and the rise of biophysical and biochemical methods, on the other. The driving force behind the first wave was the discovery of the cell culture by Enders, Robbins and Weller in 1948; this technique was reached its height from 1950 to 1965. In 1948, a mere 20 human viruses had been recognized of which only nine were established in the laboratory. In only one decade, by 1958, this number had tripled; about 70 additional human viruses had been established and studied in the laboratory. To the best of our knowledge, over the cell culture era, isolations of hitherto unknown viruses were not described in the Netherlands besides the isolation in suckling mice of several arboviruses achieved by Metselaar during his relatively short stay in Suriname in 1962. As far as we could investigate, cell culture was first introduced in Dutch research laboratories by the beginning of the 1950s and later at few diagnostic laboratories. In this way, the cell culture technique provided an important impetus to laboratory diagnosis of virus infection. This method also opened the way to the production of polio vaccine and the large-scale preparation of viral antigens for serological tests, which revolutionized the field of medical virology. Henceforth, a much smaller number of monkeys were then needed for the production of this particular vaccine.

Severe poliomyelitis epidemics occurred in the course of the 1950s in the Netherlands (1952 and 1956). These epidemics triggered the government to advocate mass vaccination. Initially, the vaccine was purchased abroad, first in the US and following the Cutter incident, in Belgium; but by the decision of the government in 1957, RIV was to produce the vaccine itself. Vaccine production thus was not conceded to a commercial company. Although there were two competing schools advocating for the attenuated Sabin vaccine (OPV) that could be administered orally or for the inactivated Salk vaccine (IPV), administered intramuscularly, respectively, the choice was made for the latter. This decision was in line with the already existing production of inactivated diphtheria-tetanus-pertussis (DTP) vaccine. A new combined DTP-polio vaccine had to be formulated so that the combined vaccine could be incorporated without problems in the existing immunization scheme. In hindsight, it might be said that in the Netherlands, polio vaccination using the inactivated Salk vaccine took place rapidly and was successful. Explanations that can be put forward are: a well-functioning health service organization, the national production of the vaccine, and the drive of the head of the state production facility, H. Cohen, and of the head of the RIV Laboratory for Virology, R. Gispen, to combine the inactivated polio vaccine with the already developed diphtheria-pertussis-tetanus vaccine. It must be noted that together with the Netherlands, only the Nordic countries (Denmark, Finland, Iceland, Norway, and Sweden) chose the IPV over the OPV, and in all these countries the immunization schemes were immediately successful (Böttiger, 1993).

The next era, starting in the 1960s and ongoing until the 1980s, was marked by the rise of visualization and immunological techniques. Electron microscopy using the technique of negative staining as described by Brenner and Horne in 1959 made important contributions to knowledge of uncultivable viruses. The electron microscope developed by J.B. le Poole during World War II was subsequently produced by a national company, becoming a commercial success. Nevertheless, this instrument was rarely employed at Dutch clinical virological laboratories. According to several experts interviewed for this book, the main objections were financial reasons and the lack of specifically trained technicians (G. van Doornum, personal communication, 2019). By contrast, when immunofluorescent techniques for the rapid diagnosis of virus infections became available, these were readily applied on clinical specimens as well as on cell culture monolayers.

Introduction of the enzyme immunoassay methodology in the 1970s revolutionized yet once again the serological detection of either virus antigens or specific antibodies against viruses. Since the discovery of Köhler and Millstein in 1975, monoclonal as well as polyclonal antibodies could be used in these tests. An advantage of the monoclonal antibodies is the continuity of supply. The Dutch scientists Van Weemen and Schuurs at the pharmaceutical company Organon contributed greatly to the practical exploitation of the enzyme immunoassay methodology. As R. Lequin wrote (2005): 'Today, fully automated instruments in medical laboratories around the world use the immunoassay principle with an enzyme as the reporter label for routine measurements of innumerable analytes in patient samples.'

The serologic virus diagnostic methods using enzyme immunoassay methodology were applied in diagnostic virological facilities and were well suited for routine laboratories in general hospitals. For instance, the EIA test for the diagnosis of hepatitis B surface antigen that replaced the assays using the format of the radioimmunoassay could be implemented without the disadvantages associated with the use of radioisotopes. As a consequence, staff members of these general bacteriology laboratories felt the need for further training in virology and they were gradually welcomed at the meetings of the Dutch Working Group for Clinical Virology, where they received continuing education.

One of the most significant advances of long-ranging impact that ushered virology in the new era of molecular revolution was the invention of the polymerase chain reaction (PCR) technique. This took place in the beginning of the 1980s, parallel to the emerging AIDS pandemic. We would like to argue that the development of the molecular revolution was a long evolution with pivotal moments rather than a revolution characterized by rapid and radical changes. Indeed, it started with the rising field of biochemistry in the 1930s. The symposia on viruses which were organized by the Netherlands Chemistry Society in 1939 and 1948 reflect the interest in the Netherlands in this subject throughout that period. The deciphering of the structure of

DNA occurred during the 1950s, followed by the discovery of the transfer of information from DNA by messenger RNA to ribosomes for protein production, and later by the discovery of the reverse transcriptase. Medical virology would benefit from all the accompanying insights and techniques. Since 1984, the PCR technique was introduced in research laboratories in the Netherlands. Technological advances (such as automation in closed systems) made it possible for other types of laboratories, such as those in teaching hospitals and, later, in general hospitals, to introduce nucleic acids technology-based assays over the 1990s.

Another advance was the ability of real-time amplification technology developed over the 1990s to quantitatively detect viral agents. This turned out to be a useful tool for the management of HIV, HBV, HCV, EBV, CMV, and HSV infections. Dutch virologists made a significant contribution to the setup of the European external quality control scheme QCMD.

There were also consequences for the application of the cell culture technique. Within fifteen years after the introduction of the PCR technology, virus isolation by cell culture lost ground in daily diagnostics practice, because the automated nucleic acid amplification instruments provided ample opportunity for virus diagnostics laboratories to employ these new techniques. In this respect, Dutch virologists contributed to the interpretation and clinical significance of the information obtained with these new assays on the presence of viruses in cerebrospinal fluid, respiratory, faecal, or urine specimens.

The clear demarcation of virology into a separate discipline in the 1950s had consequences for the organization of its practitioners, namely the virologists. The growing subset of virology-oriented members of the Netherlands Society for Microbiology, recognized for organizing meetings that included virologist from various backgrounds, began to convene so-called 'Virology Day'. A letter dated 18 March 1968 undersigned by J.D. Verlinde from Leiden to the council of the Netherlands Society of Microbiology (NVvM) spelled out a plan to include members of other scientific societies. In the planning of the virology meetings, they would take into account the planning of the general meeting of the society to avoid organizational conflicts. Besides Verlinde, a veterinarian working in a medical setting, the other three organizers were medical virologists. Finally, in 1977, the structure of the NVvM was officially changed to include all upcoming specializations in microbiology. Since that time, the society has had five sections: technical microbiology, food microbiology, virology, medical microbiology, and molecular microbiology, including ecology and genetics. Each section committee organized the planning and programme of its own sections and meetings. The first members of the virology committee's council comprised representatives of veterinary, molecular, medical, and plant virology. It must be noted that the planning of the virology meetings was carried out since 1992 mainly by two staff members of the Laboratory for Virology of the Veterinary Faculty in Utrecht. The combination with the presentation of the Beijerinck Awards made the meetings, now named the Dutch Annual Virology Symposium, very successful. These meetings provide excellent opportunities for researchers to keep abreast of the developments in areas that they are not involved in on a daily basis.

Another more clinical virology- and epidemiology-focused working group had been established by M.F. Polak, epidemiologist at RIV, in 1964. He organized monthly meetings gathering virologists of RIV and virologists associated with laboratories where clinical or epidemiological research was carried out. Their meetings were part epidemiological, part clinical, part technical. Again, here appear the same names of the virologists who took the initiative of the Virology Days (Verlinde, Dekking, and Van der Veen), besides the staff members of the RIV Laboratory for Virology. The group was later expanded with virologists of the Regional Public Health Laboratory in Rotterdam, and representatives from the Medical Microbiology Laboratory of the University of Groningen and the Veterinary Faculty in Utrecht. At the end of the 1970s, these closed meetings were widened with representatives from general hospital bacteriology laboratories where virology tests were performed. This working group focused on diagnostic virology and epidemiology and worked under the wing of the Netherlands Society of Medical Microbiology.

External quality control schemes and laboratory accreditation were developed since the 1980s and 1990s, respectively. Molecular biologists appeared around 1990 in virus diagnostics laboratories. With the foresight that molecular biology would also be introduced in the fields of bacteriology and parasitology, the Working Group for Molecular Diagnostics of Infectious diseases was established in 1997, mainly by molecular biologists from the Dutch Working Group for Clinical Virology.

This pattern of distinct organizations of the different branches of medical or clinical virology and experimental virology is also observed yet in a somewhat different way in other European countries and in North America. It is a matter of formation and transformation of scientific networks. Distinctions can be drawn between the technical and the social in scientific practice, between spheres of professional practice and jurisdiction, and so on. For a more general and elaborate reflection, we refer to the papers of De Chadarevian and Kamminga, and Sturdy in De Chadarevian and

Kamminga (eds), *Molecularizing biology and medicine: New practices and alliances, 1910s-1970s* (1998).

Medical virology was served in its early years by the laboratories of tropical medicine in Amsterdam and Leiden and by the laboratory of the Institute for Preventive Hygiene in Leiden. Medical virology made a start at the laboratory of the Medical Faculty in Utrecht, but appeared to come to an end following the sudden death of the head of the laboratory in 1938. Soon after World War II, the picture changed, although the number of tests that could be offered remained rather limited by 1953. Clinical virology was then mainly practised in three laboratories; two public health laboratories, and one academic research laboratory: RIV (Utrecht), IPG (Leiden), and the Laboratory for Hygiene (Amsterdam), respectively. The limitations in the number of available tests were an international phenomenon, although according to the famous pioneer in diagnostic virology, J.E. Smadel, in those days, the range of serologic tests for viral and rickettsial diseases could be satisfactory, provided that the diagnostic antigens were made generally available. In his opinion, complement fixation assays and agglutination tests could be performed in any hospital laboratory in which Wassermann tests and bacterial agglutination tests were done (1948). However, in the Netherlands and elsewhere, this development did not occur. In the Netherlands, by the 1960s, a great part of diagnostic virology was performed by the RIV Laboratory for Virology for the general hospitals. When, in 1958, RIV moved from Utrecht to nearby Bilthoven, it continued performing virological diagnostic services for the Academic Hospital in Utrecht and other hospitals in the country. In this respect, the situation was similar to that in England and Wales where most virological investigations were carried out by the Public Health Service laboratories.

The number of research and diagnostic laboratories increased from the 1950s onwards. First, besides the existing four medical faculties, two new medical faculties were established at the Free University in Amsterdam (1950) and Radboud University in Nijmegen (1951). Second, in 1966, a seventh medical faculty was established in Rotterdam and in 1974 the eighth medical faculty was inaugurated in Maastricht, in the south of the Netherlands. Masurel moved in 1969 from Leiden to Rotterdam, where he was appointed in 1971 professor of virology. The Department of Virology in Rotterdam developed most fruitfully over the last decade of the twentieth century since the appointment of Osterhaus as successor to Masurel in 1993 and thanks to recruiting staff who became pivotal in the expansion of the virology research laboratory. The influenza laboratory of the Department of Internal Medicine in Leiden closed operations towards the end of the 1960s, unable to survive the double blows of Mulder's sudden death in 1965 and Masurel's departure to the new medical faculty in Rotterdam. Verlinde's laboratory at the IPG in Leiden became part of the Medical Faculty in 1960 and performed clinical virology diagnostics for the Academic Hospital. Meanwhile, the head of the Laboratory for Medical Microbiology of the University of Groningen, appointed in 1970, established a virus diagnostic laboratory located at the Municipal Public Health Laboratory.

The AIDS pandemic quickly marshalled epidemiological, clinical and biomedical research in the Netherlands. It is not surprising that Dutch HIV research was centred in Amsterdam, where a large community of men who have sex with men (MSM) live. The prospective Amsterdam Cohort Studies (ACS) on HIV infection and AIDS started in 1984. The results of the ACS contributed considerably to insights into the epidemiology, viral and host factors during infection, as well as antiretroviral therapy. The research practised within the ACS was not just following trends from abroad – it set the tone internationally. The power of the ACS approach was also the value brought by all the samples and data collected and stored from the beginning of the study onwards, which could be used to be tested if new insights or assays came up.

The HIV research that was performed at the Special Department of Immunobiology at the National Institute for Public Health and the Environment (since 1984 RIVM instead of RIV) moved, together with the other work groups of Osterhaus's Special Department, to Erasmus MC in Rotterdam in 1992. Over the last decade of the nineteenth century, Osterhaus and his staff members laid the building blocks for successful and diverse research lines on respiratory viruses, emerging viruses, herpes viruses, and a well-equipped virus diagnostic laboratory.

The major change in diagnostic virology services in the Netherlands over the second half of the twentieth century might be inferred from the following numbers. In 1953, virological services were offered by ten laboratories of which only three performed tests for six or more virus infections. Laboratory diagnosis for measles, rubella, chickenpox, common cold, epidemic hepatitis and serum hepatitis was not performed in the Netherlands; external quality control was unknown in the country, although at every laboratory internal procedures implemented many control steps.

At the end of the twentieth century, about 20 laboratories provided diagnostic facilities for virology, executing a full range of diagnostic procedures, including cell culture or nucleic acid amplification techniques, serology, and rapid diagnostic test for detection of a variety of respiratory viruses. All laboratories participated in external quality control schemes and provided weekly epidemiological information to the public health centre at RIVM. Furthermore, reference services for the laboratory diagnosis of emerging diseases and influenza viruses were present at the Erasmus MC in Rotterdam and at RIVM in Bilthoven. In the great majority of the diagnostic laboratories, one consultant clinical virologist and a staff member molecular biologist were employed. In the virology centres of the university laboratories and reference laboratories, at least two posts of consultant clinical virologists and several posts for scientists with appropriate expertise were filled.

This picture differs from that in the UK, where the UK Clinical Virology Network was established by a series of 20 laboratories in 2001 to co-ordinate the activities of the nation's clinical virology services. Their aim was to provide best practice to all parts of the UK by sharing laboratory protocols and epidemiological information using a dedicated website. However, one of the main drivers was poor representation of clinical virology across the country at the time with only around 25 clinical consultants in post (C. Aitkin and P. Griffiths, personal communication, 2018; Griffiths, 2002). The provision of virology advice fell largely to consultant medical microbiologists, few of whom had received specialist training in virology (Cartwright, 2001; Zuckerman et al., 2001). A cry of distress was expressed to the authorities and the Parliament. This illustrates well the need to maintain sufficient training posts in clinical virology and biomedical science.

It might be of interest to review the developments of medical virology in the former Dutch colonies in the East and West Indies when Indonesia, Suriname and the Dutch Antilles were units of the Dutch colonial empire. We could not escape the impression that the Netherlands authorities paid more attention to the East Indies than to the West Indies. It appeared to us to be apposite to investigate general public health measures, epidemiology or immunization program for some specific diseases as smallpox, rabies, yellow fever and other arboviruses.

A general picture was that before the 1890s, colonial medicine was predominantly military and aimed at securing the health of Europeans (Worboys, 1989). It may seem surprising that after the introduction of vaccination in 1804, not only Europeans, but also Javanese and slaves were vaccinated. However, the household slaves lived in close contact with their master's families. Some of the Javanese belonged to high-ranking members of the Javanese aristocracy, but others were ordinary people who were vaccinated in order to transport the vaccine fluid in the vesicles on their body to other places. During the last decades of the nineteenth century, there were significant changes and the government in the Netherlands started to accept their ethical responsibility for the health of the inhabitants of the colonies.

When the political independence of Indonesia was declared by Sukarno in 1945 and officially recognized by the Netherlands in 1949, Dutch medical doctors specialized in tropical medicine started gradually to relocate their work to Africa. In the beginning of the 1960s, O. Kranendonk, head of the Department Public Health and Microbiology of the Institute for Tropical Hygiene of the Royal Tropical Institute was charged to reconnoitre an appropriate country in Africa for a research centre. In March 1966, a Medical Research Centre was inaugurated in Kenya by President Mzee Jomo Kenyatta. Therefore, some projects and activities of Dutch virologists, epidemiologist or clinicians in Africa are also described in this book.

The search for the origin of cancer followed several paths, with the molecurization of cancer aetiology emerging in different places at different times. At the NKI-AVL, a line of research stemmed from genetic research on mouse mammary cancer in the 1930s. The results showed that besides a genetic factor, an extrachromosomal factor also played a role. Later, at the end of the 1940s, this extrachomosomal factor was recognized as the mouse mammary tumour virus (MMTV). The confirmation of the presence of tumour viruses relied on ultracentrifugation and electron microscopy (Cardiff and Kenney, 2007, 2011).

Then, over the 1960s, Bentvelzen and Daams hypothesized, after consultation of the 1965 Nobel Prize winners F. Jacob and A.M. Lwoff, that a double-stranded DNA copy of the single stranded MMTV RNA could be integrated in chromosomal mouse DNA. Evidence of this hypothesis was given by R. Nusse and H. Varmus in 1982. The pioneering work of Nusse was an impetus for a new field of research, because they demonstrated that the integration locus *int-1* was homologous with the wingless gene in fruit flies. The *int-1* gene was renamed *Wnt-1*. Years later, in 2012, Nusse and Varmus noted with satisfaction the growth of the *Wnt* field from the finding of a single cancer gene in a mouse model to a rich system branching out to fields as diverse as embryogenesis, growth of organs, regeneration of injured organs, and maintenance of stem cells. Ironically, a human mammary tumour virus has never been found, but genetic factors were demonstrated indeed.

Dutch cancer researchers are an outstanding lot. The work of Bentvelzen and Nusse demonstrated that the origin of a greater part of tumours is rooted in DNA changes. They had also an impact on similar research elsewhere in the Netherlands, for example, at the groups of Bloemendal, Bloemers and Berns in Nijmegen.

Another line of research was started in Leiden by Van der Eb on transformation caused by adenoviruses, as well as in Amsterdam by Van der Noordaa, who used SV 40 as a model. It was on the initiative of Mühlbock

Figure 29   Roel Nusse and Harold Varmus as enthusiastic cyclists

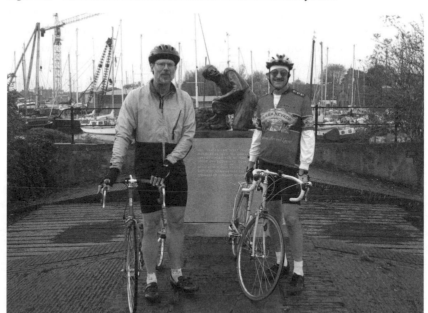

The photo was taken at the statue of Hans Brinkers at the Woerdersluis in Spaarndam, The Netherlands. Reproduction courtesy R. Nusse

at the NKI-AVL in Amsterdam that the Working Group on Persistent Virus Infections and Oncogenesis was established and initially funded by the Queen Wilhelmina Fund, a charitable institution that also financed a great part of the biochemical research of the NKI-AVL. Within the working group, researchers consulted on projects to be submitted and actually decided on the allocation themselves. This practice differed from the American National Cancer Institute (NCI) cancer virus program that was based on public debates in the manner of congressional hearings. As Gaudillière describes it, at the end of the 1960s, 'the NCI was spending over \$40 million per year on tumor virus studies' (1998, p. 150). The virus program was managed by a standard system of contract partners, half of them with profit-making companies.

An important aspect of the development and production of virus vaccines in the Netherlands was the 1957 decision of the government to produce vaccines within the public sector. Although we had to draw a line and wanted to end the book story at the turn of the twentieth century, we deliberately crossed over into the twenty-first century in order to describe the sale of the public vaccine-production facilities to a private corporation, in 2012 (the Serum Institute of India Ltd). After completing the narrative of our book, our attention was brought Stuart Blume's (2017) article 'The erosion of public sector vaccine production: The case of the Netherlands'. For a complete overview of the rise and fall of public sector virus and bacterial vaccines production, we refer to this article. We much agree with his conclusion that in the 1960s and 1970s the Dutch Institute of Public Health was a significant and internationally respected participant in vaccine development and production. An ideological (and, as a consequence, also a political) shift took place – the growing influence of free-market economics – that provided conceptual support for the giant corporations' attempts to capture global markets (Blume, 2017, p. 167). After the sale of the production part of the vaccine division to the Serum Institute of India in 2012, the last part of the former Vaccine Division of RIVM remained. This was the Institute for Translational Vaccinology (Intravacc), which accommodated vaccinology research and development. According to J.T. Hendriks, an expert in vaccinology and public health, Intravacc's mission included 'the fostering of global health through international partnerships in innovative vaccinology. Projected activities will include training courses and curricula, capitalizing on various currently established platform technologies and the legacy of previous "producer-producer" collaborations between the RIVM and emerging manufacturers over the past 40 years' (2017, p. 70). We doubt whether the wish he expressed in his thesis will be fulfilled. It is to be hoped that the conditions set by the government for the pending privatization of Intravacc, originally planned for 2017, will ensure at least the partial continuation of global public good creation from Bilthoven as has been done so successfully in the past decades (Hendriks, 2017, p. 156). However, very recently, on 1 February 2019, the website of Intravacc reads the following: 'Intravacc announced today the establishment of Intravacc B.V. This is an important step in the anticipated privatization of Intravacc and the sale of its activities to private partners.'[121]

The increase in the number of antivaccination campaigns over the last decade of the twentieth century (involving individuals beyond the known group of refusers on religious grounds) is a worrying trend. As a consequence, there will be more clusters or an increase in the distribution of unvaccinated children and adults over the country, a development that will require new and different approaches to ensure public health.

Nothing is more difficult than predicting the future. In fact, matters such as the emergence of new epidemic infectious diseases as well as developments in technology in the broad sense of the word are stimuli for new

---

121 https://www.intravacc.nl/, latest access February 2019.

developments. We have just to point out the tests building on next-generation sequencing and sequence analysis. At important junctures, promotion by government agencies or private funds may direct research strategies and associations representing patients or vaccination hesitancy groups may support or counter the implementation of advances and novel opportunities. Above all, what remains is that personal interest and perseverance of scientists are of fundamental importance.

To conclude our book, twentieth-century Dutch medical virology has witnessed the conversion of a hardly noticeable group of interested bacteriologists into a flourishing scientific community. The twenty-first century has already brought and will surely continue to bring new challenges and exciting developments in the never-ending fight against viral diseases.

List of institutes and laboratories

Amsterdam
Amsterdam Cohort Studies on HIV infection and AIDS
Central Laboratory of the Netherlands Red Cross Blood Transfusion Service
(CLB, since 1998 Sanquin), Laboratory of Viro-Immunology
Free University Amsterdam: Laboratory of Medical Microbiology, Department of Medical Virology
Free University in Amsterdam, VUmc, Department of Pathology
Laboratory of the Department for Tropical Hygiene of the Colonial Institute
Municipal Health Service of Amsterdam, Regional Public Health Laboratory
National Antiviral Therapy Evaluation Centre (NATEC), AMC
Nederlands Kanker Instituut-Antoni van Leeuwenhoek Ziekenhuis
(NKI-AVL)
Red Cross Blood Bank of Amsterdam
State Veterinary Research Institute (SVRI)
University of Amsterdam AMC, Department of Retrovirology
University of Amsterdam AMC, Department of Virology
University of Amsterdam, Laboratory for Hygiene

Bilthoven
RIV, National Institute of Public Health, relocated from Utrecht to Bilthoven
through 1953-1965
RIV, Central vaccinia production
RIV, Laboratory for serum and vaccine control
RIV, Laboratory for serum and vaccine production
RIV, Laboratory for viral diseases and rickettsial infections
RIVM, Laboratory for inactivated virus vaccines
RIVM, Laboratory for live virus vaccines
RIVM, Laboratory for Virology
RIVM, National Institute for Public Health and the Environment, since 1984
RIVM, Special Department for Immunobiology
RIVM, Unit control of virus vaccines

Boxtel
Organon Teknika

Delft
Delft Diagnostic Laboratories (DDL) since 1994, moved to Rijswijk in 2003
Diagnostic Centre SSDZ Department for Molecular Biology

Netherlands Yeast and Spirit Works
Polytechnical School, Laboratory for Microbiology
Technical University Delft since 1986

Groningen
Municipal Health Service of Groningen: Regional Public Health Laboratory
Regional Public Health Laboratory Groningen
State University of Groningen, Laboratory for Hygiene
State University of Groningen, Laboratory of Molecular Virology
UMC Groningen, Laboratory of Clinical Virology
UMC Groningen, Laboratory of Medical Microbiology

Leiden
Academic Hospital Leiden, Central Clinical Virology Laboratory
Academic Hospital Leiden, Respiratory Viruses Laboratory of the Clinic of
    Internal Medicine
Crucell
Laboratory for Tropical Hygiene
Leiden University Laboratory of Bacteriology
Leiden University Medical Centre, Department of Medical Microbiology
Netherlands Institute for Preventive Medicine, Department of Bacteriology
    and Experimental Pathology

Lelystad
Central Veterinary Institute: Laboratory for Molecular Recognition
Institute for Animal Science and Health, Department of Mammalian Virology
Pepscan

Maastricht
Maastricht University Medical Centre, Department of Medical Microbiology

Nijmegen
Radboud University, Laboratory for Biochemistry, Department of
    Biochemistry
Radboud University Medical Center, Department of Medical Microbiology

Rijswijk
Medical-Biological Laboratory (Medisch-Biologisch Laboratorium) of TNO-RVO
Radiobiological Institute TNO (RBI)
TNO Primatencentrum, since 1994 Biomedical Primate Research Centre (BPRC)

Rotterdam

Academisch Ziekenhuis Rotterdam, Laboratory of Virology

Daniel den Hoed Clinic, merged with Academisch Ziekenhuis Rotterdam in 1993

Dijkzigt Ziekenhuis, Laboratory of Medical Microbiology

Erasmus MC, Department of Virology

Regional Public Health Laboratory of the Municipal Health Service of Rotterdam

State Veterinary Research in Rotterdam

Viroclinics

Tilburg

Laboratory for Bacteriology, Immunology and Virology and Regional Public Health Laboratory (since 1969)

Regional Laboratory for Public Health Tilburg, Laboratory for Medical Microbiology and Immunology (since 2001)

St Elisabeth Hospital Bacteriology and Serology Laboratory (1951)

Utrecht

Central Laboratory of the National Institute of Public Health (RIV) Utrecht

Laboratory of Physiological Chemistry, Utrecht University

Rijks Instituut voor de Volksgezondheid (RIV), relocated from Utrecht to Bilthoven through 1953-1965

Stads- en Academisch Ziekenhuis Utrecht (SAZU)

State University of Utrecht, Laboratory for Hygiene

State University of Utrecht, Laboratory for Microbiology

UMC Utrecht, Laboratory for Medical Microbiology

University of Utrecht, Veterinary Faculty: Laboratory for Virology

Veterinary School (Rijks-Veeartsenij School)

Wageningen

Agricultural Experimental Station in Wageningen

Agricultural School

Wageningen University and Research, Laboratory for Virology

Weesp

Philips Duphar

References

Aaij C, Borst P. 1972. The gel electrophoresis of DNA. Biochim Biophys Acta 269:192-200.

Aalberse PJM. 1918-1919. Aanhangsel II van het Verslag van de Handelingen der Tweede Kamer 1918-1919. Vel 30, pp. 61-62.

Ackerknecht EH. 2009. Anticontagionism between 1821 and 1867. The Fielding H. Garrison Lecture. Int J Epidemiol 38:7-21.

ACS. 1992. Amsterdam Cohort Studies on HIV infection and AIDS in homosexual men: A summary of the results (1984-1992). Amsterdam, Amsterdam University Press.

ACS. 1996. Amsterdam Cohort Studies on HIV infection and AIDS: A summary of the results (1984-1995). Amsterdam, Amsterdam Cohort Studies.

ACS. 2001. Amsterdam Cohort Studies on HIV infection and AIDS: A summary of the results (1996-2000). Amsterdam, Amsterdam Cohort Studies.

ACS. 2009. Amsterdam Cohort Studies on HIV infection and AIDS: A summary of the results (2001-2009). Amsterdam, Amsterdam Cohort Studies.

Adhin JH. 1960. In memoriam Prof. Dr W.A. Collier. New West Indian Guide/Nieuwe West-Indische Gids 41:1-3.

Alberda AT, Van Os HC, Schalm SW, Rothbarth PhH, Heijtink RA, Zeilmaker GH. 1989. Hepatitis B-virusinfectie bij vrouwen behandeld met in vitro-fertilisatie. Ned Tijdschr Geneeskd 133:20-25.

Aldershoff H, Pot AW. 1929. Onderzoekingen naar den aard van het virus van hier te lande voorgekomen 'alastrim'-gevallen. Ned Tijdschr Geneeskd 73(II):4232-4238.

Ali Cohen L. 1864a. De voornaamste uitkomsten van de waarnemingen betreffende de hondsdolheid, in Rijnland gedurende 1861 en 1862 gedaan. Ned Tijdschr Geneeskd 8:406-407.

Ali Cohen L. 1864b. Over hondsdolheid uit het oogpunt der gezondheidsleer en der gezondheidspolitie. Ned Tijdschr Geneeskd 8:485-486.

Ali Cohen L. 1889. Over Pasteur's inenting tegen de hondsdolheid. Ned Tijdschr Geneeskd 33:369-372.

Allard HA. 1914. Review of investigations of the mosaic disease of tobacco, together with a bibliography of the more important contributions. Bulletin of the Torrey Botanical Club 41:435-458.

Allicock OM, Lemey P, Tatem AJ, Pybus OG, Bennett SN, Mueller BA, Suchard MA, Foster JE, Rambaut A, Carrington CV. 2012. Phylogeography and population dynamics of dengue viruses in the Americas. Mol Biol Evol 92:1533-1543. DOI: 10.1093/molbev/msr320.

American Philosophical Society. 1843. Transactions of the Historical and Literary Committee of the American Philosophical Society, Volume III, part I. List of members. Carey and Hart, Philadelphia, PA.

Anderson MJ, May RM. 1992. Infectious diseases of humans: Dynamics and control. Oxford University Press, Oxford.

Andrewes C. 1935. Christmas fairy-story for oncologists' sent by Christopher Andrewes with a 1935 letter to Peyton Rous.

Andriesse CD. 2008. Dutch messengers: A history of science and science publishing 1930-1980. Brill, Leiden.

Anon. 1948. Vereeniging Instituut voor Tropische Geneeskunde Rotterdam-Leiden. Acta Leidensia, edita cura et sumptibus. Scholae Medicinae Tropicae 19:1-13.

Archief Nederlandse Kankerbestrijding/Koningin Wilhelmina Fonds, Noord-Hollands Archief, Haarlem: 426, 701.

Arends A, Hadders HN, Van Rijssel, TG. 1961. In memoriam Prof. J.J.Th. Vos. Ned Tijdschr Geneeskd 105:513-515.

Arita, I. 1988. Smallpox vaccine and vaccination in the intensified smallpox eradication programme, pp. 539-592. *In* F Fenner, DA Henderson, I Arita, Z Ježek, ID Ladnyi (eds) Smallpox and its eradication. World Health Organization, Geneva.

Avrameas S. 1969. Coupling of enzymes to proteins with glutaraldehyde: Use of conjugates for the detection of antigens and antibodies. Immunochemistry 104:93-99.

Axelsson P. 2009. Do no teat those apples; They've been on the ground! Polio epidemics and preventive meausures, Sweden 1880s-1940s. Asclepio: Revista de Historia de la Medicina y de la Ciencia LXI:23-38.

Bakker S, Taal B, Valdés Olmos R (eds). 2015. Het Antoni van Leeuwenhoek Toen en Nu. Een eeuw visuele momenten toegelicht. Het Nederlands Kanker instituut-Antoni van Leeuwenhoek Ziekenhuis, Amsterdam.

Ballot AM. 1871. Overzicht van de epidemieën van pokken, roodvonk en mazelen van 1778-1811 en van 1815-1870. Ned Tijdschr Geneeskd 15(I):309-314.

Balter M. 1998. The Netherlands. Access to patients is key to success of Dutch quartet. Science 280(5371):1859. DOI: 10.1126/science.280.5371.1859.

Banatvala, JE, Kennedy EA, Best JM. 1967. Clinical virology: A year's experience. Br Med J 3:609-612.

Bänffer JRJ, Kooy P, Schaap GJP, Schönfeld JK. 1979. In memoriam H. Esseveld. Ned Tijdschr Geneeskd 123:25.

Barnard JE, Elford WJ. 1931. The causative organisms in infectious ectromelia. Proc Roy Soc B109:360-375.

Barnes K. 2016. Milestone 4. Making antibodies work. Nature S8(2). DOI: 10.1038/ni.3603.

Baron W. 2006. Het belang en de welvaart van alle ingezetenen: Gezondheidszorg in de stad Groningen, 1800-1870. Van Gorcum, Assen.

Barré-Sinoussi F, Chermann JC, Rey F, Nugeyre MT, Chamaret S, Gruest J, Dauguet C, Axler-Blin C, Vézinet-Brun F, Rouzioux C, Rozenbaum W, Montagnier L. 1983. Isolation of a T-lymphotropic retrovirus from a patient at risk for acquired immune deficiency syndrome (AIDS). Science 220(4599):868-871.

Barteling SJ, Vreeswijk J. 1991. Developments in foot-and-mouth disease vaccines. Vaccine 9:75-88.

Baumann ED. 1924. Over de hondsdolheid in de oudheid. Ned Tijdschr Geneeskd 68:458-481.

Bawden FC, Pirie NW. 1937. The isolation of and some properties of liquid crystalline substances from solanaceous plants infected with three strains of tobacco mosaic virus. Proc R Soc London, Ser B Biol 123:274-320.

Bazin H. 1999. The eradication of smallpox: Edward Jenner and the first and only eradication of human infectious disease. Academic Press, San Diego, CA.

Beale N, Beale E. 2005. Evidence based medicine in the eighteenth century: The Ingen Housz-Jenner correspondence revisited. Med Hist 49:79-98.

Beijerinck MW. 1898a. Over een contagium vivum fluidum als oorzaak van de vlekziekte der tabaksbladen. Versl. Gewone Vergad. Wis- en Natuurk Afdeling. Kon Akad v Wet Amsterdam, Deel VII:229-235.

Beijerinck MW. 1898b. Ueber ein contagium vivum fluidum als Ursache der Fleck-enkrankheit der Tabaksblätter. Verhandelingen der Kon Akad v Wet Amsterdam 65(2):3-21.

Beijerinck MW. 1899a. Bemerkung zu dem Aufsatz von Herrn Iwanowsky über die Mosaikkrankheit der Tabakspflanze. Centrbl Bakt Parasitenk 5:310-311.

Beijerinck MW. 1899b. On a contagium vivum fluidum causing the spotdisease of the tobacco-leaves, pp. 170-176. Royal Netherlands Academy of Arts and Sciences (KNAW), Proceedings 1, 1898-1899, Amsterdam.

Beijerinck MW. 1899c. Ueber ein contagium vivum fluidum als Ursache der Fleckenkrankheit der Tabaksblätter. Centrbl Bakt Parasitenk 5:27-33.

Beijerinck MW. 1913. De infusies en de ontdekking der bakteriën. Jaarboek der Koninklijke Akademie van Wetenschappen. Amsterdam, pp. 1-28.

Beijerinck MW. 1922. Pasteur en de ultramicrobiologie. Chemisch Weekblad 19:525-527.

Beijerinck MW. 1942/1898. Concerning a contagium vivum fluidum as cause of the spot disease of tobacco leaves. Translated by J Johnson. Phytopathological Classics 7:33-52. Original: Ueber ein contagium vivum fluidum als Ursache der Fleckenkrankheit der Tabaksblätter. Verhandelingen der Koninklyke Akademie van Wetenschappen te Amsterdam 65(2):3-21.

Beijerinck MW. 1961/1899. A contagium vivum fluidum as the cause of the mosaic disease of tobacco leaves. Translated by TD Brock, pp. 153-157. *In* TD Brock (ed. and trans.) Milestones in microbiology, 1546 to 1940. Prentice Hall International, London. Original: 1899.

Belcaid Z, Lamfers MLM, Van Beusechem VW, Hoeben RC. 2014. Changing faces in virology: The Dutch shift from oncogenic to oncolytic viruses. Human gene therapy 25:875-884.

Bemelmans E. 1919. De 'griep' en hare bestrijding. Ned Tijdschr Geneeskd 64:184-187.

Benison S, Rivers T. 1967. Tom Rivers: Reflections on a life in medicine and science. An oral history prepared by S. Benison. MIT Press, Cambridge, MA.

Benjamins HD, Snelleman JF. 1914-1917. Encyclopaedie van Nederlandsch West-Indië. Martinus Nijhoff, Den Haag/E.J. Brill, Leiden.

Bennett AH, Jupnik H, Osterberg H, Richards OW. 1946. Phase microscopy. Trans. Amer. micr. Soc., 65:99-131.

Benot Y. 2013. Denis Diderot. Voyage en Hollande. Introduction and notes by Yves Benot. La Découverte/Poche, Paris.

Bentvelzen PA. 1968. Genetical control of vertical transmission of the Mühlbock mammary tumor virus in the GR-mouse strain. Hollandia Publishing House, Amsterdam.

Bentvelzen P. 1975. Kanttekeningen bij kranteberichten over een leukemia virus. Ned Tijdschr Geneeskd 119:842-843.

Bentvelzen P. 1980. RNA tumour viruses: Interesting interactions with the host genome. *In* F Cleton F, JWIM Simons (eds) Genetic origins of tumor cells: Developments in oncology. Martinus Nijhoff, The Hague.

Bentvelzen P. 1982. Interaction between host and viral genomes in mouse mammary tumors. Ann Rev Genet 16:273-295.

Bentvelzen P, Daams JH. 1969. Hereditary infections with mammary tumor viruses in mice. J Nat Cancer Inst 43:1025-1035.

Bentvelzen P, Timmermans A, Daams JH, Van der Gugten A. 1967. Genetic transmission of Mammary tumor inciting viruses in mice: Possible implications for murine leukemia. *In* Proc. 3rd int. Symp. comp. Leukemia Res. Paris; Bibl. haemat. 31:101-103, Karger, Basel/New York, 1968.

Berkhout B, Bukrinsky M. 2015. Jan van der Noordaa (1934-2015): A virologist *pur sang*. Viruses 7(9):5016-5017. DOI: 10.3390/v7092859.

Bernard C. 1865. Introduction à l'étude de la médecine expérimentale. J.B. Baillière et Fils, Paris.

Betsch C. 2017. Advocating for vaccination in a climate of science denial. Nat Microbiol. 2017 Jun 27;2:17106. doi: 10.1038/nmicrobiol.2017.106.

Beukers H. 1986. Een nieuwe werkplaats in de geneeskunde: De opkomst van laboratoria in de geneeskundige faculteiten. Tdsch. Gnk. Natuurw. Wisk. Techn 9:266-277.

Beukers H. 1989. The development of tropical medicine in Leiden. Acta Leidensia 58(1):3-43.

Beyer WEP, Masurel N. 1983. Influenza-vaccinatie: De baten worden nog steeds onderschat. Ned Tijdschr Geneeskd 127:1979-1980.

Beylon D. 1921/1779. Korte aantekening wegens eene algemeene ziekte doorgaans genaamd Knokkel-koorts. Javasche Boekhandel en Drukkerij, Rijswijk. Original: d'E Compagnies Boek-drukkerij, Egbert Heemen, Batavia, 1780.

Biel SS, Gelderblom HR. 1999. Diagnostic electron microscopy is still a timely and rewarding method. J Clin Virol 13: 105-119.

Biel SS, Madeley D. 2001. Diagnostic virology – the need for electron microscopy: A discussion paper. J Clin Virol 22:1-9.

Bijkerk H, Draaisma FJ, Van der Gugten AC, Van Os M. 1979. De poliomyelitis-epidemie in 1978. Ned Tijdschr Geneeskd 123:1700-1714.

Bijl JP. 1954. Een kwart eeuw Nederlands Instituut voor Praeventieve Geneeskunde. H.E. Stenfert Kroese N.V., Leiden.

Bijlmer L. 1943. Aetiologie der influenza, de isolering van het influenza-virus tijdens de epidemie van 1941 te Groningen. H.E. Stenfert Kroese's Uitgevers-Mij N.V. Leiden.

Bijlsma R. 1982. David de Is. C. Nassy. Author of the 'Essai Historique sur Surinam'. In R Cohen (ed.), The Jewish nation in Surinam: Historical essays. S. Emmering, Amsterdam.

BioPharm. 2011. Johnson & Johnson acquires vaccine developer Crucell, 8 March. http://www.biopharminternational.com/johnson-johnson-acquires-vaccine-developer-crucell.

Bittner JJ. 1936. Some possible effects of nursing on the mammary gland tumor incidence in mice. Science 84:162.

Bittner JJ. 1939. Relation of nursing to the extra-chromosomal theory of breast cancer in mice. Am J Cancer. 1939 Jan 35(1):90-97.

Bittner JJ, Little CC. 1937. The transmission of breast and lung cancer in mice. Journal of Heredity 28(3):117-121, https://doi.org/10.1093/oxfordjournals.jhered.a104326.

Bleck TP, Rupprecht CE. 2005. Rhabdoviruses. In GL Mandell, JE Bennett, R Dolin (eds) Mandell, Douglas, and Bennett's principles and practice of infectious diseases, 6th ed. Elsevier, Churchill Livingstone, Philadelphia, PA.

Bloemers P. 1998. Hans Bloemendal en Sjoerd Bonting. In H Corman (ed.), Nijmeegse Gezichten. Vijfenzeventig jaar Katholieke Universiteit. Uitgeverij KU Nijmegen.

Blume S. 2006. Antivaccination movements and their interpretations. Social Science & Medicine 62:628-642.

Blume S. 2017. The erosion of public sector vaccine production: The case of the Netherlands. *In* C Holmberg, S Blume, P Greenough (eds.), The politics of vaccination: A global history. Manchester University Press, Manchester.

Blume S, Tump J. 2010. Evidence and policymaking: The introduction of MMR vaccine in the Netherlands. Social Science & Medicine 71:1049-1055.

Boerhaave H. 1728. Aphorismi de Cognoscendis et Curandis Morbis, pp. 327-336. (Editio Leydensis quarta auctior). Samuel Luchtmans & Theodoor Haak. Lugduni Batavorum.

Bonne C. 1936. De ontwikkeling der geneeskundige wetenschappen in Nederlandsch-Indië in de periode 1911-1935, pp. 16-44. *In* Feestbundel 1936. Geneesk Tijdschr Ned-Indië. Vereniging tot Bevordering der Geneeskundige Wetenschappen in Nederlands-Indië, Batavia.

Bontius J. 1931. Tropische geneeskunde/On tropical Medicine. Edited by MA van Andel. Opuscula Selecta Neerlandicorum De Arte Medica, no. 10. Geneeskundig tijdschrift voor Geneeskunst, Amsterdam.

Boom R, Sol CJ, Salimans MM, Jansen CL, Wertheim-van Dillen PM, Van der Noordaa J. 1990. Rapid and simple method for purification of nucleic acids. J Clin Microbiol 28:495-503.

Boomgaard P. 1989a. Pokken en pokkenvaccinatie op Java; medische gegevens als bron voor demografische geschiedenis, pp. 115-129. *In* AM Luyendijk-Elshout, GM van Heteren, A de Knecht-van Eekelen, MJD Poulissen (eds) Nederlandse geneeskunde in de Indische Archipel. Rodopi, Amsterdam.

Boomgaard P. 1989b. Smallpox and vaccination on Java, 1780-1860: Medical data as source for demographic history, pp. 119-131. *In* AM Luyendijk-Elshout, GM van Heteren, A de Knecht-van Eekelen, MJD Poulissen (eds) Dutch medicine in the Malay Archipelago, 1816-1942; Articles presented at a symposium held in honor of Prof. Dr D. de Moulin on the occasion of his retirement from the professorship of the History of Medicine at the Catholic University of Nijmegen, 30 September 1989. Rodopi, Amsterdam.

Boomgaard P. 1996. Dutch medicine in Asia 1600-1900. Clio Med 5:42-64.

Boomgaard P. 2003. Smallpox, vaccination, and the Pax Neerlandica, Indonesia, 1550-1930. Bijdragen tot de Taal-, Land- en Volkenkunde 159(4):590-617.

Booss J, August MJ. 2013. To catch a virus. ASM Press, Washington, DC.

Boot LM. 1980. Obituary Otto F.E. Mühlbock 1906-1979. Cancer Research 40:190.

Bordet J. 1922. Concerning the theories of the so-called bacteriophage. Br Med J 2(3216):296.

Bordet J. 1923. The Cameron Prize Lecture on microbic transmissible autolysis. Br Med J 1(3240):175-178.

Bordet J. 1931. Croonian lecture: The theories of the bacteriophage. Proceedings of the Royal Society of London. Series B, containing papers of a biological character 107(752):398-417.

Bornebroek A. 2006. Een heer in een volkspartij. Theodoor Heemskerk (1852-1932), minister-president en minister van justitie. Aksant, Amsterdam.

Borst P. 2004a. Disciplines en wetenschapsbeleid, pp. 148-153. *In* E Homburg, L Palm (eds) De geschiedenis van de scheikunde in Nederland 3. De ontwikkeling van de chemie van 1945 tot het begin van de jaren tachtig. Delft University Press, Delft.

Borst P. 2004b. Het Koningin Wilhelminafonds als financier van biochemisch onderzoek, pp. 146-148. *In* E Homburg, L Palm (eds) De geschiedenis van de scheikunde in Nederland 3. De ontwikkeling van de chemie van 1945 tot het begin van de jaren tachtig. Delft University Press, Delft.

Bos L. 1999. Beijerinck's work on tobacco mosaic virus: Historical context and legacy. Phil Trans R Soc London. Series B: Biological Sciences 354(1383):675-685.

Bos L. 2000. 100 years of virology: From vitalism via molecular biology to genetic engineering. Trends Microbiol 82(8):82-87.

Bos P, Theunissen B (eds). 1995. Beijerinck and the Delft school of microbiology. Delft University Press, Delft.

Bosgra O, Roerink JHG. 1967. Preparation of virus vaccines by means of tissue cultures. Philips Techn Rev 3/4:81.

Böttiger M. 1993. The elimination of polio in the Scandinavian countries. Public Health Rev 21(1-2):27-33.

Böttiger M, Zetterberg B, Salenstedt C-R. 1972. Seroimmunity to poliomyelitis in Sweden after the use of inactivated poliovirus vaccine for 10 years. Bull Wld Hlth Org 46:141-149.

Boycott AE. 1928. The transition from live to dead: The nature of filterable viruses. Proceedings of the Royal Society of Medicine XXII:55-69.

Braat P. 1937. Middelen tegen hondsdolheid. Ned Tijdschr Geneeskd 82:2293-2295.

Brabers J. 2009. Hippocrates op Heyendael. Ontstaan en ontplooiing van de Faculteit der Medische Wetenschappen van de Nijmeegse universiteit, 1951-2001. Valkhof Pers, Nijmegen.

Bradstreet CMP, Pereira MS, Andrews BE. 1964. The development of a national virological diagnostic service. Prog Med Virol 6:149-174.

Bradstreet CMP, Pereira MS, Pollock TM. 1973. The organization of a national virological diagnostic service. Progr Med Virol 16:241-268.

Brandwijk AC, Cohen H, Hekker AC, Hofman B, Van Ramshorst JD, Tasman A, Van Driel CB, Schaapman-Tilma B, De Vries JA. 1961. Een gecombineerd difterie-kinkhoest-tetanus-poliomyelitisvaccin (DKTP) ter immunisatie van de zuigeling. Ned Tijdschr Geneeskd 105:1331-1337.

Brans LM. 1959. Modern methods of preparation and use of smallpox vaccine derived from the calf. Ned Tijdschr Geneeskd 103(10):495-450.

Brenner S, Horne RW. 1959. A negative staining method of high resolution electron microscopy of viruses. Biochim Biophys Acta 34:103-110.

British Medical Journal. 1894. Epidemic influenza in Holland [editorial]. Br Med J 17(March):599-600.

Brock TD. 1988. Robert Koch. A life in Medicine and bacteriology. Science Tech, Madison, WI/Springer, Berlin.

Brown CS, Salimans MM, Noteborn MH, Weiland HT. 1990. Antigenic parvovirus B19 coat proteins VP1 and VP2 produced in large quantities in a baculovirus expression system. Virus Res 15:197-211.

Brown F. 1984. The nature of viruses. *In* G Wilson, AM Miles, MT Parker (eds) Topley and Wilson's Principles of bacteriology, virology and immunity, vol. 4, 7th ed., Edward Arnold, London.

Bruins LH. 1951. Leven en werken van Geert Reinders, de grondlegger van de immunologie. PhD thesis, Groningen.

Buck HM, Koole LH, Van Genderen MHP, Smit L, Geelen JLMC, Jurriaans S, Goudsmit J. 1990. Phosphate-methylated DNA aimed at HIV-1 RNA loops and integrated DNA inhibits viral infectivity. Science 248(4952):208-212.

Buiter H. 2012. Hightech systemen: Elektronenmicroscoop. *In* H Lintsen (ed.), Tachtig jaar TNO. TNO (Delft) en Stichting Historie der Techniek, Eindhoven.

Bull Carroll G. 1925. Bacteriophage. Physiol Revs 5(1):95-111.

Buonaguro FM, Tornesello ML, Buonaguro L. 2015. The XIX century smallpox prevention in Naples and the risk of transmission of human blood-related pathogens. J Transl Med 13:33. DOI 10.1186/s12967-015-0400-9.

Burgmeijer R, Hoppenbrouwers K, Bolscher N. 2007a. Handboek Vaccinaties. Deel A. Theorie en uitvoeringspraktijk. Van Gorcum, Assen.

Burgmeijer R, Hoppenbrouwers K, Bolscher N. 2007b. Handboek Vaccinaties. Deel B. Theorie en uitvoeringspraktijk. Van Gorcum, Assen.

Burnet FM. 1936. The use of the developing egg in virus research. Medical Research Council Special Reports 220.

Burnet FM. 1953a. Virology as an independent science. Med J Aust 40(II):809-813.

Burnet FM. 1953b. Virology as an independent science. Med J Aust 40(II):841-845.

Bush DL. 1961. Epizootic rabies in Surinam. Effectiveness of a mass field immunization program. J Am Vet Assoc 138:363-365.

Bynum WF. 1994. Science and the practice of medicine in the nineteenth century. Cambridge University Press, Cambridge.

Bynum WF. 2008. The history of medicine: A very short introduction. Oxford University Press, Oxford.

Calisher CH, Horzinek MC (eds). 1999. 100 Years of virology. Springer, Wien.

Camper P. 1774. Les avantages de l'inoculation et la meilleure méthode de l'administrer, ouvrage traduit de la dissertation latine, couronnée par l'Académie Royale des Sciences, Inscriptions et Belles Lettres de Toulouse. Veuve J.P. Robert, Toulouse.

Cardiff RD, Kenney N. 2007. Mouse mammary tumor biology: A short history. Adv Cancer Res. 98:53-116. DOI: 10.1016/S0065-230X(06)98003-8.

Cardiff RD, Kenney N. 2011. A compendium of the mouse mammary tumor biologist: From the initial observations in the house mouse to the development of genetically engineered mice. Cold Spring Harb Perspect Biol 3(6). pii: a003111. DOI: 10.1101/cshperspect.a003111.

Carrel A. 1912. Pure cultures of cells. J Exp Med 16(2):165-168.

Cartwright K. 2001. Consultant workload and staffing in medical microbiology and virology. Report of a working group of the Royal College of Pathologists, London.

Casimir HBG. 1983. Het toeval van de werkelijkheid. Een halve eeuw natuurkunde. Meulenhoff Informatief, Amsterdam.

Catrin M. 1891. Les lésions histologiques de la peau dans la rougeole. C R Hebd Séances Acad Sci 112:538.

Catrin M. 1897. Un cas de contagion de la rougeole après la période éruptive. Bull et Xlé Mem Soc Méd Hôp Paris.

Cello J, Paul AV, Wimmer E. 2002. Chemical synthesis of poliovirus cDNA: Generation of infectious virus in the absence of natural template. Science 297:1016-1018.

Chastel C. 1992. Histoire des virus, de la variole au SIDA. Société Nouvelle des Éditions Boubée, Paris.

Chernesky M. 2000. The organizational meeting for the Pan American Group for Rapid Viral Diagnosis (PAGRVD) and the first ten years (1977-1987). J Clinic Virol 16:S3-S8.

Chippaux A, Deubel V, Moreau JP, Reynes JM. 1993. Current situation of yellow fever in Latin America. Bull Soc Pathol Exot 86(5 Pt 2):460-464.

Claas EC, Osterhaus AD, Van Beek R, De Jong JC, Rimmelzwaan GF, Senne DA, Kruss S, Schortridge KF, Webster RG. 1998. Human influenza A H5N1 virus related to a highly pathogenic avian influenza virus. Lancet 351:472-477.

Clavel F, Guetard D, Brun-Vezinet F, Chamaret S, Rey MA, Santos-Ferreira MO, Laurent AG, Dauget C, Katlama C, Rouzioux C. 1986. Isolation of a new human retrovirus from West African Patients with AIDS. Science 233:343-346.

Cleland JB, B Bradley. 1918. Dengue fever in Australia.Its history and clinical course, its experimental transmission byStegomyia fasciata, and the results of inoculation and other experiments. J Hyg (Lond) 16(4):317-418.

Cleton F, Simons JWIM (eds). 1980. Genetic origins of tumor cells. Developments in oncology. Martinus Nijhoff, The Hague.

Clewley JP. 1986. Diagnosis by viral genome detection. In PP Mortimer, Public Health virology, 12 reports. Public Health Laboratory Service, London.

Cocchi F, DeVico AL, Garzino-Demo A, Arya SK, Gallo RC, Lusso P. 1995. Identification of RANTES, MIP-1 alpha, and MIP-1 beta as the major HIV-suppressive factors produced by CD8+ T cells. Science 270:1811-1815.

Cockburn WC. 1964. The programme of the World Health Organization in medical virology. Progr Med Virol 6:175-192.

Cockburn WC. 1973. The programme of the World Health Organization in medical virology.Virus Diseases Unit, World Health Organization, Geneva. Progr Med Virol 15:159-204.

Codell Carter K. 1982. Nineteenth-century treatments for rabies as reported in the Lancet. Med Hist 26:67-78.

Cohen HH. 1987. Sabin and Salk poliovirus vaccine: Vice versa. Acta Leiden 56:65-83.

Cohen HH, Hofman R. 2002. Letter to the editor. Ned Tijdschr Geneeskd 146:2454.

Cohen HH, Kampelmacher EH. 2001. In memoriam prof.dr. R. Gispen. Ned Tijdschr Geneeskd 145:238.

Cohen R. 1991. Jews in another environment: Surinam in the second half of the eighteenth century. E.J. Brill, Leiden.

Collier LH. 1954. The preservation of vaccinia virus. Bacteriol Rev 18(1):74-86.

Collier WA. 1952. Vaccins antivarioliques secs. Preparation du vaccine d'Otten à l'Institut Pasteur de Bandoeng, Indonesie. Bull Wld Hlth Org 5:127-147.

Collier WA, Tiggelman-van Krugten VAH. 1955. De vleermuizen-lyssa in Suriname. Tijdschr Diergeneesk 80:723.

Collier WA, Winckel WE, Kafiluddi S. 1954. Coxsackie infections (pseudopoliomyelitis) in Surinam. Doc Med Geogr Trop 6:97-105.

Compton J. 1991. Nucleic acid sequence-based amplification. Nature 350(6313):91-92.

Cook HJ. 2007. Matters of exchange. Yale University Press, New Haven, CT.

Correns, C., 1950. G. Mendel's law concerning the behavior of progeny of varietal hybrids. Genetics, 35(5, pt 2): 33-41. Originally published as: Correns, C. 1900. G. Mendels Regel Über das Verhalten der Nachkommenschaft der Rassenbastarde. Berichte der Deutschen Botanischen Gesellschaft, 18: 158-168. Reprinted in: Carl Correns Gesammelte Abhandlungen zur Vererbungswissenschaft aus periodischen Schriften 1899-1924. (Fritz v. Wettstein, ed.) Berlin, Julius Springer, 1924, pp. 9-16.

Cossart YE, Field AM, Cant B, Widdows D. 1975. Parvovirus-like particles in human sera. Lancet I:72-73.

Coutinho RA, Lelie PN, Albrecht-van Lent P, Stoutjesdijk L, Huisman J, Kuipers H, Schut LJT, Reerink-Brongers EE, Reesink HW, Van Aken WG. 1983. Efficacy of heat-inactivated hepatitis B vaccine (CLB) in male homosexuals in the Netherlands. Second WHO/IABS symposium on viral hepatitis: Standardization in immunoprophylaxis of infections by hepatitis viruses, Athens, Greece, 1982. Develop Biol Standard 54:287-292.

Creager ANH. 2002. The life of a virus: Tobacco mosaic virus as an experimental model, 1930-1965. University of Chicago Press, Chicago.

Creager ANH. 2014. 'Happily ever after' for cancer viruses? Stud Hist Philos Biol Biomed Sci 48:260-262.

Croon JJ, Wolff HL. 1980. The inhibition of yellow fever virus multiplication by suramin: A preliminary note. Acta Leiden 48:5-8.

Crucell. 2006. Press release. Crucell files for cancellation of remaining Berna Biotech minority shares. Leiden, the Netherlands/Berne, Switzerland, 12 April.

Cunningham A, Williams P. 1992 Introduction. *In* A Cunningham, P Williams (eds), The laboratory revolution in medicine. Cambridge University Press, Cambridge.

Daniels-Bosman MSM, De Villeneuve VH. 1963. Cytomegalie bij een pasgeborene, bevestigd door virologisch onderzoek. Ned Tijdschr Geneeskd 107:241-242.

Darvishian M, Dijkstra F, Van Doorn E, Bijlsma J, Donker GA, De Lange MMA, Cadenau LM, Hak E, Meijer A. 2017. Influenza vaccine effectiveness in the Netherlands from 2003/2004 through 2013/2014: The importance of circulating influenza virus types and subtypes. PLoS ONE 12(1):e0169528. DOI:10.1371/journal.pone.0169528.

De Bruyn PHH. 1942. The cultivation of filterable viruses in vitro. Antonie van Leeuwenhoek 8:19-31.

De Bruyn WM. 1949. Werkgemeenschap voor Weefselkweek. Ned Tijdschr Geneeskd 93:3366.

De Bruyn WM. 1961. In Memoriam Dr Remmert Korteweg. Jaarboek voor Kanker-onderzoek en Kankerbestrijding in Nederland, NKI 11:21-31.

De Chadarevian S, Kamminga, H (eds). 1998. Molecularizing biology and medicine: New practices and alliances, 1910s-1970s. Routledge, New York.

De Feyfer PMG. 1928. Overheidszorg bij hondsdolheid in de achttiende eeuw. Ned Tijdschr Geneeskd 72:1708-1710.

Degkwitz R. 1920. Über Masernrekonvaleszentenserum. Zeitschr f Kinderheilk 27:171-194.

De Groot W. 1951. Scientific research of Philips' Industries from 1891 to 1951. Philips Techn Rev July-August:3-47.

De Haan. 1896. Genees-serum bij mazelen. Ned Tijdschr Geneeskd 40:359.

De Haan J. 1924. Het kweeken van weefsels buiten het lichaam door middel van een doorstromingsmethode. Ned Tijdschr Geneeskd 68:2108-2117.

De Haas RA. 1971. Studies on the distribution of polioviruses in Surinam. Arch Gesamte Virusforsch 33:72-76.

De Haas RA, De Kruyf HA. 1971. Isolation of Guama-group viruses in Surinam. Trop Geogr Med 23:268-271.

De Haas RA, Jonkers AH, Heinemann DW. 1966. Kwatta virus, a new agent isolated from Culex mosquitos in Surinam. Am J Trop Med Hyg 15:954-957.

De Haas RA, Oostburg BF, Sitalsing AD, Bellot SM. 1971. Isolation of yellow fever virus from a human liver obtained by autopsy in Surinam. Trop Geogr Med 23:59-63.

De Jong J, Akhtar W, Badhai J, Rust AG, Rad R, Hilkens J, Berns A, Van Lohuizen M, Wessels LFA, De Ridder J. 2014. Chromatin landscapes of retroviral and transposon integration profiles. PLoS Genet 10(4):e1004250. DOI: 10.1371/journal.pgen.1004250.

De Jong JC, Claas ECJ, Osterhaus ADME, Webster RG, Lim WL. 1997. A pandemic warning? Nature 389:554.

De Jong JC, Wermenbol AG, Verweij-Uijterwaal MW, Slaterus KW, Wertheim-van Dillen P, Van Doornum GJJ, Khoo SH, Hierholzer JC. 1999. Adenoviruses from human immunodeficiency virus-infected individuals, including two strains that represent new candidate serotypes Ad50 and Ad51 of species B1 and D, respectively. J Clin Microbiol 37:3940-3945.

De Jong JC, Wigand R, Kidd AH, Wadell G, Kapsenberg JG, Muzerie CJ, Wermenbol AG, Firtzlaff RG. 1983. Candidate adenoviruses 40 and 41: Fastidious adenoviruses from human infant stool. J Med Virol 11:215-231.

De Jong M. 2010. Inaugural lecture. Vossiuspress, UvA, Amsterdam.

De Jong RN, Van der Vliet PC. 1999. Mechanism of DNA replication in eukaryotic cells: Cellular host factors stimulating adenovirus DNA replication. Gene 236:1-12.

De Jongh CL. 1953. Acute infectieziekten. Elsevier, Amsterdam.

Dekking F. 1953. Aetiologie en diagnostiek van virusziekten. Ned Tijdschr Geneeskd 97:1857-1861.

Dekking F. 1968. Hic sunt leones. Inaugurele rede. A. Oosthoek's Uitgeversmaatschappij N.V., Utrecht.

De Knecht-van Eekelen A. 1984. Abraham Pieter Fokker (1840-1906) en de serumtherapie bij difterie. Tsch Gesch Gnk Natuurw Wisk Techn 7(1984) 4:161-171.

De Knecht-van Eekelen A. 1989. The interaction of Western and tropical medicine. In GM van Heteren, A De Knecht-van Eekelen, MJD Poulissen, AM Luyendijk-Elshout (eds) Dutch medicine in the Malay archipelago, 1816-1942. Rodopi, Amsterdam.

De Knecht-van Eekelen A. 1991. Intree-redes en het beeld van het medisch onderwijs in de Heel- en Verloskunde in Nederland 1865-1900. Tschr Gnk Natuurw Wisk Techn 14:119-149.

De Lange C. 1906. Vaccine-lichaampjes. H. Aldershoff. Dissertatie Groningen. Ned Tijdschr Geneeskd 50:1080-1082.

Delprat CC, Kummer A. 1965. De wording en geschiedenis van het Genootschap ter Bevordering van Natuur-, Genees- en Heelkunde te Amsterdam, 1790-1915 ... Vervolg 1915-1965. Amsterdam.

De Melker HE, Van den Hof S, Berbers GAM, Conyn-van Spaendonck MAE. 2003. Evaluation of the national immunisation programme in the Netherlands: Immunity to diphtheria, tetanus, poliomyelitis, measles, mumps, rubella and Haemophilus influenzae type b. Vaccine 21:716-720.

Den Dooren de Jong LE. 1954. Virussen en hun gedrag in de levende cel. Ned Tijdschr Geneeskd 98:2546-2557.

Den Dooren de Jong LE. 1983. Beijerinck, the Man. *In* G van Iterson, LE den Dooren de Jong, AJ Kluyver, Martinus Willem Beijerinck: His life and his work. Science Tech, Madison, WI.

Deng H, Liu R, Ellmeier W, Choe S, Unutmaz D, Burkhart M, Di Marzio P, Marmon S, Sutton RE, Hill CM, Davis CB, Peiper SC, Schall TJ, Littman DR, Landau NR. 1996. Identification of a major co-receptor for primary isolates of HIV-1. Nature 381:661-666.

De Ruiter HI. 1939. Therapie en profylaxis van mazelen. Ned Tijdschr Geneeskd 83:1356-1361.

Dewhurst K. 1955. Sydenham on smallpox. Br Med J 4936:432-433.

Dewhurst K. 1959. Sydenham's original treatise on smallpox with a preface, and dedication to the Earl of Shaftesbury, by John Locke. Med Hist 3:278-302.

D'Herelle F. 1916. Contribution à l'étude de l'immunité. C R Hebd Séances Acad Sci Tome 162:570-573.

D'Herelle F. 1917. Sur un microbe invisible antagoniste des bacilles dysentériques. Note présentée par M. Roux. C R Acad Sci Paris 165:373-375.

D'Herelle F. 1922. The nature of bacteriophage. Brit Med J 2(3216):289-293.

D'Herelle F. 1925. Verslagen Afd Natuurk Kon Akad v Wet Amsterdam 34:835.

D'Herelle F. 1926. Le bactériophage et son comportement. Masson et Cie, Paris.

D'Herelle F. 1926. The bacteriophage and its behavior. Translated by GH Smith. The Williams & Wilkins Co., Baltimore, MD.

D'Herelle F. 1928. Versl Afd Natuurk Kon Akad v Wet, Amsterdam 34:835.

Dicke WK. 1953. Mazelen. *In* CL de Jongh (ed.) Acute infectieziekten. Elsevier, Amsterdam.

Dinger JE. 1950. In Memoriam Prof. Dr W.A.P. Schüffner. Ned Tijdschr Geneeskd 95:3003-3006.

Dinger JE. 1951. Het aandeel van Nederland in de vooruitgang der geneeskundige wetenschap van 1900-1950. Tropische Hygiëne. Ned Tijdschr Geneeskd 95:3718-3723.

Dinger JE, Schüffner WAP, Snijders EP, Swellengrebel NH. 1929a. Onderzoek over gele koorts in Nederland. Ned Tijdschr Geneeskd 73:3255-3257.

Dinger JE, Schüffner WAP, Snijders EP, Swellengrebel NH. 1929b. Onderzoek over gele koorts in Nederland (Tweede mededeling). Ned Tijdschr Geneeskd 73:4378-4384.

Dinger JE, Schüffner WAP, Snijders EP, Swellengrebel NH. 1929c. Onderzoek over gele koorts in Nederland (Derde mededeling). Ned Tijdschr Geneeskd 73:5982-5991.

Dobson AP, Carper ER. 1996. Infectious diseases and human population history. Bioscience 46:115-126.

Dobson M. 2015. Murderous contagion: a human history of disease. Quercus Publishing, 2015, Kindle location 5035.

Doerr R. 1938. Die Entwicklung der Virusforschung und ihrer Problematik, pp. 1-21. In R Doerr, C Hallauer (eds) Handbuch der Virusforschung. Erste Hälfte, Springer, Wien.

Doerr R, Hallauer C (eds). 1938. Handbuch der Virusforschung. Erste Hälfte. Springer, Wien.

Doerr R, Hallauer C (eds). 1939. Handbuch der Virusforschung. Zweite Hälfte. Springer, Wien.

Doerr R, Hallauer C (eds). 1944. Handbuch der Virusforschung. I. Ergänzungsband. Springer, Wien.

Doerr R, Hallauer C (eds). 1950. Handbuch der Virusforschung. II. Ergänzungsband. Springer, Wien.

Dragic T, Litwin V, Allaway GP, Martin SC, Huang Y, Nagashima KA, Cayanan C, Maddon PJ, Koup RA, Moore JP, Paxton WA. 1996. HIV-1 entry into CD4$^+$ cells is mediated by the chemokine receptor CC-CKR-5. Nature 381:667-673.

Drielsma A. 1861. De ziektekundig-ontleedkundige veranderingen in de longen na mazelen. Ned Tijdschr Geneeskd 5:179-180.

Dubos R. 1986/1950. Louis Pasteur, free lance of science. Da Capo Press, New York. Original edition: 1950.

Duckworth DH. 1976. Who discovered bacteriophage? Bacteriol Rev 40:793-802.

Dulbecco R. 1974. Oncogenic viruses: The last twelve years. Cold Spring Harb Symp. Quant Biol 39:1-7.

Dulbecco R, Vogt M. 1954. Plague formation and isolation of pure line with polio-myelitis viruses. J Exp Med 99:167-182.

Dumas AM, Geelen JL, Weststrate MW, Wertheim P, Van der Noordaa J. 1981. XbaI, PstI, and BglII restriction enzyme maps of the two orientations of the varicella-zoster virus genome. J Virol 39:390-400.

Editorial JAMA. 1932. Crystallized filtrable virus. JAMA 99:656.

Eijgenraam F. 1991. Dutch AIDS researchers feel heat of publicity. Science 251:1422-1423.

Einstein A, Mühsam H. 1923. Experimentele Bestimmung der Kanalweite von Filtern. Dtsch Med Wochenschr 49:1012.

Elford WJ. 1933. The principles of ultrafiltration as applied in biological studies. Proc Roy Soc B 112:384-406.

Elford WJ, Andrewes CH. 1932. The sizes of different bacteriophages. Brit J Exp Path 13:446-456.

Elkeles G. 1934. Experimentelle Untersuchungen zur Aetiologie der Influenza. Mededeelingen uit het Instituut voor Praeventieve Geneeskunde 1934:60-79.

Elkeles G. 1971. Über 30 Jahre Artz. Therapie der Gegenwart 110(10):1541-1564.

Emmelot P, Bentvelzen P (eds). 1972. RNA viruses and host genome in oncogenesis. Proceedings of a conference. North-Holland Publishing Co., Amsterdam.

Enders JF. 1961. Letter, New York Times, 1 October.

Enders JF, Peebles TC. 1954. Propagation in tissue cultures of cytopathogenic agents from patients with measles. Proc Soc Exp Biol Med 86:277-286.

Enders JF, Robbins FC, Weller TH. 1954. The cultivation of the poliomyelitis viruses in tissue culture. Nobel Lecture, 11 December. NobelPrize.org. https://www.nobelprize.org/prizes/medicine/1954/enders/lecture/.

Enders JF, Weller TH, Robbins FC. 1949. Cultivation of the Lansing strain of polio-myelitis virus in various human embryonic tissues. Science 109:85-87.

Endtz LJ. 1986. Over het moeizame begin van de pokkenpreventie. Ned Tijdschr Geneeskd 130:929-930.

Engvall E, Perlmann P. 1971. Enzyme linked immunosorbent assay (ELISA): Quantitative assay of IgG. Immunochemistry 8:871.

Entrop M. 2003. Verliefde ogen zien Mondriaan. Uit het dagboek van Eva de Beneditty. De Parelduiker, 2003/1. Uitgeverij Bas Lubberhuizen, Amsterdam.

Eriksen A. 2013. Cure or protection? The meaning of smallpox inoculation, ca 1750-1775. Med Hist 57:516-536. DOI: 10.1017/mdh.2013.37.

Erkoreka A. 2009. Origins of the Spanish influenza pandemic (1918-1920) and its relation to the First World War. J Mol Genet Med 3(2):190-194.

Erkoreka A. 2010. The Spanish influenza pandemic in occidental Europe (1918-1920) and victim age. Influenza and Other Respiratory Viruses 4(2):81-89.

Eykman C. 1900. Over Pasteur's methode der preventieve behandeling van rabies en haar resultaten. Ned Tijdschr Geneeskd 44:1009-1030.

Feng Y, Broder CC, Kennedy PE, Berger EA. 1996. HIV-1 entry cofactor: Functional cDNA cloning of a seven-transmembrane, G protein-coupled receptor. Science 272:872.

Fenner F. 1988a. Early efforts at control: Variolation, vaccination and quarantine, pp. 253-256. In F Fenner, DA Henderson, L Arita, Z Ježek, ID Ladnyi (eds) Smallpox and its eradication. World Health Organization, Geneva.

Fenner F. 1988b. The history of smallpox and its spread around the world, pp. 235-236. In F Fenner, DA Henderson, L Arita, Z Ježek, ID Ladnyi (eds) Smallpox and its eradication. World Health Organization, Geneva.

Fenner F, Gibbs A (eds). 1988. Portraits of viruses: A history of virology. Karger, Basel

Fenner F, Henderson DA, Arita L, Ježek Z, Ladnyi ID (eds). 1988. Smallpox and its eradication. World Health Organization, Geneva.

Field AM. 1986. The contribution of the electron microscope. In PP Mortimer (ed.) Public health virology, 12 reports, Public Health Laboratory Service, London.

Flu PC. 1910. Gelbfieber in Paramaribo, Suriname, 1908-1909. Z Hyg Infektionskr 65:17-54.

Flu PC. 1928. Over filtreerbare en onzichtbare stadia bij microörganismen. Ned Tijdschr Geneeskd 72:4764-4774.

Flu PC. 1929. Immunisering van ratten tegen pest door middel van geconcentreerde bacteriophaaglysaten uit virulente pestbacteriën. Ned Tijdschr Geneeskd 73(II):4010-4020.

Flu PC. 1937.Enkele beschouwingen over de gele koorts in Suriname. Geneesk Tijdschr Ned-Indië 77:1411-1422.

Flu PC. 1940. Het ultravirus als ziekte-oorzaak, zijn eigenschappen en een critisch overzicht van de opvattingen omtrent zijn aard. Ned Tijdschr Geneeskd 84:3198-3211.

Flu PC, Renaux E. 1932. Le phénomène de Twort et la bactériophage. Ann l'Inst Pasteur 48:15-18.

Flu PK. 2018. Paul Christiaan Flu: Leven en Werk, 1884-1945. Carbona Uitgeverij, Rotterdam.

Fokker AP. 1891. Mazelen. Ned Tijdschr Geneeskd 35:691-692.

Fokker AP. 1899. De serumtherapie der diphtheria. Ned Tijdschr Geneeskd 43:322-325.

Foster SO, El Sid AGH, Deria A. 1978. Spread of smallpox among a Somali nomadic group. Lancet 14(2):831-833.

Fouchier RA, Rimmelzwaan GF, Kuiken T, Osterhaus AD. 2005. Newer respiratory virus infections: Human metapneumovirus, avian influenza virus, and human coronaviruses: Review. Curr Opin Infect Dis 18(2):141-146.

Fox JP, Hall CE. 1980. Viruses in families. Surveillance of families as a key to epidemiology of virus infections. PSG Publishing Co., Littleton, MA.

Frenkel HS. 1939. Het kweeken van ultrafiltreerbare smetstoffen. Chemisch Weekblad 36(40):688-691.

Frenkel HS. 1957. Het kweken van vaccinia-virus in geëxplanteerd epitheelweefsel afkomstig uit de diepe lagen van rundertongslijmvliesepitheel. Ned Tijdschr Geneeskd 101:2413-2416.

Frenkel HS. 1961. Letter to Dr Albert B. Sabin, 17 June.

Frenkel HS. 1963. Zijn virussen levend? Acta Leiden 32:83-87.

Frenkel HS, Julius HW. 1932. Die Züchtung von Vakzin-Virus in Vitro mittels des Durchströmungsapparates. Acta Brev Neerl 2:116-118.

Frenkel HS, Kapsenberg JG. 1954. Het kweken van vaccinia-virus in geëxplanteerd huidweefsel van de runder- en schapenfoetus. Ned Tijdschr Geneeskd 98:991-996.

Frenkel HS, Van Waveren GM. 1934. Verslag over de werkzaamheden van het Staats Veeartsenijkundig Onderzoekingsinstituut 1933-1934. Uitg. Alg. Landsdrukkerij, 's Gravenhage.

Frenkel HS, Van Waveren GM. 1935. Over het kweeken van mond- en klauwzeer-smetstof in vitro. 1e mededeling. Uitg. Alg. Landsdrukkerij, 's Gravenhage.

Frerichs L. 2014. Geheime geliefden. Brieven aan Ada Prins en Jenne Clinge Doorenbos. Van Oorschot, Amsterdam.

Freundlich MM. 1963. Origin of the electron microscope. Science 142(3589):185-188.

Galama JMD. 2001. Virussen en de paradox van preventie. Inaugural Lecture, Katholieke Universiteit Nijmegen.

Galassi FM, Habicht ME, Rühli FJ. 2017. Poliomyelitis in Ancient Egypt? Neurol Sci 38(2):375. DOI: 10.1007/s10072-016-2720-9.

Galjaard H. 1977. Professor P.J. Gaillard met emeritaat. Ned Tijdschr Geneeskd 121:1532.

Gallo RC, Sarin PS, Gelmann EP, Robert-Guroff M, Richardson E, Kalyanaraman VS, Mann D, Sidhu GD, Stahl RE, Zolla-Pazner S, Leibowitch J, Popovic M. 1983. Isolation of human T-cell leukemia virus in acquired immune deficiency syndrome (AIDS). Science 220(4599):865-867.

Gard S. 1954. Award presentation speech. The Nobel Prize in Physiology or Medicine. NobelPrize.org. https://www.nobelprize.org/prizes/medicine/1954/ceremony-speech/.

Gardner PS. 1978. European Group for Rapid Laboratory Diagnosis. Amsterdam Symposium on Rapid Diagnosis. J Gen Virol 39:201-203.

Gardner PS, McQuillin J. 1980. Rapid virus diagnosis. 2nd ed. Butterworths, London.

Garfield E. 1990. Will the Lowry method ever be obliterated? The most-cited papers of all time, SCI 1945-1988. Part 1A. The SCI Top 100. Current Contents 7:3-14.

Gaudillière J-P. 1998. The molecularization of cancer etiology in the postwar United States: Instruments, politics and management, pp. 139-170. In S de Chadarevian, H Kamminga (eds) Molecularizing biology and medicine: New practices and alliances 1910s-1970s. Routledge, New York.

Geison GL. 1995. The private science of Louis Pasteur. Princeton University Press, Princeton, NJ.

Geist-Hofman AM, Meininger JV, Verkroost CM. 1972. Zinking, zinkingskoorts en zinkingsziekte. Ned Tijdschr Geneeskd 116:23-30.

Geysen HM, Meloen RH, Barteling SJ. 1984. Use of peptide synthesis to probe viral antigens for epitopes to a resolution of a single amino acid. Proc Nat Acad Sci USA 81:3998-4002.

Gezondheids Organisatie TNO. 1952. Verslag over het jaar 1951. Nederlandse
    Organisatie voor Toegepast-natuurwetenschappelijk Onderzoek ten behoeve
    van de Volksgezondheid, 's-Gravenhage.

GGD Amsterdam, Archief. 1956. Gemeentelijke Geneeskundige en Gezondheids-
    dienst, Amsterdam. Jaarverslag.

GGD Amsterdam, Archief. 1957. Jaarverslagen van de Geneeskundige en
    Gezondheidsdienst.

GGD Amsterdam, Archief. 1956. Streeklaboratorium voor de Volksgezondheid.
    GG&GD, Amsterdam. Jaarverslag.

GGD Amsterdam, Archief. 1959. Streeklaboratorium voor de Volksgezondheid.
    GG&GD, Amsterdam. Jaarverslag.

GGD Amsterdam, Archief. 1965. Streeklaboratorium voor de Volksgezondheid.
    GG&GD, Amsterdam. Jaarverslag.

Gildemeister E, Haagen E, Waldmann O. 1939a. Handbuch der Viruskrankheiten.
    Erster Band. Verlag von Gustav Fischer in Jena.

Gildemeister E, Haagen E, Waldmann O. 1939b. Handbuch der Viruskrankheiten.
    Zweiter Band. Verlag von Gustav Fischer in Jena.

Gillett MC. 2009. The Army Medical Department 1917-1941. Center of Military
    History, US Army, Washington, DC.

Girard M. 1988. The Pasteur Institute's contributions to the field of virology. Ann
    Rev Microbiol 42:745-763.

Gispen R. 1951. Het aandeel van Nederland in de vooruitgang der geneeskun-
    dige wetenschap van 1900 tot 1950. Microbiologie. Ned Tijdschr Geneeskd
    95:830-839.

Gispen R. 1953. Inenting tegen pokken, pp. 131-183. *In* CL de Jongh (ed.), Acute
    infectieziekten. Elsevier, Amsterdam.

Gispen R. 1957. Vaccinatie tegen poliomyelitis. Ned Tijdschr Geneeskd 101:1813-1818.

Gispen R. 1961. Vaccinatie tegen poliomyelitis met niet vermeerderingsvatbaar virus.
    Verslag van het poliomyelitis-symposium. Excerpta Medica Amsterdam, pp. 9-16.

Gispen R. 1975. Vosserabies aan deze zijde van de grens. Ned Tijdschr Geneeskd
    119:800-802.

Gispen R, Schmittmann GJP, Saathof B. 1965. Rabies vaccine derived from suckling
    rabbit brain. Arch Ges Virusforsch 15:366-376.

GNGH. 1845 Archief van het Genootschap ter bevordering van Natuur- Genees- en
    Heelkunde, Stadsarchief Amsterdam, toegangsnummer 819, inv. nr. 1.1.2:99-100.
    Jaarvergadering 1845.

GNGH. 1859-1895. Archief van het Genootschap ter bevordering van Natuur- Genees-
    en Heelkunde, Stadsarchief Amsterdam, toegangsnummer 819, inv. nr. 1.1.19.
    Presentielijsten voor aanwezigen op vergaderingen 1859-1895.

GNGH. 1924. Archief van het Genootschap ter bevordering van Natuur- Genees- en Heelkunde, Stadsarchief Amsterdam, toegangsnummer 819, inv. nr. 3.9.608. Werken van het Genootschap. 2^e serie, Deel 11. Afl. 1.

GNGH. 1926. Archief van het Genootschap ter bevordering van Natuur- Genees- en Heelkunde, Stadsarchief Amsterdam, toegangsnummer 819, inv. nr. 3.9.608. Werken van het Genootschap. 2^e serie, Deel 11. Afl. 3.

GNGH. 1928. Archief van het Genootschap ter bevordering van Natuur- Genees- en Heelkunde, Stadsarchief Amsterdam, toegangsnummer 819, inv. nr. 3.9.608. Werken van het Genootschap. 2^e serie, Deel 12. Afl. 3.

GNGH. 1931. Archief van het Genootschap ter bevordering van Natuur- Genees- en Heelkunde, Stadsarchief Amsterdam, toegangsnummer 819, inv. nr. 3.9.608. Werken van het Genootschap. 2^e serie, Deel 13. Afl. 2.

Gorter E, De Graaff WC. 1915. Klinische diagnostiek. Bacteriologische, Serologische en Chemische onderzoekingsmethoden. 1915. S.C. van Doesburgh, Leiden.

Gorter E, De Graaff WC. 1949. Klinische diagnostiek. 6^e druk. Stenfert Kroese's Uitgevers-Mij, Leiden.

Gorter HW. 2014. Brief aan Ada, Bern, 2 november 1918, pp. 350-351. *In* L Frerichs. Geheime geliefden. Brieven aan Ada Prins en Jenne Clinge Doorenbos. Van Oorschot, Amsterdam.

Goslinga CC. 1979. A short history of the Netherlands Antilles and Surinam. Martinus Nijhoff, The Hague.

Goudsmit J, Debouck C, Meloen RH, Smit L, Bakker M, Asher DM, Wolff AV, Gibbs Jr CJ, Gajdusek CD. 1988. HIV type 1 neutralization epitope with conserved architecture elicits early type-specific antibodies in experimentally infected chimpanzees. Proc Natl Acad Sci USA 85:4478-4482.

Gradmann C. 2014. A spirit of scientific rigour: Koch's postulates in twentieth-century medicine. Microbes and Infection 16:885-892.

Grafe A. 1991. A history of experimental virology. Springer, Berlin.

Graham FL. 1988. This Week's Citation Classic. Current Contents 46:16.

Graham FL, Van der Eb AJ. 1973. A new technique for the assay of infectivity of human adenovirus 5 DNA. Virology 52:456-467.

Gratia A. 1938. Nature des ultravirus, pp. 109-157. *In* C Levaditi, P Lépine et al., Les ultravirus des maladies humaines. Maloine, Paris.

Gratia A. 1945. La conception endo-exogène des virus et des bactériophages et la théorie infra-cellulaire de la vie. Bull Acad R Med Belg 10:139-150.

Griffiths P. 2002. Science and Technology Committee, House of Lords. Minutes of evidence, session 2002-03. Examination of Witnesses, 2002, Question 225. (www.Parliament.UK > Parliamentary business > Publications and Records > Committee Publications > All Select Committee Publications > Lords Select

Committees > Science and Technology > Science and Technology. Minutes of Evidence).

Griffiths PD, Panjwani DD, Stirk PR, Ball MG, Ganczakowski M, Blacklock HA, Prentice HG. 1984. Rapid diagnosis of cytomegalovirus infection in immuno-compromised patients by detection of early antigen fluorescent foci. Lancet 2(8414):1242-1245.

Groen J, Veening MM, Leentvaar-Kuipers A, Osterhaus AD. 1998. A case of human rabies in the Netherlands. Infection 26:196.

Grosheide PM, Klokman-Houweling JM, Conyn-van Spaendonck MAE, and the National Hepatitis B Steering Committee. 1995. Programme for preventing perinatal hepatitis B infection through screening of pregnant women and immunisation of infants of infected mothers in the Netherlands, 1989-92. Brit Med J 311:1200-1202.

Grosheide PM, Van Osand HC, Schalm SW, Heijtink RA. 1991. Immunoprophylaxis to limit a hepatitis B epidemic among women undergoing in vitro fertilization. Vaccine 9:682-687.

Guatelli JC, Whitfield KM, Kwoh DY, Barringer KJ, Richman DD, Gingeras TR. 1990. Isothermal, in vitro amplification of nucleic acids by a multienzyme reaction modeled after retroviral replication. Proc Natl Acad Sci USA 87(5):1874-1878.

Haakma Tresling T. 1872. Aantekeningen over mazelen te Winschoten in de jaren 1861, 1865 en 1871. Ned Tijdschr Geneeskd 16:228-256.

Haakma Tresling T. 1893. Rapport van de commissie voor de geneeskundige statistiek. Iets over mazelen te Winschoten en een woord over de prophylaxis. Ned Tijdschr Geneeskd 37:32-40.

Haalboom AF. 2014. Spanish flu and army horses: What historians and biologists can learn from a history of animals with flu during the 1918-1919 influenza pandemic. Studium 7:124-139.

Haalboom AF. 2017. Negotiating zoonoses: Dealings with infectious diseases shared by humans and livestock in the Netherlands (1898-2001). PhD thesis, Utrecht University.

Haeseker B. 2002. Karl Landsteiner (1868-1943) en de specificiteit van serologische reacties, honderd jaar geleden en nu. Ned Tijdschr Geneeskd 146:575-579.

Haex AJC. 1965. In memoriam Prof. Dr. J. Mulder. Ned Tijdschr Geneeskd 109:2161-2163.

Halifax Chronicle Herald. 1989. Obituary of Dr Clennel van Rooyen. Halifax Chronicle Herald, 17 March.

Hallewas G-J. 1981. De gezondheidszorg in Suriname. PhD thesis, University of Groningen.

Haneveld GT. 2004. Het besloten Utrechts Geneeskundig Gezelschap Matthias van Geuns als historie- en inspiratiebron. Ned Tijdschr Geneeskd 148:2602-2606.

Hankins CA, Wainberg MA, Weiss RA. 2014. In tribute to Joep Lange. Retrovirology 11:82.

Hanlo J. 1880. De sterfteverhouding aan mazelen en roodvonk. Ned Tijdschr Geneeskd 23:570-571.

Havenga M, Vogels R, Zuijdgeest D, Radosevic K, Mueller S, Sieuwerts M, Weichold F, Damen I, Kaspers J, Lemckert A, Van Meerendonk M, Van der Vlugt R, Holterman L, Hone D, Skeiky Y, Mintardjo R, Gillissen G, Barouch D, Sadoff J, Goudsmit J. 2006. Novel replication-incompetent adenoviral B-group vectors: High vector stability and yield in PER.C6 cells. J Gen Virol 87:2135-2143. DOI 10.1099/vir.0.81956-0.

Hawkes RA. 1979. General principles underlying laboratory diagnosis of viral infections. In EH Lennette, P Halonen, FA Murphy (eds) Laboratory diagnosis of infectious diseases: Principles and practice, Volume II: Viral, rickettsial and chlamydial diseases. Springer, New York.

Health Council of the Netherlands. 2001. Universal vaccination against hepatitis B. Publication no. 2001/03. Health Council of the Netherlands, The Hague.

Health Inspectorate. Mededelingen en Bekendmakingen. 1953. Kinkhoest-Diphtherie-Tetanusvaccinatie van Kinderen. Ned Tijdschr Geneeskd 93:695-696.

Heine J von. 1840. Beobachtungen über Lähmungzustände der unteren Extremitäten und deren Behandlung. Köhler, Stuttgart.

Heine J von. 1860. Spinale Kinderlähmung. Cotta.

Hekker AC. 1962. De antigeniteitsbepaling van geïnactiveerd poliomyelitisviriusvaccin. Academic thesis, University of Leiden.

Hekker AC. 1982. Van cbr en har via IF naar Elisa: de Virologie vandaag. Inaugural Lecture. University of Utrecht, 18 May.

Hekmeijer FC. 1867. Over een algemene rationele wet op het houden van honden ter voorkoming van hondsdolheid en de verspreiding van deze ziekte. Ned Tijdschr Geneeskd 11:248-250.

Henderson DA, Ježek Z. 1988. Somalia and Djibouti, pp. 1037-1068. In F Fenner, DA Henderson, L Arita, Z Ježek, ID Ladnyi (eds) Smallpox and its eradication. World Health Organization, Geneva.

Hendriks JT. 2017. Societal vaccinology: The Netherlands public sector vaccine development, production and technology transfer in the context of global health. PhD thesis, University of Amsterdam.

Henle J. 1938. On miasmata and contagia. Translated by G Rosen. Johns Hopkins Press, Baltimore, MD.

Herderschêe D. 1910. School en besmettelijke ziekten. Ned Tijdschr Geneeskd 54:279-295.

Herderschêe D, Wolff LK. 1924. De geneeskrachtige waarde van den typhusbacterio-phaag bij lijders aan typhus abdominalis. Ned Tijdschr Geneeskd 68:2706-2714.

Hermanides CH. 1911. Gevallen van de ziekte van Heine-Medin (epidemische kinderverlamming) te Noordwijk. Ned Tijdschr Geneeskd 55:681-693.

Hermans PH. 1963. In memoriam Dr Sandor Weidinger. Chemisch Weekblad 59:537.

Hers JFP, Mulder J. 1961. Broad aspects of the pathology and pathogenesis of human influenza. Am Rev Resp Diseases 83:84-97.

Hers JF, Van der Kuip L, Masurel N. 1968. Rapid diagnosis of influenza. Lancet 7541:510-511.

Heston WE, Parks WP. 1977. Mammary tumors and mammary tumor virus expression in hybrid mice of strains C57BL and GR. J Exp Med 146:1206-1220.

Hillen HFP. 2017. De hofarts, de dominee, een geleerd genootschap en de pokken. Ned Tijdschr Geneeskd 161:D111.

Himawan S. 1995. The history of pathology in Indonesia. Med J Indones 4:4-11.

Hippocrates. [1923]. English translation by WHS Jones. Harvard University Press, Cambridge, MA.

Hoeben RC, Valerio D, Van der Eb AJ, Van Ormondt H. 1992. Gene therapy for human inherited disorders: Techniques and status. Crit Rev Oncol Hematol 13:33-54.

Hofman B. 1967. Poliomyelitis in the Netherlands before and after vaccination with inactivated polio vaccine. J Hyg 65:547-557.

Hofman B. 1972. Poliomyelitis in the Netherlands 1958-69: The influence of a vaccination programme with inactivated poliovaccine. Bull Wld Hlth Org 46:735-745.

Hofman B, Wilterdink JB. 1960. Poliomyelitis antibodies in sera from the Netherlands, Curaçao, Surinam, St Eustatius and Netherlands New Guinea. Antonie van Leeuwenhoek 20:397-406.

Holmberg C, Blume S, Greenough P (eds). 2017. The politics of vaccination: A global history. Manchester University Press, Manchester.

Hoogendoorn D. 1948. Over de diphtherie in Nederland. Epidemiologie en prophy-laxe. PhD thesis, University of Utrecht.

Houwaart ES. 1991. De Hygiënisten. Artsen, staat & volksgezondheid in Nederland, 1840-1890. Historische Uitgeverij, Groningen.

Houweling H, Heisterkamp SH, Van Wijngaarden JK, Wiessing LG, Coutinho RA, Jager JC. 1994. Analyse van de AIDS-epidemie in Nederland, 1982-1993. Ned Tijdschr Geneeskd 138:1954-1959.

Huebner RJ. 1957. Implications of recent viral studies. Public Health Reports 72:377-380.

Huebner RJ. 1959. 70 Newly recognized viruses in man. Public Health Reports 74:6-12.

Huisman J. 2002a. Pokkenvaccinatie. In Gezondheidsraad A08/08, 2002:4-5 (pokkenvaccinatie).

Huisman J. 2002b. Poliovaccinatie. *In* Gezondheidsraad A08/08, 2002:3 (polio vaccinatie).

Huët GJ. 1951. Het rapport over de mazelenprophylaxe. Maandschr. v. Kindergeneesk, 19:509.

Hüsken-Nillissen HWM, De Moulin D. 1986. De Dienst der Volksgezondheid in Nederlands-Indië: een terugblik. Ned Tijdschr Geneeskd 130:2356-2360.

Huygelen C. 1997. The immunization of cattle against Rinderpest in eighteenth-century Europe. Med Hist 41:182-196.

Illy J. 2012. The practical Einstein: Experiments, patents, inventions. Johns Hopkins University Press, Baltimore, MD.

Ingen Housz JM, Beale N, Beale E. 2005. The life of Dr Jan Ingen Housz (1730-99), private counsellor and personal physician to Emperor Joseph II of Austria. J Med Biogr 13:15-21.

International Poliomyelitis Congress. 1952. Poliomyelitis: Papers and discussions presented at the Second Poliomyelitis Conference, 1951, Copenhagen. J.B. Lippincott, Philadelphia, PA.

Ivanovski D. 1903. Uber die Mosaikkrankheit der Tabakspflanze [On the mosaic disease of tobacco plant]. Z. Pflanzenkr. 13:1-41.

Ivanowski D. 1942/1892. On the mosaic disease of the tobacco plant. Translated by J Johnson. Phytopathological Classics 7:27-30. Original: Ueber die Mosaikkrankheit der Tabakspflanze. St Peters. Acad Imp Sci Bull 35:67-70.

Jansen J. 1951. Richard Shope: Doctor medicinae honoris causa Medicinae Veterinarae. Tijdschr Diergeneesk 76:209.

Janssen LW. 1939. Inleiding tot het virusprobleem met mond- en klauwzeer als voorbeeld. Symposium 'Het ultrafiltreerbare virus'. Nederlandse Vereniging voor Biochemie, 1 juli 1939 te Wageningen. Chemisch Weekblad 36(40):684-688.

Janssen LW. 1940. Viruseiwitten en hun productie door de cel. Ned Tijdschr Geneeskd 84:3220-3239.

Janssen LW. 1948. Experimenteel en theoretisch virusonderzoek. *In* Symposium over virussen. Nederlandse Vereniging voor Biochemie. 13 december 1947 en 14 februari 1948. D.B. Centen's Uitgevers-Maatschappij N.V., Amsterdam.

Jansz HS. 1968. Replicatie in vitro, rede uitgesproken bij de aanvaarding van het ambt van gewoon hoogleraar in de Fysiologische Chemie aan de Rijksuniversiteit te Utrecht op 22 april 1968. Uitgeverij A. Oosthoek, Utrecht.

Janzen JW, Wolff LK. 1923a. Bacteriophaag-studies II. Ned Tijdschr Geneeskd 67:2107-2112.

Janzen JW, Wolff LK. 1923b. Bacteriophaag-studies III. Ned Tijdschr Geneeskd 67:147-150.

Javier RT, Butel, JS. 2008. The history of tumor virology. Cancer Research 68:7693-7706.

Jeanselme E. 1929. L'oeuvre de J. Bontius, pp. 209-222. Paper presented at the Sixth International Congress of History of Medicine, Leiden-Amsterdam, 18-25 July 1927. De Vlijt, Anvers.

Jeffery K, Aarons E. 2009. Diagnostic approaches, p. 3. In AJ Zuckerman, JE Banat-vala, BD Schoub, PD Griffiths, P Mortimer (eds) Principles & Practice of Clinical Virology, 6th ed. Wiley-Blackwell.

Jenkins JS. 1999. The English inoculator: Jan Ingen-Housz. J R Soc Med 92:534-537.

Jenner E. 1801. The origin of the vaccine inoculation. D.N. Shury, London.

Johnson HN. 1959. Rabies, pp. 405-431. In TM Rivers, FL Horsfall (eds) Viral and rickettsial infections of man. J.B. Lippincott, Philadelphia, PA.

Johnson J (ed. and trans.). 1942. Phytopathological Classics 7.

Johnson N, Vos A, Freuling C, Tordo N, Fooks AR, Müller T. 2010. Human rabies due to lyssavirus infection of bat origin. Vet Microbiol 142:151-159.

Joly R. 1964a. Hippocrate, medicine grecque. Des airs, des eaux, des lieux. Editions Gallimard.

Joly R. 1964b. Hippocrate, medicine grecque. Épidémies. Editions Gallimard.

Jongkees LBW. 1963. Het Nederlandse Kanker-Instituut 50 jaar. Ned Tijdschr Geneeskd 107:1589-1592.

Jonkers AH, Metselaar D, Homobono Pães de Andrade A, Tikasingh ES. 1967. Restan virus, a new group C arbovirus from Trinidad and Surinam. Am J Trop Med Hyg 16:74-78.

Josephus Jitta NM. 1937. In memoriam Professor Dr. H. Aldershoff. Ned Tijdschr Geneeskd 81:4034-4035.

Kaadan, AN. 2000. Al Raz's book on smallpox and measles. Qatar Medical Journal 7. DOI: 10.5339/qmj.2000.2.7.

Kalwij, AS. 1959. De epidemiologie van de poliomyelitis in Nederland. Van Gorcum, Assen.

Kamerbeek E, Van Gilde PHG, Hildernisse LW. 1947. Rubeola als oorzaak van aangeboren afwijkingen. Ned Tijdschr Geneeskd 91:966-967.

Kamerbeek EHM. 1953. Rode hond, pp. 184-201. In CL de Jongh (ed.) Acute infectie-ziekten. Elsevier, Amsterdam.

Kamp AF, La Rivière JWM, Verhoeven W (eds). 1959. Albert Jan Kluyver: His life and his work. North-Holland Publishing Co., Amsterdam/Interscience, New York.

Kaplan C. 1971. Rabies vaccines: An assessment. Proc R Soc Med 64:228-231.

Kapsenberg JG. 1975. Wetenschappelijke achtergronden in de ontwikkeling van de medische virologische diagnostiek. Ned Tijdschr Geneeskd 119:1946-1951.

Kapsenberg JG. 1988a. In memoriam prof.dr. A.C. Hekker. Ned Tijdschr Geneeskd 132:512.

Kapsenberg JG. 1988b. Picornaviridae: The enteroviruses (Polioviruses, Coxsacki-
eviruses, Echoviruses), p. 713. *In* EH Lennette, P Halonen, FA Murphy (eds)
Laboratory diagnosis of infectious diseases: Principles and practice, Volume
II: Viral, rickettsial and chlamydial diseases. Springer, New York.

Kapsenberg JG. 2002. [private] Brief aan Werkgroep Klinische Virologie.

Kast WM, Offringa R, Peters PJ, Voordouw AC, Meloen RH, Van der Eb AM, Melief
CJM. 1989. Eradication of adenovirus E1-induced tumors by E1A specific cytotoxic
T lymphocytes. Cell 59:603-614.

Kemeny DM, Challacombe SJ. 1988. An introduction to ELISA, pp. 1-29. *In* DM
Kemeny, SJ Challacombe (eds) ELISA and other solid phase immunoassays:
Theoretical and practical aspects. John Wiley & Sons, Chichester.

Kersten AE. 1996. Een organisatie van en voor onderzoekers. De Nederlandse
organisatie voor Zuiver-Wetenschappelijk Onderzoek (Z.W.O.) 1947-1988. Van
Gorcum & Comp. B.V., Assen.

Kievits T, Van Gemen B, Van Strijp D, Schukking R, Dircks M, Adriaanse H, Malek
L, Sooknanan R, Lens P. 1991. NASBA isothermal enzymatic invitro nucleic acid
amplification optimized for the diagnosis of HIV-1 infection. J Virol Methods
35:273-286.

Kirschner L. 1936. De Landskoepokinrichting en het Instituut Pasteur 1890-1935.
Geneesk Tijdschr Ned-Indië. Feestbundel:258-274.

Klein AJ, Hertzberger E. 1951. The manufacture of virus vaccine against influenza.
Philips Techn Rev 12(10):273-304.

Kluyver AJ. 1937. Life's fringes. Handelingen XXV[ste] Nederlandsch Natuur- en
Geneeskundig Congres 82.

Kluyver AJ. 1983. Beijerinck, the Microbiologist, pp. 99-154. *In* G van Iterson, LE
den Dooren de Jong, AJ Kluyver, Martinus Willem Beijerinck: His life and his
work. Science Tech, Madison, WI.

Knegtmans PJ. 2007. From Illustrious School to University of Amsterdam. Amsterdam University Press, Amsterdam.

Knudson AG. 1971. Mutation and cancer: Statistical study of retinoblastoma. Proc
Natl Acad Sci USA 68:820-823.

Köhler G, Milstein C. 1975. Continuous cultures of fused cells secreting antibody
of predefined specificity. Nature 256:495-497.

Kok GJPCM. 1957. Infectious respiratory diseases by adenoviruses among military
recruits using the cell culture technique. PhD thesis, Radboud University,
Nijmegen.

Kok PW, Leeuwenburg J, Tukei P, Van Wezel AL, Kapsenberg JG, Van Steenis G,
Galazka A, Robertson SE, Robinson D. 1992. Serological and virological assess-
ment of oral and inactivated poliovirus vaccines in a rural population in Kenya.
Bull Wld Hlth Org 70 (1):93-103.

Korteweg R. 1933. Experimenteel onderzoek aangaande de erfelijkheid van kanker. Ned Tijdschr Geneeskd 77:4034-4050.

Korteweg R. 1934a. Proefondervindelijke onderzoekingen aangaande erfelijkheid van kanker. Ned Tijdschr Geneeskd 78:240-242.

Korteweg R. 1934b. Chromosomale invloeden op den groei en extra-chromosomale invloeden op het ontstaan van kanker bij de muis. Ned Tijdschr Geneeskd 78:13.

Korteweg R. 1935. De vierde bijeenkomst van de Leeuwenhoekvereeniging gehouden te Amsterdam op 5, 6 en 7 juni 1935. Ned Tijdschr Geneeskd 79:5084.

Korteweg R. 1936a. De erfelijke factoren, welke de dispositie voor kanker van de borstklier bij de muis bepalen. Ned Tijdschr Geneeskd 80:4008-4014.

Korteweg R. 1936b. On the manner in which the disposition to carcinoma of the mammary gland is inherited in mice. Genetica 18:350-371.

Korteweg R. 1937a. Les facteurs hereditaires déterminants la predisposition au cancer de la mamelle chez la souris. Acta de l'Union Internationale contre le Cancer 2:136-143.

Korteweg R. 1937b. Nieuwe gezichtspunten op het gebied van het experimenteele kankeronderzoek. Ned Tijdschr Geneeskd 81:6154.

Korteweg R. 1946. Kanker van de borstklier bij de muis. Ned Tijdschr Geneeskd 90:780-783.

Korteweg R. 1948. Indrukken en gedachten naar aanleiding van een studiereis naar Amerika. Ned Tijdschr Geneeskd 92:1486-1489.

Kramer PH. 1930. Mededeelingen over pokken, naar aanleiding van 118 behandelde gevallen. Ned Tijdschr Geneeskd 74:2366-2382.

Kranendonk O. 1967. L'Institut d'Hygiène Tropicale, Amsterdam. Département de l'Institut Royal des Tropiques. Acta Trop. XXIV(2):151-157.

Kroes CM. 1922. Voorbehoeding tegen mazelen door serum-inspuiting. Ned Tijdschr Geneeskd 66:1746-1747.

Kropveld SM. 1923. Studies over den bacteriophaag tegen staphylocokken. Ned Tijdschr Geneeskd 67:1228-123.

Kruit P, Schapink FW, Geus JW, Verkleij AJ, Hulstaert CE. 1996. Electron microscopy in the Netherlands. 2.10B Developments since the 1950s, pp. 287-299. In T Mulvey (ed.) Advances in imaging and electron physics: The growth of electron microscopy. Academic Press, San Diego, CA.

Kühler KP. 1953. Jan van Geuns: zijn betekenis voor de geneeskundige wetenschap en het geneeskundig onderwijs. PhD thesis, University of Amsterdam.

Laidlaw PP. 1935. Epidemic influenza: A virus disease. Lancet 225(5828):1118-1124.

Lampe PHJ. 1927. Suriname. Sociaal-hygiënische beschouwingen. Koninklijke Vereeniging Koloniaal Instituut, Amsterdam. Mededeling no. XXIII, Afdeeling Tropische Hygiëne no. 14. Uitgave van het Instituut. Druk J.H. de Bussy, Amsterdam.

Lampe PHJ. 1936. De gezondheidszorg in Nederlandsch West-Indië. Geneesk Tijdschr Ned-Indië. Feestbundel:320-347.

Landsteiner K, Popper E. 1909. Uebertragung der Poliomyelitis acuta auf Affen. Z. Immunitatsforsch. Orig., 2:377-390.

Lange JMA. 1987. Serological markers in HIV infection. Rodopi, Amsterdam.

Lange JMA. 1993. HIV-related morbidity and mortality in sub-Saharan Africa: Opportunities for prevention. AIDS 7(12):1675-1676.

Langeveld JPM, Casal JI, Osterhaus ADME, Cortés E, Swart R de, Vela C, Dalsgaard K, Puijk WC, Schaaper WMM. Meloen R. 1994. First peptide vaccine providing protection against viral infection in the target animal: Studies of canine parvovirus in dogs. J Virol 68:4506-4513.

Lavigne R, Robben J. 2012. Professor Dr Richard Bruynoghe. Bacteriophage 2(1):1-4. DOI: 10.4161/bact.20024.

Lechevalier H. 1972. Dmitri Iosifovich Ivanovski (1864-1920). Bacteriological Reviews 36:135-145.

Lechevalier HA, Solotorovsky M. 1974. Three centuries of microbiology. Dover, New York.

Lee DN, Papes M, Van Den Bussche RA. 2012. Present and potential future distribution of common vampire bats in the Americas and the associated risk to cattle. PLoS ONE 7(8):e42466. DOI: 10.1371/journal.pone.0042466.

Le Goff J-M. 2011. Diffusion of influenza during the winter of 1889-1890 in Switzerland. Genus 67(2):77-99.

Le Goff J-M, Bühlmann F, Camenisch M, Giudici F, Tettamanti M. 2009. The diffusion of influenza in Switzerland in 1889-90. IUSSP, session 223, Marrakech.

Lelie PN, Reesink HW, De Jong-van Manen ST, Dees PJ, Reerink-Brongers EE. 1984. Immunogenicity and safety of a plasma-derived heat-inactivated hepatitis B vaccine (CLB). Studies in volunteers at a low risk of infection with hepatitis B virus. Am J Epidemiol 120:694-702.

Lennette EH, Halonen P, Murphy FA (eds). 1988. Laboratory diagnosis of infectious diseases: Principles and practice, Volume II: Viral, rickettsial and chlamydial diseases. Springer, New York.

Lennette EH, Schmidt NJ (eds). 1979. Diagnostic procedures for viral, rickettsial and chlamydial infections, 5th ed. American Public Health Association, Washington, DC.

Lenoir T. 1992. Laboratories, medicine and public life in Germany 1830-1849: Ideological roots of the institutional revolution, pp. 1-14. In A Cunningham, P Williams (eds) The laboratory revolution in medicine. Cambridge University Press, Cambridge.

Le Poole JB. 1947/1948. A new electron microscope with continuously variable magnification. Philips Techn Rev 9:33-45.

Lequin R. 2005. Enzyme Immunoassay (EIA)/Enzyme-Linked Immunosorbent Assay (ELISA). Clin Chem 51:2415-2418.

Lesterhuis J, Houwaart ES. 2000. Bringing the inbred-mouse to Europe: The Neth-
    erlands Cancer Institute within the context of international cancer research
    1913-1950. *In* WU Eckart (ed.) 100 Years of organized cancer research/100 Jahre
    organisierte Krebsforschung. Georg Thieme Verlag, Stuttgart.
Levaditi C. 1922. Ectodemoses neurotropes. Poliomyélite, encephalite, herpes.
    Masson et Cie, Éditeurs, Paris.
Lie KT. 1960. Poliomyelitis in Indonesia, a serological survey for neutralizing
    antibodies against polio viruses, 1957-1959. Trop Geogr Med 12:293-302.
Lindner U, Blume SS. 2006. Vaccine innovation and adoption: Polio vaccines in
    the UK, the Netherlands and West Germany, 1955-1965. Med Hist 50:425-446.
Lodder WJ, Vinjé J, Van der Heide R, De Roda Husman AM, Leenen EJ, Koopmans
    MP. 1999. Molecular detection of Norwalk-like caliciviruses in sewage. Appl
    Environ Microbiol 65(12):5624-5627.
Loeffler F, Frosch P. 1898. Berichte (I-III) der Kommission zur Erforschung der
    Maul- und Klauenseuche bei dem Institut für Infektionskrankheiten in Berlin.
    Zbl Bakt Parasitenkr I(23):371-391.
Löffler F, Frosch P. 1961/1898. Report of the commission for research on the foot-and-
    mouth disease., p. 152. *In* TD Brock (ed. and trans.) Milestones in microbiology,
    1546 to 1940. Prentice Hall International, London. Original: 1898.
Löwy, I. 1990. Variances in meaning in discovery accounts: The case of contemporary
    biology. Hist Stud Phys Biol Sci 21 (1):87-121.
Lustig A, Levine AJ. 1992. One hundred years of virology. J Virol 66:4629-4631.
Lutz H, Koopmans M, Osterhaus A, Rottier P. 2016. Prof. Dr Dr h.c. mult. Marian
    Horzinek, Obituary. http://www.abcdcatsvets.org/obituary/.
Luyendijk-Elshout AM, Van Heteren GM, De Knecht-van Eekelen A, Poulissen
    KJD (eds). 1989. Dutch medicine in the Malay Archipelago 1816-1942. Rodopi,
    Amsterdam.
Lvov DK. 1993. Centenary of virology, pp. 3-14. *In* BWH Mahy and DK Lvov (eds)
    Concepts in virology: From Ivanovsky to the present. Harwood Academic
    Publishers, Chur, Switzerland.
Lwoff A. 1957. The concept of virus: The Third Marjory Stephenson Memorial
    Lecture. J Gen Microbiol 17:239-253.
Lwoff A, Tournier P. 1966. The classification of viruses. Annu Rev Microbiol 20:45-74.

Maddox J. 1990. Dutch cure for AIDS is discredited. Nature 347:411.
Madeley CR. 1992. Virus diagnosis and the electron microscope, pp. 53-67. *In*
    AJ Scheffer (ed.) Liber amicorum voor prof. dr. J.B. Wilterdink. Universiteits-
    drukkerij, Groningen.
Madeley CR. 2001. Who needs clinical virologists anyway? Ned Tijdschr Med
    Microbiol 9:38-42.

Mahy BWJ. 1997. A dictionary of virology, 2nd ed. Academic Press, San Diego, CA.

Mandema E. 2002. Levensbericht A. Querido, pp. 73-82. *In* Levensberichten en herdenkingen, Amsterdam.

Masurel N. 1962. Studies on the content of haemagglutination inhibiting antibody for swine influenza virus A. PhD thesis, Leiden.

Masurel N. 1969. Serological characteristics of a 'new' serotype of influenza A virus: The Hong Kong strain. Bull Wld Hlth Org 41:461-468.

Masurel N. 1971. Adreswijziging Nationaal Influenza Centrum van de WHO. Ned Tijdschr Geneeskd 115:975.

Masurel N. 1979. Immunisatie van bejaarden met H1N1-influenzavirus bevattend subunit- en totaal-virusvaccin. Ned Tijdschr Geneeskd 123:196-199.

Masurel N, Anker WJ. 1978. Influenza A during the winter season 1977-78 caused by the 'old' H3N2-virus and the 'new' H1N1-virus. Ned Tijdschr Geneeskd 122(11):383-384.

Mathiot CC, Grimaud G, Garry P, Bouquety JC, Mada A, Daguisy AM, Georges AJ. 1990. An outbreak of human Semliki Forest virus infections in Central African Republic. Am J Trop Med Hyg 42:386-393.

Matijević M. 2011. Ein vergrößerndes Transfersystem für ein Cs-korrigiertes Phasenkontrast-Transmissions-Elektronenmikroskop. PhD dissertation, Eberhard-Karls-Universität.

Matthews REF. 1979. The classification and nomenclature of viruses: Summary of results of meetings of the International Committee on Taxonomy of Viruses in The Hague, September 1978. Intervirology 11:133-135.

Mayer A. 1942/1886. Concerning the mosaic disease of tobacco. Translated by J Johnson. Phytopathological Classics 7:11-24. Original: Über die Mosaikkrankenheit des Tabaks: Die landwirtschaftlichen Versuchs-Stationen 32:451-467.

Medisch Contact. 1958. Advertisement. Medisch Contact, nos 6 and 1.

Meijer van Putten JB. 1998. Prof. Dr A.J. van der Eb over adenovirussen en kanker. Ned Tijdschr Geneeskd 142(25):1478-1479.

Melief CJM, Scheper RJ, De Vries IJM. 2014. Scientific contributions toward successful cancer immunotherapy in the Netherlands. Immunology Letters 162:121-126.

Melnick JL. 1988. The picornaviruses, pp. 147-188. *In* F Fenner, A Gibbs (eds) Portraits of viruses: A history of virology. Karger, Basel.

Melnick JL, Rennick V, Molina Lozano MG. 1962. Serological epidemiology of poliomyelitis in Surinam. Arch Environm Hlth 4:202.

Meloen RH. 2001. Gerobotiseerde chemie, pp. 102-104. *In* H Bekkum, J Reedijk, S Rozendaal (eds). Chemie achter de dijken: Uitvindingen en uitvinders in de eeuw na Van 't Hoff. KNAW, KNCV, Amsterdam.

Meloen RH, Casall JI, Dalsgaard K, Langeveld JPM. 1995. Synthetic peptide vaccines: Success at last. Vaccine 13:885-886.

Meloen RH, Langeveld JPM, Schaaper WMM, Slootstra JW. 2001. Synthetic peptide vaccines: Unexpected fulfilment of discarded hope? Biologicals 29:233-236.

Mérieux C, Lambrichs LL. 1988. Charles Mérieux. Le virus de la découverte. Robert Laffont SA, Paris.

Méthot P-O. 2016. Writing the history of virology in the twentieth century: Discovery, disciplines, and conceptual change. Studies in History and Philosophy of Biological and Biomedical Sciences XXX:1-9.

Metselaar D. 1966. Isolation of arboviruses of group A and group C in Surinam. Trop Geogr Med 18:137-142.

Metselaar D. 1976. Selection of virulent poliovirus strains in developing countries? A hypothesis. Ned Tijdschr Geneeskd 120:1990-1995.

Metselaar D. 1977. Medical research in Kenya. I. Virology. Trop Geogr Med 29:S9-17.

Metselaar D. 1978. Poliomyelitis: Epidemiology and prophylaxis. 6. Geographic synchronism in poliomyelitis epidemics in Kenya. Bull Wld Hlth Org 56(4):649-651.

Metselaar D, Awan AM, Ensering HL. 1976. Acute haemorrhagic conjunctivitis and enterovirus 70 in Kenya. Trop Geogr Med 28(2):131-136.

Metselaar D, McDonald K, Gemert W, Nottay B, Muli JM. 1977a. Poliomyelitis: Epidemiology and prophylaxis 4. Serological and virological surveys conducted after a mass vaccination campaign for the control of a threatening poliomyelitis epidemic. Bull Wld Hlth Org 55(6):747-753.

Metselaar D, McDonald K, Gemert W, Van Rens MM, Muller AS. 1977b. Poliomyelitis: Epidemiology and prophylaxis 5. Results of a two- and three-dose vaccination experiment. Bull Wld Hlth Org 55(6):755-759.

Metselaar D, Robin Y. 1976. Akabane virus isolated in Kenya. Vet Rec 99(5):86.

Metselaar D, Simpson DIH. 1982. Practical virology, for medical students and practitioners in tropical countries. Oxford University Press, Oxford.

Metselaar D, Verlinde JD, Versteeg J. 1964a. Paramaribo virus: Properties of a group A arbovirus isolated from human blood in Surinam. Arch F gesamm Virusforsch XIV:336-343.

Metselaar D, Wilterdink JB, Verlinde JD. 1964b. Virological and serological observations made during the development and control of an outbreak of poliomyelitis in Surinam. Trop Geogr Med 2:129-134.

M'Fadyean J. 1900. African horse-sickness. J Comp Pathol Ther 13:1-20.

M'Fadyean J. 1908. The ultravisible viruses. J Comp Pathol Ther 21:232-242.

Middeldorp JM, Meloen RH. 1988. Epitope-mapping on the Epstein-Barr virus major capsid protein using systematic synthesis of overlapping oligopeptides. J Virol Methods 21:147-159.

Minister van Volksgezondheid, Welzijn en Sport. 2003. Kamerstukken. Brief van de minister van Volksgezondheid, Welzijn en Sport d.d. 27 mei 2003. KST68325, 0203tkkst28920-1. ISSN 0921-7371. Sdu Uitgevers, 's-Gravenhage 2003.

Mollaret HH. 1983. Contribution à la connaissance des relations entre Koch et Pasteur. NTM 20(1):57-65.

Moody HM, Quaedflieg PJ, Koole LH, Van Genderen MH, Buck HM, Smit L, Jurriaans S, Geelen JL, Goudsmit J. 1990. Inhibition of HIV-1 infectivity by phosphate-methylated DNA: Retraction. Science 250(4977):125-126.

Mortimer P. 2009. Classic paper: How monolayer cell culture transformed diagnostic virology: A review of a classic paper and the development that stemmed from it. Rev Med Virol 19:241-249.

Moscona A. 1952. Cell suspensions from organ rudiments of chick embryos. Exp Cell Res 3:535-539.

Mühlbock O. 1965. Note on a new inbred mouse-strain GR-A. Eur J Cancer 1(2):123-124.

Mühlbock O. 1968. Letter to executive committee of the Queen Wihlhelmina Fund, 23 February. Archive Nederlandse Kankerbestrijding/Koningin Wilhelmina Fonds te Amsterdam. 1968. Noord-Hollands Archief, Haarlem: 426, 295 and 296. Stukken betreffende de oprichting en samenstelling van de Studiegroep 'Oncogene Virussen'.

Mulder DW. 1996. The epidemiology of HIV-1 in a rural Uganda population. PhD thesis, Erasmus University.

Mulder J. 1937. Haemophilus influenza (Pfeiffer) als ubiquitaire verwekker van acute en chronische bronchitis. PhD dissertation, Groningen.

Mulder J. 1947. Influenza-onderzoek in Amerika. Ned Tijdschr Geneeskd 91:2767-2770.

Mulder J, Bijlmer L, Van Tuinen L. 1941. De antigene structuur van den in februari 1939 in Groningen geïsoleerde stam van influenza-virus. Ned Tijdschr Geneeskd 85:1743-1747.

Mulder J, Masurel N. 1958. Pre-epidemic antibody against 1957 strain of Asiatic influenza in serum of older people living in the Netherlands. Lancet 1(7025):810-814.

Mulder J, Van den Berg R, Van Kollem R. 1940. De influenza-epidemie van februari-maart 1939 in het garnizoen te Groningen. II (Bacteriologie). Ned Tijdschr Geneeskd 84:214-224.

Mulders M, Reimerink JHJ, Koopmans MGP, Van Loon AM, Van der Avoort HGAM. 1997. Genetic analysis of wild-type poliovirus importation into the Netherlands (1979-1995). J Infect Dis 176:617-624.

Muller AS, Ouma JH, Mburu FM, Blok PG, Kleevens JW. 1977. Machakos project studies. Agents affecting health of mother and child in a rural area of Kenya. I. Introduction: Study design and methodology. Trop Geogr Med 29:291-302.

Mullis KB. 1993. Nobel Lecture, 8 December. The Nobel Prize in Chemistry. NobelPrize.org. https://www.nobelprize.org/prizes/chemistry/1993/mullis/lecture/.

Munk K. 1995. Virologie in Deutschland. Die Entwicklung eines Fachgebietes. Karger, Basel.

Muntendam P. 1909. Spinale kinderverlamming in Nederland. Ned Tijdschr Geneeskd, 53:1170.

Müri W. 1986. Der Artz im Altertum. Artemis Verlag, München.

Murphy FA. 2018. The foundations of virology: Discoverers and discoveries, inventors and inventions, developers and technologies. Infinity Publishing, West Conshohocken, PA.

Murray WS, Little CC. 1935. The genetics of mammary tumor incidence in mice. Genetics 20:466-496.

Mutinelli F, Stankov S, Hristovski M, Seimenis A, Theoharakou H, Vodopija I. 2004. Rabies in Italy, Yugoslavia, Croatia, Bosnia, Macedonia, Albania and Greece. *In* AA King, AR Fooks, M Aubert, AI Wandeler (eds) Historical perspective of rabies in Europe and the Mediterranean Basin: A testament to rabies by Dr Arthur A. King. OIE, Paris.

Nakano J. 1979. Poxviruses, p. 267. *In* EH Lennette, NJ Schmidt (eds) Diagnostic procedures for viral, rickettsial and chlamydial infections, 5th ed. American Public Health Association, Washington, DC.

Nassy D. 1793. Epidemic disorder, prevalent in Philadelphia. M. Carey, Philadelphia, PA.

Nassy D de Isaac Cohen, Brandon SH, De Leon MP, De la Parra SJV, De la Parra J. 1789. Essai historique sur la colonie de Surinam. Hendrik Gartman, Amsterdam.

Nassy JG. 1918. Verduurzaming van 'Virus fixe' in verband met de bestrijding der hondsdolheid in de tropen [Preservation of 'virus fixe' with regard to the fight against rabies in the tropics]. PhD thesis, Amsterdam.

Nathanson N, Langmuir AD. 1963. The Cutter incident: Poliomyelitis following Formaldehyde-inactivated poliovirus vaccinationin the United States during the spring of 1955, II: Relation of poliomyelitis to the Cutter vaccine. Am J Hyg 78:29-60.

Nederlandse Kankerbestrijding/Koningin Wilhelmina Fonds te Amsterdam. 1968. Noord-Hollands Archief, Haarlem: 426, 701. Stukken betreffende de werkzaamheden van de FUNGO Deelwerkgemeenschap 'Persisterende virusinfecties en oncogenese', 1984-1989. NHA, Haarlem.

Netherlands Staten-Generaal. 1889. Handelingen Tweede Kamer. Verslag van de 24[e] vergadering, 10 December. Vel 116:446-449.

Netherlands Staten-Generaal. 1893. Handelingen Tweede Kamer. Verslag van de 26[e] vergadering, 14 December. Vel 128:481, 484, 495.

New York Times. 1923. Climbing Mount Everest is work for supermen. New York Times, 18 March.

Nicholson KG, Webster RG, Hay AJ. 1998. Textbook of influenza. Blackwell Science Ltd., Oxford.

Niesters HG. 2002. Clinical virology in real time. J Clin Virol 25 Suppl 3:S3-12.

Nieuwenhuis I. 2014. Onder het mom van satire. Laster spot en ironie in Nederland, 1780-1800. Verloren, Hilversum.

NKI-AVL Annual Reports (A). 1914-1968. Jaarverslag Vereeniging Het Nederlands Kankerinstituur. Netherlands Cancer Institute, Amsterdam.

NKI-AVL Annual Reports (B). 1969-1996. Jaarverslag Vereniging Het Nederlands Kanker Instituut, Stichting Antoni van Leeuwenhoek Ziekenhuis, vols 56 to 83.

NKI-AVL Annual Reports (C). 1997-2005. Jaarverslag Het Nederlands Kanker Instituut-Antoni van Leeuwenhoek Ziekenhuis.

NKI-AVL Annual Reports (D). 1974-1995. Annual Report. The Netherlands Cancer Institute: Cancer Research Laboratory, and Cancer Hospital.

NKI-AVL Annual Reports (E). 1996-2000. Scientific Report. The Netherlands Cancer Institute: Cancer Research Laboratory and Cancer Hospital.

NKI-AVL Annual Reports (F). 2001-2017. Scientific Annual Report. The Netherlands Cancer Institute: Cancer Research Laboratory and Cancer Hospital.

NKI-AVL Annual Reports (G). 1979-1996. Werkplannen. Het Nederlands Kanker Instituut-Antoni van Leeuwenhoek Ziekenhuis.

NKI-AVL Annual Reports (H). 1996-1997. Scientific Program. The Netherlands Cancer Institute – Cancer Research Laboratory and Cancer Hospital.

Nobel Foundation. N.d. a. Arne Tiselius – Nominations. NobelPrize.org. https://www.nobelprize.org/prizes/chemistry/1948/tiselius/nominations/, latest access October 2019.

Nobel Foundation. N.d. b. Ernest W. Goodpasture. Nobel Prize.org. http://www.nobelprize.org/nomination/archive/show_people.php?id=3545, latest access October 2019.

Nobel Foundation. N.d. c. The Svedberg: Biographical. NobelPrize.org. https://www.nobelprize.org/prizes/chemistry/1926/svedberg/biographical/, latest access October 2019.

Nolen W. 1889. Influenza (Griep). Ned Tijdschr Geneeskd 33:772-774.

Nusse R. 1980. Mouse mammary tumour virus proteins: mechanism of synthesis and antigenic expression in experimental animals. Academic thesis, University of Amsterdam.

Nusse R, Varmus H. 1982. Many tumors induced by the mouse mammary tumor virus contain a provirus integrated in the same region of the host genome. Cell 31:99-109.

Nusse R, Varmus H. 2012. Three decades of Wnts: A personal perspective on how a scientific field developed. EMBO J 31:2670-2684.

Office for National Statistics. 2017. Overview of the UK population: November 2015.

Offit PA. 2005. The Cutter incident, 50 years later. N Engl J Med 352(14):1411-1412.

Offringa C. 1971. Van Gildestein naar Uithof: 150 jaar diergeneeskundig onderwijs in Utrecht, deel I. s'Rijksveeartsenijschool (1821-1918). Veeartsenijkundige Hoogeschool (1918-1925). Rijksuniversiteit te Utrecht. Faculteit der Diergeneeskunde, Utrecht.

Offringa C. 1981. Van Gildestein naar Uithof: 150 jaar diergeneeskundig onderwijs in Utrecht, deel II. Faculteit der veeartsenijkunde (1925-1956). Faculteit der diergeneeskunde (1956-1971). Rijksuniversiteit te Utrecht. Faculteit der diergeneeskunde van de Rijksuniversiteit te Utrecht.

Oostvogel PM, Van Wijngaarden JK, Van der Avoort HG, Mulders MN, Conyn-van Spaendonck MA, Rümke HC, Van Steenis G, Van Loon AM. 1994. Poliomyelitis outbreak in an unvaccinated community in the Netherlands, 1992-1993. Lancet 344:665-670.

Osterhaus AD, Yang H, Spijkers HE, Groen J, Teppema JS, Van Steenis G. 1985. The isolation and partial characterization of a highly pathogenic herpesvirus from the harbor seal (Phoca vitulina). Arch Virol 86:239-251.

Osterhaus AD, Groen J, De Vries P, UytdeHaag FG, Klingeborn B, Zarnke R. 1988. Canine distemper virus in seals. Nature 35:403-404.

Osterhaus AD, Vos MC, Balk AH, De Man RA, Mouton JW, Rothbarth PH, Schalm SW, Tomaello AM, Niesters HG, Verbrugh HA. 1998. Transmission of hepatitis B virus among heart transplant recipients during endomyocardial biopsy procedures. J Heart Lung Transplant 17(2):158-166.

Osterhaus ADME, Vedder EJ. 1988. Identification of virus causing recent seal deaths. Nature 335:20.

Osterholm MT, Kelley NS, Sommer A, Belongia EA. 2012. Efficacy and effectiveness of influenza vaccines: A systematic review and meta-analysis. Lancet Infect Dis 12:36-44.

Otten L. 1926. Droge vaccine. Geneesk Tijdschr Ned-Indië 66:642-670.

Otten L. 1927. Trockenlymphe. Z Hyg Infektionskr 107:677-696.

Otten L. 1947. Investigations into rabies II. Antonie van Leeuwenhoek 13:101-127.

Otten-van Stockum MJ. 1941. Rabies research in the Netherlands Indies. Mededelingen van den Dienst der Volksgezondheid in Nederlandsch-Indië 30: 269-279.

Oudschans Dentz F. 1943. Maatregelen tegen de pokken en de toepassing van Jenner's koepokstof in Suriname in het begin van de negentiende eeuw. Ned Tijdschr Geneeskd 87 II (23):1020-1021.

Packard R. 2016. 'Break-bone' fever in Philadelphia, 1780: Reflections on the history of disease. Bull Hist Med 90:193-221.

Pais A. 1982. The science and the life of Albert Einstein. Oxford University Press, Oxford.

Palm L. 1999. Christiaan Eijkman 1858-1930. *In* K van Berkel, A van Helden, L Palm (eds) A history of science in the Netherlands: Survey, themes and reference. Brill, Leiden.

Parkin DM. 2006. The global health burden of infection-associated cancers in the year 2002. Int J Cancer 118:3030-3044. http://dx.doi.org/10.1002/ijc.21731.

Parsons HF. 1891a. The influenza epidemics 1889-90 and 1891 and their distribution in England and Wales. Br Med J 2(1597):303-308.

Parsons HF. 1891b. Report on the epidemic of 1889-90. HMSO, London.

Pasteur L. 1882. Discours de réception de M. Pasteur prononcé dans la séance publique du 24 avril 1882, en venant prendre sa place de M. Littré. Académie Française. Imprimerie de l'Institut de France, 1885.

Patterson KD, Pyle GF. 1991. The geography and mortality of the 1918 influenza pandemic. Bull Hist Med 65(1):4-21.

Paul JR. 1971. A history of poliomyelitis. Yale University Press, New Haven, CT.

Peeters MF. 2001. 50 Jaar Bacteriologisch-Serologisch Laboratorium. De geschiedenis van het Laboratorium voor Medische Microbiologie en Immunologie. Tilburg.

Pekelharing CA. 1909. Toespraak gehouden bij de opening van het 12[de] Nederlands Natuur- en Geneeskundig Congres te Utrecht. Ned Tijdschr Geneeskd 53:1244-1256.

Pereira HG, Huebner RJ, Ginsberg HS, Van der Veen J. 1963. A short description of the adenovirus group. Virology 20(4):613-620.

Pereira MS. 1986. 40 Years of virology in the PHLS, pp. 6-13. *In* PP Mortimer (ed.) Public health virology: 12 reports. Public Health Laboratory Service, London.

Persing DH, Landry ML. 1989. In vitro amplification techniques for the detection of nucleic acids: New tools for the diagnostic laboratory. Yale J Biol Med 62:159-171.

Pfeiffer R. 1892a. I – Preliminary communication on the exciting causes of influenza. Br Med J 1 (1620):128.

Pfeiffer R. 1892b. Vorläuffiger Mitteilungen über den Erreger der Influenza. Dtsch Med Wochenschr 18:28.

Pharmaletter. 2000. Dutch firms IntroGene and U-BiSys merge. Pharmaletter, 3 July. https://www.thepharmaletter.com/article/dutch-firms-introgene-and-u-bisys-merge.

PharmaTimes. 2006. Crucell expands in vaccines with SBL buy. PharmaTimes, 21 November. http://www.pharmatimes.com/news/crucell_expands_in_vaccines_with_sbl_bu.

Pinkster H. 2003. Woordenboek Latijn/Nederlands. Tweede herziene druk. Amsterdam University Press, Amsterdam.

Ploem JS. 1976. The use of vertical illuminator with interchangeable dichroic illuminators for fluorescence microscopy with incident light. Z wiss Mikrosk 68:129.

Plotkin SA, Vidor E. 2008. Poliovirus vaccine-inactivated, p. 605. *In* S Plotkin, W Orenstein, P Offit (eds) Vaccines, 5th ed. Saunders Elsevier, Amsterdam.

Polak MF. 1944/1945. Vraagstukken der gele koorts. Epidemiologie en vaccinatie. Noord-Hollandsche Uitgevers Maatschappij, Amsterdam.

Polak MF. 1964. Voorbehoedende behandeling tegen rabies in het jaar 1886. Ned Tijdschr Geneeskd 108:36-40.

Polak MF, Beunders BJ, Van der Werff AR, Sanders EW, Van Klaveren JN, Brans LM. 1963. A comparative study of clinical reaction observed after application of several smallpox vaccines in primary vaccination of young adults. Bull Wld Hlth Org 29:311-322.

Polak MF, Brans LM. 1962. Onderzoek naar het succes der pokkenvaccinatie bij zuigelingen. Ned Tijdschr Geneeskd 106:1793-1799.

Polak MF, Swart-van der Hoeven JT, Smeenk C, Pel JZS, Van Stalborch WC, Pasdeloup F. 1964. Vergelijking van twee vaccinia-stammen bij enting van zuigelingen. Ned Tijdschr Geneeskd 108:458-465.

Pondman A. 1952. Oorzaak en verspreiding, serologische diagnose en prophylaxe van vlektyphus. Ned Tijdschr Geneeskd 96:926-931.

Porter JA. 1973. Some correspondence of Pasteur. ASM News 39:8-15.

Potter CW. 1998. Chronicle of influenza pandemics. In KG Nicholson, RG Webster, AJ Hay (eds) Textbook of influenza. Blackwell Science Ltd., Oxford.

Prakken JR. 1975. Een scheepschirurgijn over chocolaadziekten. Ned Tijdschr Geneeskd 119:198-201.

Proust A. 1892. Rapport sur l'enquête concernant l'épidémie de grippe de 1884-1890. Bulletin de l'Académie de Médicine:510-531 and 552-596.

Proust M. 1981. Remembrance of things past, Volume 3: Time regained. Translated by CK Scott Moncrieff, T Kilmartin, A Mayor. Chatoo & Windus, London.

Proust M. 1986. A la recherche du temps perdu. Le temps retrouvé. Édition du texte par Bernard Brun. GF Flammarion, Paris.

QCMD. N.d. Quality Control for Molecular Diagnostics website. https://www.qcmd. org/, latest access August 2019.

Quanjer AAJ. 1921. De griep in Nederland, 1918 tot 1920. Centrale Gezondheidsraad, 's Gravenhage.

Querido A. 1971. Mechanisms for the conservation and efficient use of iodine in man. In J Monod, E Borek (eds) Les microbes et la vie/Of microbes and life. Columbia University Press, New York.

Querido A. 1990. De binnenkant van de geneeskunde, een autobiografie. Meulenhoff, Amsterdam.

Quinn TC. 2001. AIDS in Africa: A retrospective. Bull Wld Hlth Org 79:1156-1158.

Quint WGV. Endogenous murine leukaemia viruses: germline transmission and involvement in generation of recombinant viruses. Academic Thesis, Radboud University, Nijmegen, 1984.

Raben R. 2013. A new Dutch imperial history? Low Countries Historical Review 128:5-30.

Rahamat-Langendoen J. 2008. De constructie van influenza tijdens influenzaepidemieën in Nederland 1880-1970. MA thesis, VUmc, Amsterdam.

Reed W, Carroll J, Agramonte A, Lazear JW. 1900. The etiology of yellow fever: A preliminary note. Public Health Papers and Reports 26:37-53.

Reerink-Brongers EE, Lelie PN, Reesink HW, Dees PJ, Brummelhuis HGJ, Van Aken WG. 1983. Immunogenicity and safety of heat-inactivated hepatitis B vaccine (CLB) in low risk human volunteers and in patients treated with chronic haemodialysis in the Netherlands. Second WHO/IABS Symposium on viral hepatitis: Standardization in immunoprophylaxis of infections by hepatitis viruses, Athens, Greece, 1982. Develop Biol Standard 54:197-203.

Remlinger P. 1903. Le passage du virus rabique à travers les filtres. Ann Inst Pasteur, Paris 17:834-849.

Rhazes. 1848. A treatise on the small pox and measles, by Abu Becr Mohammed Ibn Zacariya Ar-Razi (commonly called Rhazes). Translated by William Alexander Greenhill. Sydenham Society, London.

Rida A. 1964. La paralysie infantile aux temps de pharaons. Cahiers d'Alexandrie, série II, fascicule 4:69-77.

Riddiough MA, Sisl JE, Bell JC. 1983. Influenza vaccination. JAMA 249:3189-3195.

Rigter RBM. 1992. Met raad en daad. De geschiedenis van de Gezondheidsraad 1902-1985, PhD thesis, Erasmus University.

Rigter R. 1996. De integratie van preventieve gezondheidszorg in Nederland (1890-1940). Gewina 19:313-327.

Rivers TM. 1927. Filterable viruses: A critical review. J Bacteriol 14:217-258.

Rivers TM. 1932. The nature of viruses. Physiological Reviews 12(3):423-452.

Rivers TM, Horsfall FL. 1959. Viral and rickettsial infections of man, 3rd ed. J.B. Lippincott, Philadelphia, PA.

RIVM. 1988. Berichten uit het RIVM. 1989. Rijksinstituut voor Volksgezondheid en Milieu (RIVM), Bilthoven.

RIVM. 2014. Vaccinatiegraad. Rijksvaccinatieprogramma Nederland. Verslagjaar 2014. Report no. 150202003. Rijksinstituut voor Volksgezondheid en Milieu (RIVM), Bilthoven.

Rodhain F, Ardoin P, Metselaar D, Salmon AM, Hannoun C. 1975. An epidemiologic and serologic study of arboviruses in Lake Rudolf basin. Trop Geogr Med 27(3):307-312.

Rose W. 1914. Yellow fever: Feasibility of its eradication. October 27, 1914, Hench Reed collection, Historical collections, CMHSL, University of Virginia, http://etext. lib.virginia.edu/etcbin/fever-browse?id=00757001, latest access 25 July 2012.

Rosen G. 1993/1958. A history of public health. Johns Hopkins University Press, Baltimore MD. Original edition: 1958.

Rothbarth PH, Diepersloot RJ, Metselaar HJ, Nooyen Y, Velzing J, Weimar W. 1987. Rapid demonstration of cytomegalovirus in clinical specimens. Infection 15:228-231.

Rothbarth PH, Habova JKJ, Masurel N. 1988. Rapid diagnosis of infections caused by respiratory syncytial virus. Infection 16:252.

Rous P. 1911. A sarcoma of the fowl transmissible by an agent separable from the tumor cells. J Exp Med 13(4):397-411.

Rous P, Kidd JG, Beard JW. 1936. Observations on the relation of the virus causing rabbit papillomas to the cancers deriving therefrom: I. The influence of the host species and of the pathogenic activity and concentration of the virus. J Exp Med 64(3):385-400.

Roux E. 1903. Sur les microbes dits invisibles. Bull Inst Pasteur 1:7-12.

Roux E, Yersin A. 1888. Contribution à l'étude de la diphtérie. Annales de l'Institut Pasteur 2(12):629-661.

Rubin H. 2011. The early history of tumor virology: Rous, RIF, and RAV. Proc Natl Acad Sci USA 108:14389-14396.

Ruijsch WP, Van Asch van Wijck HAM. 1915. Inenting tegen dollehondsbeet. Ned Tijdschr Geneeskd 59:625.

Ruitenberg EJ. 1984. Vaccinbereiding. Micro-organismen in macro produktie. Natuur & Techniek 52:978-991.

Rümke HC, Cohen HH. 1996. In memoriam Ch.A. Hannik. Ned Tijdschr Geneeskd 140:579.

Rümke HC, Oostvogel PM, Van Steenis G, Van Loon AM. 1995. Poliomyelitis in the Netherlands: a review of population immunity and exposure between the epidemics in 1978 and 1992. Epidemiol Infect 115:289-298.

Rümke HC, Visser HKA. 2004. Vaccinaties op de kinderleeftijd anno 2004. I. Effectiviteit en acceptatie van het Rijksvaccinatieprogramma. Ned Tijdschr Geneeskd 148:356-363.

Ruska E. 1987. The development of the electron microscope and of the electron microscopy. Biosci Rep 7(8):607-629.

Ruska H, Von Borries B, Ruska E. 1939/1940. Die Bedeutung der Übermikroskopie für Virusforschung. Arch gesamte Virusforsch 1:155-169.

Rutten W. 1997. De vreselijkste aller harpijen. Pokkenepidemieën in Nederland in de 18e en 19e eeuw. HES Uitgevers, Houten.

Rutten W. 2010. Dreigen, dwingen, verleiden en belonen. Het succes achter de pokkenvaccinatie in de negentiende eeuw, pp. 29-46. In J van Steenbergen, CT Bakker (eds) Infectieziektenbestrijding, het leeft onder de bevolking. Maatschappelijke aspecten van de infectieziektebestrijding vroeger en nu. Het Zuiden, Hoensbroek.

Ruys AC. 1960. In memoriam Prof. Dr W.A. Collier. Ned Tijdschr Geneeskd 104:2199-2200.

Sabin A. 1957. Letter from Sabin, Albert B. to Verlinde, J.D. dated 1957-04-09. University of Cincinnati, Hauck Center for the Albert B. Sabin Archives.

Salzmann, JG. 1734. Dissertatio medica sistens plurium pedis musculorum defectus. Argentorati: Johannis Henrici Heitzii.

Sanders EJ, Messele T, Wolday D, Dorigo-Zetsma W, WoldeMichael T, Geyid A, Coutinho R. 2003. Development of research capability in Ethiopia: The Ethio-Netherlands AIDS Research Project (ENARP), 1994-2002: Achievements, scientific findings and project goals. Ethiop Med J 41, Suppl 1:11-23.

Sanders EJ, Rinke de Wit TF, Fontanet AL, Goudsmit J, Miedema F, Coutinho RA. 2001. Ethiopia-Netherlands AIDS research project. Ned Tijdschr Geneeskd 145:1261-1265.

Sankaran N, Van Helvoort T. 2016. Andrewes's Christmas fairy tale: Atypical thinking about cancer aetiology in 1935. Notes Rec R Soc Lond 70(2):175-201. DOI: 10.1098/rsnr.2015.0062.

Sas GJ. 1954. Klinische en epidemiologische waarnemingen tijdens de pokkene-pidemie te Tilburg in 1951. PhD thesis, Leiden University. Drukkerij Antoine, Geertruidenberg.

Scheltema Beduin L. 1886. Berichten Binnenland. Ned Tijdschr Geneeskd 30:470-471.

Scherer WF, Syverton JT, Gey GO. 1953. Studies on the propagation in vitro of poliomyelitis viruses. J Exp Med 97(5):695-710.

Schim van der Loeff MF. 2003. HIV-2 in West Africa: Epidemiological studies. PhD thesis, University of Amsterdam.

Schimmel WC. 1889. Rabies in Nederlandsch-Indië. Ned Tijdschr Geneeskd 33:733.

Schippers EI. 2016. Uitwerking voornemen verzelfstandiging Intravacc. Brief van de minister aan de Tweede Kamer. Kenmerk: 1061393-159046-BPZ, 22 December. Den Haag.

Schippers JC. 1925. Voorbehoeding tegen mazelen door het inspuiten van reconvalescenten-serum. Ned Tijdschr Geneeskd 69:2328-2330.

Schirm J, Luijt DS, Pastoor GW, Mandema JM, Schröder FP. 1992. Rapid detection of respiratory viruses using mixtures of monoclonal antibodies on shell vial cultures. J Med Virol 38:147-151.

Schirm J, Timmerije W, Van der Bij W, The TH, Wilterdink JB, Tegzess AM, Van Son WJ, Schröder FP. 1987. Rapid detection of infectious cytomegalovirus in blood with the aid of monoclonal antibodies. J Med Virol 23:31-40.

Schmidt NJ. 1979. Cell culture techniques for diagnostic virology, pp. 65-141. In EH Lennette, NJ Schmidt (eds) Diagnostic procedures for: viral, rickettsial and chlamydial infections, 5th ed. American Public Health Association, Washington, DC.

Schmiedebach HP. 1999. The Prussian state and microbiological research. Friedrich Loeffler and his approach to the 'invisible virus'. In CH Calisher, MC Horzinek (eds.), 100 years of virology: The birth and growth of a discipline. Springer, Vienna, New York.

Scholthof K-BG, Shaw JG, and Zaitlin M. 1999. Tobacco Mosaic Virus: One Hundred Years of Contributions to Virology. American Phytopathological Society Press, St Paul, MN.

Schoute D. 1935a. Enkele volksplagen in het verleden van Nederlandsch-Indië. I. Pokken. Ned Tijdschr Geneeskd 79:42-57.

Schoute D. 1935b. Enkele volksplagen in het verleden van Nederlandsch-Indië. V. De bestrijders der plagen. Ned Tijdschr Geneeskd 79:2089-2106.

Schoute D. 1942. De reis van Jenner's koepokstof van Europa naar Oost-Azië. Ned Tijdschr Geneeskd 86 III (36):2229-2233.

Schreuder BEC, Van Keulen LJM, Vromans MEW, Langeveld JPM, Smits MA. 1996. Preclinical test for prion diseases. Nature 381:563.

Schröder FP. 1992. Van CBR tot PCR. In AJ Scheffer (ed.) Liber amicorum voor prof. dr. J.B. Wilterdink. Universiteitsdrukkerij, Groningen.

Schüffner W. 1913. Pseudotyphus in Deli. Ned Tijdschr Geneeskd 57:1141-1144.

Schuitemaker H, Kootstra NA, De Goede RE, de Wolf F, Miedema F, Tersmette M. 1991. Monocytotropic human immunodeficiency virus type 1 (HIV-1) variants detectable in all stages of HIV-1 infection lack T-cell line tropism and syncytium-inducing ability in primary T-cell culture. J Virol 65(1):356-363.

Schultz EW. 1948. The present status of viruses and virus diseases. JAMA 136:1075-1079.

Shope RE. 1931. Swine influenza. III. Filtration experiments and aetiology. J Exp Med 54:373-385.

Shope RE, Francis T. 1936. The susceptibility of swine to the virus of human influenza. J Exp Med 64(5):791-801.

Shope RE. 1951. The provocation of masked swine influenza virus by infection with human influenza virus. Tijdschrift voor Diergeneeskunde 76:414-420.

Simons RDGP. 1947. Een Collegium Medicum van 1781 in Suriname. Ned Tijdschr Geneeskd 93(I):340-342.

Singh Abhay Kumar. 2006. Modern World System and Indian Proto-Industrialization: Bengal 1650-1800 (2006), p. 682.

SKMS. 1990. Jaarverslag. Personal Archive GJJ van Doornum.

Sluiter E. 1949. Werkgemeenschap voor Weefselkweek. Ned Tijdschr Geneeskd 93:3366.

Smadel JE. 1948. The practitioner and the virus diagnostic laboratory. J Am Med Assoc 136:1079-1081.

Smith GF. 2018. Marjory Stephenson Lecture. https://microbiologysociety.org/ grants/prize-lectures/marjory-stephenson-prize-lecture.html.

Smith PG, Muller L. 2000. Daan Mulder Memorial Symposium-Introduction. Tropical Medicine and International Health 5:A1-A2.

Smith W, Andrewes CH, Laidlaw PP. 1933. A virus obtained from influenza patients. Lancet II:66-68.

Smith Hughes S. 1977. The virus: A history of the concept. Heinemann Educational Books, London/Science History Publications, New York.

Snapper I, Wolff LK. 1919. De bacteriologie van de grieppneumonie. Ned Tijdschr Geneeskd 63:1483-1488.

Snijders EP. 1925. De wisselwerking van de westersche en de tropische geneeskunde in den loop harer ontwikkeling. Inaugural Lecture. Drukkerij Portielje, Amsterdam.

Snijders EP. 1946. In memoriam Prof. Dr. P.C. Flu. Ned Tijdschr Geneeskd 90:40.

Snijders EP, Polak MF, Hoekstra J. 1947. Jungle yellow fever in Surinam. Trans R Soc Trop Med Hyg 40(6):861-868.

Sohier R. 1964. Diagnostic des maladies à virus. Editions Médicales Flammarion, Paris.

Song R, Guan S, Lee SS, Chen Z, Chen C, Han L, Xu Y, Li A, Zeng H, Ye H, Zhang F. 2018. Late or lack of vaccination linked to importation of yellow fever from Angola to China. Emerg Infect Dis 24(7). DOI: 10.3201/eid2407.171868.

Speijer N. 1946. De poliomyelitisepidemie in het 'Kamp Westerbork' augustus-december 1943. Ned Tijdschr Geneeskd 90:130-135.

Sprenger MJW, Masurel N. 1992. Influenzavaccinatie en de Postbus51-campage. Ned Tijdschr Geneeskd 136:1968-1970.

Staff Roscoe B. Jackson Memorial Laboratory, Little CC. 1933. The existence of non-chromosomal influence in the incidence of mammary tumors in mice. Science 78(2029):465-4667. DOI: 10.1126/science.78.2029.465.

Stanley WM. 1935. Isolation of a crystalline protein possessing the properties of tobacco-mosaic virus. Science 81:644-645.

Stanley WM. 1938. The nature of viruses. Trans N Y Acad Sci 1 (2 Series II):21-24.

Stenfert Kroese HE. 1999. In memoriam mr.dr. M.F. Polak. Ned Tijdschr Geneeskd 143:756-757.

Stephan BH. 1885. Over de aetiologie der tabes dorsalis. Ned Tijdschr Geneeskd 29:1057-1066.

Stephan BH. 1895. Epidemieën van acute kinder-paralyse. Ned Tijdschr Geneeskd 39:1216.

Stichting Bibliotheek van het Boekenvak bij de Amsterdamse Universiteitsbibliotheek – Bijzondere Collecties. 2007. Jaarverslag 2005-2006. Amsterdam.

Stirk PR, Griffiths PD. 1988. Comparative sensitivity of three methods for the diagnosis of cytomegalovirus lung infection. J Virol Methods 20:133-142.

Stoel G. 1931. De weefselcultuur in vitro als hulpmiddel in de bacteriologie. PhD thesis, Amsterdam. G. Naeff, 's-Gravenhage.

Stoker M. 1967. Aspects of medical virology. Br Med Bull 23(2):105-108.

Straub M. 1889. Brieven uit Parijs. I. Het Instituut Pasteur. Ned Tijdschr Geneeskd 33:709-712.

Summers WC. 1999. D'Herelle and the origins of molecular biology. Yale University Press, New Haven, CT.

Suurhoff JG. 1957. Vragen, door de leden der Kamer gesteld overeenkomstig artikel 75 van het Reglement van Orde, en de daarop door de Regering schriftelijk gegeven antwoorden. Antwoord van de heer Suurhoff, Minister van Sociale Zaken en Volksgezondheid (ingezonden 29 juni 1957). Aanhangsel tot het Verslag van de Handelingen der Eerste Kamer, p. 3027.

Suzor JR. 1888. Exposé practique du traitement de la rage par la méthode Pasteur. Maloine, Paris.

Swellengrebel NH. 1955. Emilius Paulus Snijders, 1885-24 oktober 1955. Ned Tijdschr Geneeskd 99:3174-3176.

Symposium 'Het ultrafiltreerbare virus'. 1939. Nederlandse Vereniging voor Biochemie, 1 juli 1939 te Wageningen. Chemisch Weekblad 36(40):684-688.

Symposium over virussen. 1948. Nederlandse Vereniging voor Biochemie. 13 december 1947 en 14 februari 1948. D.B. Centen's Uitgevers-Maatschappij N.V., Amsterdam.

Sypkens Smit JH. 1953. Leven en werken van Matthias van Geuns M.D. 1735-1817. PhD thesis, University of Groningen. Van Gorcum & Comp. N.V.-G.A. Hak and Dr H.J. Prakke, Assen.

Tausk M. 1978. Organon. De geschiedenis van een bijzondere Nederlandse onderneming. Dekker & van de Vegt, Nijmegen.

Tellegen AOH. 1879. Waarom moeten bepalingen voor mazelen in de Wet van 4 december 1872 staatsblad N. 134 worden gewijzigd en op welke wijze dient dit te geschieden? Ned Tijdschr Geneeskd 23:370-373.

Temin HM, Mizutani S. 1970. RNA-directed DNA polymerase in virions of Rous sarcoma virus. Nature 226:1211-1213.

Temin HM, Rubin H. 1958. Characteristics of an assay for Rous sarcoma virus and Rous sarcoma cells in tissue culture. Virology 6(3):669-688.

Tersmette M, De Goede RE, Al BJ, Winkel IN, Gruters RA, Cuypers HT, Huisman HG, Miedema F. 1988. Differential syncytium-inducing capacity of human immunodeficiency virus isolates: Frequent detection of syncytium-inducing isolates in patients with acquired immunodeficiency syndrome (AIDS) and AIDS-related complex. J Virol 62:2026-2032.

Tersteeg J. 1998. De levensschets van Geert Reinders, 1737-1815. Stichting Historische Uitgaven Winsum-Obergum, Winsum.

Théodoridès J. 1986. Histoire de la rage: Cave canem. Masson, Paris.

Théodoridès J. 1989. Pasteur and rabies: The British connection. J R Soc Med 82:488-490.

Thomas S, Ballot AM. 1918. [No title], pp. 83-84. *In* PC Molhysen, PJ Blok (eds) Nieuw Nederlandsch Biografisch Woordenboek, Deel 4. A.W. Sijthoff's Uitgeversmaatschappij, Leiden.

Thomassen à Thuessink EJ. 1822. Verslag over het al of niet besmettelijke der Gele Koorts, vooral in betrekking tot het werk van den Franschen geneeskundigen Devèze. Eerste Klasse van het Koninklijk-Nederlandsche Instituut van Wetenschappen, Letterkunde en Schoone Kunsten, Pieper en Ipenbuur, n.l.

Thomson AL. 1987. Preventive medicine: Infections and infestations, pp. 108-136. *In* AL Thomson, Half a century in medical research, Vol. 2: The programme of the Medical Research Council (UK). Edward Arnold, London.

Thomson WAR. 1957. Chair of virology. Can Med Ass J 77:62.

Thung TH. 1957. Het virologisch onderzoek aan de Landbouwhogeschool, Wageningen. Tijdschrift Over Plantenziekten 63:209-221.

Tukei PM. 1988. Epidemiology and epizootiological investigations of hemorrhagic fever viruses in Kenia. Final report, 1988. Virus Research Center, Kenya Medical Research Institute, Nairobi, Kenya.

Twort F. 1915. An investigation on the nature of ultramicroscopic viruses. Lancet 11:1241.

Tyndall J. 1882. Essays on the floating-matter of the air in relation to putrefaction and infection. D. Appleteon and Co., New York.

Tyrrell D. 1998. Discovery of influenza viruses, p. 21-23. *In* KG Nicholson, RG Webster, AJ Hay (eds) Textbook of influenza. Blackwell Science Ltd, Oxford.

Union of International Associations. N.d. Yearbook of International Organizations. https://uia.org/ybio, latest access July 2018.

University of Glasgow. N.d. Website. https://www.universitystory.gla.ac.uk, latest access August 2019.

Utrechts Geneeskundig Gezelschap 'Matthias van Geuns'. N.d. a. Het Utrechts Archief, Utrecht. Toegangsnummer 713-12; inv. nr. 10-14. http://www.hetutrechtsarchief.nl/.

Utrechts Geneeskundig Gezelschap 'Matthias van Geuns'. N.d. b. Het Utrechts Archief, Utrecht. Toegangsnummer 713-12; inv. nr. 31-47. http://www.hetutrechtsarchief.nl/.

Vallery-Radot R. 1901. The life of Pasteur. London.

Van Andel MA. 1931. Introduction. *In*: Bontius J. 1931. Tropische geneeskunde/On tropical Medicine. Edited by MA van Andel. Opuscula Selecta Neerlandicorum De Arte Medica, no. 10.

Van Andel MA. 1947. Chirurgijns, vrije meesters, beunhazen en kwakzalvers. Tweede druk. P.N. van Kampen & Zoon N.V. Amsterdam.

Van Bergen L. 2007. Van koloniale geneeskunde tot internationale gezondheidszorg. KIT Publishers, Amsterdam.

Van Bergen L. 2009. De oprichting van de 'Nederlandsche Vereeniging voor Tropische Geneeskunde': een zaak van nationaal belang. Studium 2(2):92-104.

Van Berkel K. 2015. Petrus Camper and the limits of the Enlightment. *In* K van Berkel, B Ramakers (eds) Petrus Camper in context: Science, the arts, and society in the eighteenth-century Dutch Republic. Verloren, Hilversum.

Van Berkel K, Ramakers B. 2015. Petrus Camper in context: An introduction. *In* K van Berkel, B Ramakers (eds) Petrus Camper in context: Science, the arts, and society in the eighteenth-century Dutch Republic. Verloren, Hilversum.

Van Berkel K, Van Lieburg MJ, Snelders HAM. 1991. Spiegelbeeld der wetenschap. Het Genootschap ter bevordering van Natuur-, Genees- en Heelkunde, 1790-1990. Erasmus Publishing, Rotterdam.

Van Bouwdijk Bastiaanse FS, Landsteiner K. 1922. Een familiaire vorm van tubereuse sclérose. Ned Tijdschr Geneeskd 66:248-257.

Van Campen. 1859. Paralysen op kinderlijke leeftijd. Ned Tijdschr Geneeskd 3:355.

Van Delft D, Van Helvoort T. 2018. Beelden zonder weerga: De elektronenmicroscoop van Ernst Ruska tot Ben Feringa. Prometheus, Amsterdam.

Van den Brule AJ, Snijders PJ, Raaphorst PM, Schrijnemakers HF, Delius H, Gissmann L, Meijer CJ, Walboomers JM. 1992. General primer polymerase chain reaction in combination with sequence analysis for identification of potentially novel human papillomavirus genotypes in cervical lesions. J Clin Microbiol 30:1716-1721.

Van den Hof S, De Melker HE, Berbers GAM, De Haas R, Beaumont MTA, Conyn-van Spaendonck MA. 2002. Evaluatie van het Rijksvaccinatieprogramma: immuniteit van de Nederlandse bevolking tegen bof, mazelen en rodehond. Ned Tijdschr Geneeskd 145:273-277.

Van der Avoort HGAM, Ras A, Dorigo-Zetsma JW. 1998. Enterovirus surveillance in the Netherlands 1996-1998: Indications for the absence of the circulation of wild poliovirus. RIVM report 242500 005. Bilthoven.

Van der Borght S, Janssens V, Schim van der Loeff MF, Kajem A, Rijckborst H, Lange JMA, Rinke de Wit TF. 2009. The Accelerating Access Initiative: Experience with a multinational workplace programme in Africa. Bull Wld Hlth Org 87:794-798. DOI: 10.2471/BLT.08.052027.

Van der Borght SFM. 2011. Making HIV programmes work: The Heineken workplace programme to prevent and treat HIV infection 2001-2010. PhD thesis, University of Amsterdam.

Van der Heide J. 1982. Vaccinaties tegen hepatitis B: een interim-advies van de Gezondheidsraad. Ned Tijdschr Geneeskd 126:1556-1557.

Van der Heide R, Koopmans MP, Shekary N, Houwers DJ, Van Duynhoven YT, Van der Poel WH. 2005. Molecular characterizations of human and animal group A rotaviruses in the Netherlands. J Clin Microbiol 43(2):669-675.

Van der Kuyl AC, Bakker M, Jurriaans S, Back NKT, Pasternak AO, Cornelissen M, Berkhout B. 2013. Translational HIV-1 research: from routine diagnostics to new virology insights in Amsterdam, the Netherlands during 1983-2013. Retrovirology 10:93.

Van der Kuyp E. 1958. Yellow fever in Surinam. Trop Geogr Med 10:181-194.

Van der Logt JT, Heessen FW, Van Loon AM, Van der Veen J. 1982a. Hemadsorption immunosorbent technique for determination of mumps immunoglobulin M antibody. J Clin Microbiol 15:82-86.

Van der Logt JT, Van Loon AM, Van der Veen J. 1982b. Detection of parainfluenza IgM antibody by hemadsorption immunosorbent technique. J Med Virol 10:213-221.

Van der Noordaa J. 1975. Kanttekeningen bij kranteberichten over een leukemia virus. Ned Tijdschr Geneeskd 119:633-634.

Van der Pas PW. 1971. The discovery of the Brownian motion. Scientarium Historia 13:27-35.

Van der Sar A, Gonzales W, Hull B, Williams MC. 1979. Serological evidence of dengue virus activity in children on the Northern Leeward Islands (Netherlands Antilles). Trop Geogr Med 31:229-236.

Van der Steege J. 1921/1779. Geneeskundige Berichten. Javasche Boekhandel en Drukkerij, Rijswijk. Original: Kinderziekte te Batavia, tot hoeverre men met de inenting derzelve gevorderd is. Compagnies Drukkerij, Batavia, 1779.

Van der Veen J. 1984. Vaccinatie tegen bof en rubella: het advies van de Gezond-heidsraad. Ned Tijdschr Geneeskd 128:1150-1152.

Van der Veen J, Kok G. 1957. Isolation and typing of adenoviruses recovered from military recruits with acute respiratory disease in the Netherlands. Am J Hyg 65(2):119-129.

Van der Vliet PC. 2005. Levensbericht Hendrik Simon Jansz, 30 april 1927-22 juni 2003. Royal Netherlands Academy of Arts and Sciences (KNAW), Amsterdam.

Van der Zeijst B. 2011. Fascination for vaccination: About achievements and chal-lenges in the vaccine world. Hum Vaccine 7:144-148. DOI: 10.4161/hv.7.2.15131.

Van der Zeijst BAM, Dijkman MI, Kramers PGN, Luytjes W, Rümke HC, Welte R. 2000. Naar een vaccinatieprogramma voor Nederland in de 21ste eeuw. RIVM rapport 000001 001. RIVM, Bilthoven.

Van der Zwan CW, Plantinga AD, Rümke HC, Conijn-van Spaendonck MAE. 1994. Mazelen in Nederland: epidemiologie en de invloed van vaccinatie. Ned Tijdschr Geneeskd 138:2390-2400.

Van de Schootbrugge GA. 1991. Vijftig jaar TPD in beweging: een halve eeuw natuurkunde voor de praktijk. Technisch Physische Dienst TNO-TU Delft, Delft.

Van de Schootbrugge GA. 2016. Instituut voor Toegepaste Radiobiologie en Immunologie (1990-1993). www.etnos.nl.

Van Deursen A. 2005. Een hoeksteen in het verzuild bestel: De Vrije Universiteit 1880-2005. Uitgeverij Bert Bakker, Amsterdam.

Van Dooren F. 1999. Geschiedenis van de klassiek Italiaanse literatuur. Athenaeum-Polak & Van Gennep, Amsterdam.

Van Doornum G, Osterhaus A. 2017. In memoriam Jan Cornelis de Jong (1935-2017). Ned Tijdschr Med Microbiol 25:45-46.

Van Driel BM. 1921. Enting tegen hondsdolheid met dood virus. Ned Tijdschr Geneeskd 65:3282-3283.

Van Eden W, Noordzij A, Hensen EJ, Van der Zee R, Van Embden JDA, Meloen RH. 1989. A modified PEPSCAN method for rapid identification and characterization of T-cell epitopes in protein antigens, pp. 33-36. *In* RA Lerner, H Ginsberg, RM Chanock, F Brown (eds) Vaccines 89: Modern approaches to new vaccines including prevention of AIDS, Cold Spring Harbor Laboratory Press, Cold Spring Harbor, NY.

Van Erp T. 1958. An epidemic of poliomyelitis in South Sumatra. Trop Geogr Med 10:154-156.

Van Furth R. 2009. Infectieziekten in Leiden: een geschiedenis. Van Jaap Mulder tot Jaap van Dissel. LAG, Leiden.

Van Gilse PHG, Hildernisse LW. 1947. Rubeola als oorzaak van aangeboren afwijkingen. Ned Tijdschr Geneeskd 91:966-967.

Van Helvoort T. 1993a. A bacteriological paradigm in influenza research in the first half of the twentieth century. Hist Philos Life Sci 15:3-21.

Van Helvoort T. 1993b. Research styles in virus studies in the 20th century: Controversies and the formation of consensus. PhD thesis, University of Limburg.

Van Helvoort T. 1994. History of virus research in the twentieth century: The problem of conceptual continuity. Hist Sci 32:185-235.

Van Helvoort T. 1996. When did virology start? ASM News 62:142-145.

Van Helvoort T. 2004. The start of a cancer research tradition: Peyton Rous, James Ewing, and viruses as a cause of cancer, pp. 191-209. *In* DH Stapleton (ed.) Creating a tradition of biomedical research: Contributions to the history of the Rockefeller University. Rockefeller University Press, New York.

Van Helvoort T. 2014. Virus and cancer studies: Still fascinating after all these years. Stud Hist Philos Biol Biomed Sci 48:258-259.

Van Helvoort T, De Gier J, Van Kammen A, Van de Putte P, Borst P. 2004. Biochemie: molecularisering van 'het leven', pp. 131-161. *In* E Homburg, L Palm (eds) De geschiedenis van de scheikunde in Nederland 3. De ontwikkeling van de chemie van 1945 tot het begin van de jaren tachtig. Delft University Press, Delft.

Van Helvoort T, Sankaran N. 2019. How seeing became knowing: The role of the electron microscope in shaping the modern definition of virus. J Hist Biol 2019. doi.org/10.1007/s 0739-018-9530-2.

Van Hemert P, Kilburn DG, Van Wezel AL. 1969. Homogeneous cultivation of animal cells for the production of virus and virus products. Biotechnol Bioeng 11:875-885.

Van Hogendorp W. 1921/1779. Geneeskundige Propagandageschriften. Javasche Boekhandel en Drukkerij, Rijswijk. Original: Sophronisba: of, de gelukkige moeder door de inëntinge van haare dochters [Sophronisba; or, The happy mother who had her daughters inoculated]. Lodewijk Dominicus Stads-Drukker, Batavia, 1779.

Van Hogendorp W. 1921/1784. Redevoering der inentinge. Java'sche Boekhandel en Drukkerij, Weltevreden. Original: Tweede deel der Verhandelingen van het Bataviaasch Genootschap der Konsten en Wetenschappen, Reinier Arrenberg, Rotterdam en Johannes Allart, Amsterdam in 1784.

Van Hoogenhuyze CJC. 1919. De bacteriologie van de griep. Ned Tijdschr Geneeskd 63:1696-1699.

Van Itallie-van Embden W. 1940/1928. Interview with Beijerinck, pp. 190-192. *In* Verzamelde Geschriften van M.W. Beijerinck, zesde deel, Martinus Nijhoff, 's-Gravenhage. Original: 1928.

Van Iterson G, Den Dooren de Jong LE, Kluyver AJ. 1940. Martinus Willem Beijerinck: His life and his work. Delftsch Hoogeschoolfonds, Delft/Martinus Nijhoff, The Hague.

Van Iterson G, Den Dooren de Jong LE, Kluyver AJ. 1983. Martinus Willem Beijerinck: His life and his work. Science Tech, Madison, WI.

Van Iterson W. 1996. Electron microscopy in the Netherlands, earliest developments. Advances in Imaging and Electron Physics 96:271-285. doi.org/10.1016/S1076-5670(08)70051-X.

Van Kammen A. 1999. Beijerinck's contribution to the virus concept: An introduction. Arch Virol Suppl 15:1-8.

Van Kammen A. 2004. Nucleïnezuren, pp. 139-146. *In* E Homburg, L Palm (eds) De geschiedenis van de scheikunde in Nederland 3. De ontwikkeling van de chemie van 1945 tot het begin van de jaren tachtig. Delft University Press, Delft.

Van Kammen A. 2011. L.E. den Dooren de Jong and the Beijerinck Virology Fund. KNAW, Amsterdam. https://www.knaw.nl/shared/resources/actueel/bestanden/Den_Dooren_De_Jong Beijerinck_Virology_Fund_2011.pdf.

Van Leent FJ. 1881. La Guyane néerlandaise. Arch de médicine navale, t. XXXII, XXXIV, 1880, t. XXXV, Librairie J.B. Baillière et Fils, Paris.

Van Lieburg MJ. 1985. Het Bataafsch Genootschap der Proefondervindelijke Wijsbegeerte te Rotterdam, 1769-1984: Een bibliografisch en documenterend overzicht. Rodopi, Amsterdam.

Van Lieburg MJ. 1986. De ontwikkeling van het klinisch-diagnostisch laboratorium in Nederland tot omstreeks 1925. Tijdschrift Geneesk Natuurw Wisk Techn 9:278-318.

Van Lier B. 2004. De som van zorg en onderzoek. Negentig jaar Nederlands Kanker Instituut-Antoni van Leeuwenhoek Ziekenhuis. NKI-AVL, Amsterdam.

Van Loghem JJ. 1910. Gele koorts in Suriname. Ned Tijdschr Geneeskd 54:1632-1633.

Van Loghem JJ. 1931. Beyerinck en de kennis der bacterieele veranderlijkheid. Ned Tijdschr Geneeskd 75:1046-1049.

Van Loghem JJ. 1935. De behandeling tegen lyssa in het Instituut Pasteur te Bandoeng. Ned Tijdschr Geneeskd 79:3896-3899.

Van Loghem JJ. 1938. In memoriam Ludwig Karl Wolff. Ned Tijdschr Geneeskd 82:3192-3194.

Van Loghem JJ. 1943. In memoriam G. Kapsenberg. Ned Tijdschr Geneeskd 87:1771-1773.

Van Loghem JJ. 1944. Het raadsel der vira. Ned Tijdschr Geneeskd 88:284-286.

Van Loghem JJ, Ruys AC, Polak MF. 1956. Algemene gezondheidsleer. N.V. Uitgevers-Mij 'Kosmos', Amsterdam-Antwerpen.

Van Loghem Jr JJ, Van der Noordaa J. 2000. J.J. van Loghem (1878-1968), microbioloog-hygiënist, pp. 128-137. *In* CJE Kaandorp, JJE van Everdingen, A Mooij (eds) Erflaters van de geneeskunde. Belvédère/Medidact, Overveen/Alphen aan den Rijn.

Van Lookeren Campagne J. 1943. Referaten. Kindergeneeskunde. Mazelen. Ned Tijdschr Geneeskd 87:1758-1759.

Van Raalte E. 1977. Het Nederlandse Parlement. 's-Gravenhage, Staatsuitgeverij, 6e druk.

Van Ravesteijn W. 1918-1919. Vragen van Van Ravesteijn en Antwoord van Minister Aalberse. Aanhangsel II van het Verslag van de Handelingen der Tweede Kamer 1918-1919. Vol. 30, p. 61, no. 57.

Van Riemsdijk M. 1928. Rudolph Hendrik Saltet. Drukkerij De Hoop, Amsterdam.

Van Rij RP, Blaak H, Visser JA, Brouwer M, Rientsma R, Broersen SM, De Roda Husman AM, Schuitemaker H. 2000. Differential coreceptor expression allows for independent evolution of non-syncytium-inducing and syncytium-inducing HIV-1. J Clin Invest 106:1039-1052 and 1569.

Van Rooyen CE, Rhodes AJ. 1948. Virus diseases of man, rev. ed. Thomas Nelson & Sons, New York.

Van Schevichaven HDJ. N.d. Tweede vervolg der Kroniek van Nijmegen tot en met den jare 1900. www.noviomagus.nl.

Van Steenis G, Hannik A, Van Wezel AL. 1984. Dutch cell-culture rabies vaccine for use in humans. Ned Tijdschr Geneeskd 128:1810-1814.

Van Stockum MJ. 1935. New principles of anti-rabic treatment and rabies statistics. Nijhoff, The Hague.

Van Thiel PH. 1946. Life and work of Prof. Dr P.C. Flu. Acta Leidensia 10:1-11.

Van Tongeren HA. 1965. Arbovirus group B spectrum in the province of Brokopondo, Surinam: A serological survey. Trop Geogr Med 17(4):339-352.

Van Weemen BK. 2005. The rise of EIA/ELISA. Clinical Chemistry 51:2226.

Van Weemen BK, Schuurs AHWM. 1971. Immunoassay using antigen-enzyme conjugates. FEBS Letters 15:232-236.

Van Weemen BK, Schuurs AHWM. 1972. Immunoassay using hapten-enzyme conjugates. FEBS Letters 24:77-81.

Van Weemen BK, Schuurs AHWM. 1974. Oostermeijer MW, Raymakers HHT. Immunoassay using antibody-enzyme conjugates. FEBS Letters 43:215-218.

Van Wezel AL. 1967. Growth of cell-strains and primary cells on micro-carriers in homogeneous culture. Nature 216:64-65.

Van Wezel AL. 1973. Microcarrier cultures of animal cells, pp. 372-377. In PF Kruse Jr, MK Patterson Jr (eds) Tissue culture methods and applications. Academic Press, New York.

Van Wezel AL. 1985. Monolayer growth systems: homogeneous unit processes, pp. 265-282. In RE Spier, JB Griffiths (eds) Animal cell biotechnology, vol. I. Academic Press, London.

Van Wezel AL, Van Steenis G, Hannik CA, Cohen H. 1978. New approach to the production of concentrated and purified inactivated polio and rabies tissue culture vaccines. Dev Biol Stand 41:159-168.

Van Wezel AL. Van Steenis G. Hannik CA, Kapsenberg JG, Hofman B. Cohen H. 1979. Bereiding en toepassing in Nederland van geïnactiveerd vaccin tegen poliomyelitis anterior acuta. Ned Tijdschr Geneeskd 123:466-474.

Van Wijngaarden JK. 1984. Immunodeficiëntiesyndroom, verworven: AIDS: de noodzaak van een geïntegreerde benadering. Ned Tijdschr Geneeskd 128:1061-1062.

Van Woensel P. 1800. De bij-lichter, zijnde eene uitgewerkte verhandeling over de influenza, dat is: publieke verkoudheid. In't Nieuwe Licht, Amsterdam.

Van Zon H. 1990. Tachtig jaar RIVM. Rijksinstituut voor Volksgezondheid en Milieuhygiëne, Bilthoven. Van Gorcum, Assen.

Veldhuyzen WF. 1957. Honderd en vijftig jaar pokken-preventie. De geschiedenis van het Amsterdamsch Genootschap ter bevordering van de koepokinenting voor minvermogenden 1803-1953. Scheltema & Holkema, Amsterdam.

Verdoorn JA. 1981/1965. Het gezondheidswezen te Amsterdam in de 19ᵉ eeuw. SUN, Nijmegen. Original: Volksgezondheid en sociale ontwikkeling: beschouwingen over het gezondheidswezen te Amsterdam in de 19ᵉ eeuw. Het Spectrum, Utrecht, 1965.

Verhoef P. 2005. Strenge wetenschappelijkheid en practische zin: Een eeuw Nederlands centraal veterinair instituut, 1904-2004. Erasmus Publishing, Rotterdam.

Verlinde JD. 1957. Neurotrope virussen. In AC Ruys (ed.). Leerboek der microbiologie en immunologie. N.V.A. Oosthoek's Uitgevers Maatschappij, Utrecht.

Verlinde JD. 1958. Actieve immunisatie tegen poliomyelitis met een vaccin van verzwakt virus. I. Theoretische grondslag en selectie van stammen. Ned Tijdschr Geneeskd 102:1138-1143.

Verlinde JD. 1961. Problemen rond het orale poliovirusvaccin. Verslag van het poliomyelitis-symposium. Excerpta Medica Amsterdam, pp. 26-37.

Verlinde JD. 1962. Dood (type Salk) of levend (type Sabin) poliomyelitisvirusvaccin? Ned Tijdschr Geneeskd 106:2599-2604.

Verlinde JD. 1969a. Letter to the Executive Committee of the NVVM, 18 March.

Verlinde JD. 1969b. Rabies in Suriname. Verslag van de gewone vergadering der Afdeling Natuurkunde 78. Kon Nederl Akad v Wet, Amsterdam.

Verlinde JD, Kooij P, Versteeg J. 1970. Vampire-bat transmitted rabies virus from Surinam. Trop Geogr Med 22:119-122.

Verlinde JD, Kret A. 1954. De betekenis van de weefselcultuur voor de diagnose van poliomyelitis. Ned Tijdschr Geneeskd 98:3472-3476.

Verlinde JD, Li-Fo-Sjoe, Versteeg J, Dekker SM. 1975. A local outbreak of paralytic rabies in Surinam children. Trop Geogr Med 27:136-142.

Verlinde JD, Wilterdink JB, Hofman B, Kret A. 1958. Actieve immunisatie tegen poliomyelitis met een vaccin van verzwakt virus. II. Eerste mededeling over de toepassing van het Sabin-vaccin in Nederland. Ned Tijdschr Geneeskd 102:1144-1148.

Versteeg J. 1985. A colour atlas of virology. Wolfe Medical Publications, London.

Versteeg J. 1987. In memoriam prof. dr. J.D. Verlinde. Ned Tijdschr Geneeskd 131:1243.

Versteeg J. 1992. Kweek (voer voor virussen), pp. 107-110. In AJ Scheffer (ed.) Liber amicorum voor prof. dr. J.B. Wilterdink. Universiteitsdrukkerij, Groningen.

Vinjé J, Koopmans MP. 1996. Molecular detection and epidemiology of small round-structured viruses in outbreaks of gastroenteritis in the Netherlands. J Infect Dis 174(3):610-615.

Visser RP, Hakfoort C, Lintsen H, De Clercq P, Snelders HA, Verbong G, Bakker M, Visser RP, Beukers H, Van Lieburg MJ. 1986. Werkplaatsen van wetenschap en techniek. Industriële en academische laboratoria in Nederland 1860-1940. Tijdschr Geschied Geneeskd Natuurwet Wiskd Tech 9(4):143-318.

Vos JJT. 1949. Redevoeringen uitgesproken bij gelegenheid van de promotie van Remmert Korteweg tot doctor honoris causa in de geneeskunde. J.B. Wolters' Uitgeversmaatschappij N.V., Groningen.

Waardenburg JG. 1858. Verslag over de volksziekten welke in 1855 in Nederland hebben geheerscht. Ned Tijdschr Geneeskd 2:345-366.

Wabeke M. 1964. Isolatie van virus bij patiënten met rode hond (rubeola) en vijfde ziekte (erythema infectiosum). PhD thesis, University of Amsterdam. Uitgeverij L. Stafleu & Zoon, Leiden.

Wagenaar JH. 1938. Behandeling van mazelen met reconvalescentenserum. Ned Tijdschr Geneeskd 82:2426-2427.

Walig C, Walboomers JMM, Van der Noordaa J. 1974. Ultrastructural localization of concanavalin in receptors in somatic hybrids between normal mouse cells and simian virus 40-transfomed rat cells. J Cell Biology 61:553-557.

Walvoort HC. 2006. Jan Ingenhousz (1730-1799), medicus, chemicus en fysicus. Ned Tijdschr Geneeskd 150:947.

Ward MP. 2014. Rabies in the Dutch East Indies a century ago: A spatio-temporal case study in disease emergence. Prev Vet Med 114:11-20.

Warmerdam H, Zoeter T, Floor J. 1998. 75 Jaar Organon. N.V. Organon, Oss.

Waterson AP, Wilkinson L. 1978. An introduction to the history of virology. Cambridge University Press, Cambridge.

Weidinger S. 1940. Ned Tijdschr Geneeskd 84:3220-3239.

Weiland HT, Vermey-Keers C, Salimans MM, Fleuren GJ, Verwey RA, Anderson MJ. 1987. Parvovirus B19 associated with fetal abnormality. Lancet 329(8534):682-683.

Weiland HT, Williams MC, Hull B. 1978. Serologic survey of dengue and other arboviruses in Curaçao and Aruba, 1973. Bull Pan Am Health Organ 12(2):134-142.

Weindling P. 1992. Scientific elites and laboratory organization in fin de siècle Paris and Berlin. *In* A Cunningham, P Williams (eds) The laboratory revolution in medicine. Cambridge University Press, Cambridge.

Weissmann C, Borst P. 1963. Double-stranded ribonucleic acid formation in vitro by MS 2 phage-induced RNA synthetase. Science 142(3596):1188-1191.

Weller TH, Robbins FC. 1991. John Franklin Enders, February 10, 1897-September 8, 1985. Biographical Memoirs of the National Academy of Science 60:53-55.

Wertheim Salomonson JKA, De Rooy C. 1893. Rapport over de Influenza-epidemie in Nederland van 1889-1890. Ned Tijdschr Geneeskd 37:688-779.

Westendorp Boerma F. 1960. Prof. Dr A. Pondman 70 jaar. Ned Tijdschr Geneeskd 104:1008-1010.

Westendorp Boerma F. 1977. Honderd jaar Medische Microbiologie in Groningen. Centrale Reproduktiedienst Universiteit, Groningen.

Wheeler CM, Skinner SR, Del Rosario-Raymundo MR, Garland SM, Chatterjee A, Lazcano-Ponce E, Salmerón J, McNeil S, Stapleton JT, Bouchard C, Martens MG, Money DM, Quek SC, Romanowski B, Vallejos CS, Ter Harmsel B, Prilepskaya V, Fong KL, Kitchener H, Minkina G, Lim YKT, Stoney T, Chakhtoura N, Cruickshank ME, Savicheva A, Da Silva DP, Ferguson M, Molijn AC, Quint WGV, Hardt K, Descamps D, Suryakiran PV, Karkada N, Geeraerts B, Dubin G, Struyf F: VIVIANE Study Group. 2016. Efficacy, safety, and immunogenicity of the human papillomavirus 16/18 AS04-adjuvanted vaccine in women older than 25 years: 7-year follow-up of the phase 3, double-blind, randomised controlled VIVIANE study. Lancet Infect Dis 10:1154-1168. DOI: 10.1016/S1473-3099(16)30120-7.

Wilder-Smith A, Lee V, Gubler DJ. 2019. Yellow fever: Is Asia prepared for an epidemic? Lancet Infect Dis 19:241-242. DOI: 10.1016/S1473-3099(19)30050-7.

Wilder-Smith A, Leong WY. 2017. Importation of yellow fever into China: Assessing travel patterns. J Travel Med 24. DOI: 10.1093/jtm/tax008.

Wilkinson L. 1977. The development of the virus concept as reflected in corpora of studies on individual pathogens. 4. Rabies: Two millennia of ideas and conjecture on the aetiology of a virus disease. Med Hist 21:15-31.

Williams REO. 1985. Microbiology for the public health: The evolution of the Public Health Laboratory Service 1939-1980. Public Health Health Laboratory Service, London.

Wilson D. 2005. The early history of tissue culture in Britain: The interwar years. Soc Hist Med 18:225-243.

Wilterdink JB, Billiau A, De Clercq E, Dekking F, Hekker AC, Masurel N, Van der Noordaa J, Pattyn SR, Van der Veen J, Versteeg J. 1976. Medische virologie. Bohn, Scheltema & Holkema, Utrecht.

Wilterdink JB, Metselaar D, Van der Kuyp E, Verlinde JD. 1964. Report on a type-1 outbreak in 1963 and its control by trivalent oral polio virus vaccine. Trop Geogr Med 2:120-128.

Winkelstein W. 1995. A new perspective on John Snow's communicable disease theory. Am J Epidemiol 142(9):S3-S9.

Witz J. 1998. A reappraisal of the contribution of Friedrich Loeffler to the development of the modern concept of virus. Archives of Virology 143:2261-2263.

Wolbach SB. 1912. The filterable viruses, a summary. Boston Medical and Surgical Journal 167(13):419-427.

Wolff JPD. 1986. Over het moeizame begin van de pokkenpreventie. Ned Tijdschr Geneeskd 130:599-601.

Wolff JW. 1961. Obituary Dr W.A. Collier. Trop Geogr Med 13:I.

Wolff JW, Collier WA, Bonnet-De Roever H, Hoekstra J. 1958. Yellow fever immunity in rural population groups of Surinam (with a note on other serological investigations). Trop Geogr Med 10(4):325-331.

Wolff LK. 1919a. De besmettelijkheid der influenza. Ned Tijdschr Geneeskd 63:1021-1022.

Wolff LK. 1919b. Over het virus dat de veroorzaaker is der influenza. Ned Tijdschr Geneeskd 63:492-500.

Wolff LK. 1922. Bacteriophaag: Over den bacteriophaag (d'Herelle). Ned Tijdschr Geneeskd 66:479-485.

Wolff LK. 1932. Bacteriophaag en ultravirus: Levende wezens of fermenten. Ned Tijdschr Geneeskd 76:5014-5024.

Woodruff AM, Goodpasture EW. 1931. The susceptibility of the chorioallantoic membrane of chick embryos to infection with the fowlpox virus. Am J Pathology 7:209-222.

Worboys M. 1989. British colonial and tropical imperialism: A comparative study, pp. 149-163. *In* AM Luyendijk-Elshout, GM van Heteren, A de Knecht-van Ee-kelen, MJD Poulissen (eds) Dutch Medicine in the Malay archipelago. Rodopi, Amsterdam.

Worboys M. 2000. Spreading germs: Disease theories and medical practice in Britain, 1865-1900. Cambridge University Press, Cambridge.

Worboys M. 2007. Was there a Bacteriological Revolution in late nineteenth-century medicine? Stud Hist Philos Biol Biomed Sci 38(1):20-42.

Zaaijer HL. 1995. Confirmatory testing of blood-borne viral infections. PhD thesis, University of Amsterdam.

Zernike F. 1935. Das Phasenkontrastverfahren bei der mikroskopischen Beobach-tung. Z Techn Phys 16:454-457.

Zuckerman M, Aitken C, Carman B, Mortimer PP, Cartwright K. 2001. A crisis and its solution: Setting up the UK clinical virology network. Commun Dis Public Health 4(4):238-239.

Zur Hausen H. 2006. Infections causing human cancer. Wiley-VCH, KGaA, Weinheim.

Zur Hausen H. 2008. The search for infectious causes of human cancers: Where and why. Nobel Lecture, 7 December. NobelPrize.org. https://www.nobelprize.org/uploads/2018/06/hausen_lecture.pdf.

Zwick W. 1929. Influenza der Pferde (Pferdestaupe), pp. 413-422. *In* W Kolle, R Kraus, P Uhlenhuth (eds) Handbuch der pathogene Mikroorganismen. Gustav Fischer und Urban & Schwarzenberg, Jena.

Index

Index of names

Index of subjects